T0295271

mRNA Therapeutics

This book is the most comprehensive and complete treatise on nucleic acid therapeutic products, including mRNA vaccines, their manufacturing, formulations, and testing for safety and efficacy. Details include cGMP-compliant manufacturing and regulatory filing steps. A new concept of "biosimilar" mRNA vaccine is presented to secure fast approval of copies of mRNA vaccines. Projections of financial plans to establish RNA manufacturing facilities are provided, along with details of supply chain management. Finally, the future of nucleic acid products in gene therapy and other newer applications is presented, along with a perspective that all new vaccines will be the nucleic acid type that will further provide first-time prevention of autoimmune disorders. It is projected that both big pharma and start-ups will enter this field, and we can expect significant additions to our drug armamentarium soon.

mRNA Therapeutics

Fast-to-Market Strategies

Sarfaraz K. Niazi

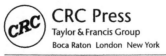

CRC Press
Taylor & Francis Group
Boca Raton London New York

CRC Press is an imprint of the
Taylor & Francis Group, an **informa** business

First edition published 2022
by CRC Press
6000 Broken Sound Parkway NW, Suite 300, Boca Raton, FL 33487-2742

and by CRC Press
4 Park Square, Milton Park, Abingdon, Oxon, OX14 4RN

CRC Press is an imprint of Taylor & Francis Group, LLC

ISBN: 9781032163444 (hbk)
ISBN: 9781032163482 (pbk)
ISBN: 9781003248156 (ebk)

DOI: 10.1201/9781003248156

Typeset in Times
by Deanta Global Publishing Services, Chennai, India

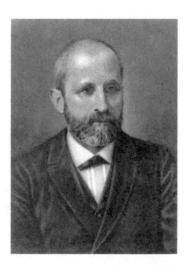

To: Johannes Friedrich Miescher (13 August 1844–26 August 1895), a Swiss physician and biologist who first isolated nucleic acid in 1869, paving the way for the identification of DNA as the carrier of inheritance as he suggested a possible role of the nucleic acids in heredity and evolution. The Nobel Prize was not established then, and it is not given posthumously.

Contents

Preface and Perspective

Chapter 1: The Genome Machine. The genome machine is a creation of the evolution of the universe. Starting from what we do not know, the fundamental particles and the rules of physics have formed that lead to chemistry and then to biology. Life, as we feel, is merely a set of chemical and physical reactions, all governed by physics; the formation of life is best described as a cellular automata that depended on the charge and size of the molecule. Carbon being the smallest and with the least charge, led the trail. Self-replication came driven by the charge interactions as demonstrated in the famous The Game of Life, also known simply as Life, a cellular automaton devised by the British mathematician John Horton Conway in 1970. It is a zero-player game, meaning that its evolution is determined by its initial state, requiring no further input. One interacts with the Game of Life by creating an initial configuration and observing how it evolves. It is Turing complete and can simulate a universal constructor or any other Turing machine. Any live cell with two or three live neighbors survives; any dead cell with three live neighbors becomes a live cell. All other live cells die in the next generation. Similarly, all other dead cells stay dead. The initial pattern constitutes the seed of the system. The first generation is created by applying the above rules simultaneously to every cell in the seed, live or dead; births and deaths co-occur, and the discrete moment at which this happens is sometimes called a tick. Each generation is a pure function of the preceding one. The rules continue to be applied repeatedly to create further generations [https://playgameoflife.com/]. This game teaches us how cells replicate, how a polypeptide chain turns into a three-dimensional protein, and how genes are mutated. Despite its instability, the RNA started life as it got tagged with other molecules. Now, after the incident that happened almost four billion years ago, we are returning to finding the solutions to all ailments of life through RNA, as it formed the life a long while ago.

Chapter 2: The Nucleic Acids. Nucleic acid is a five-carbon sugar, with a phosphate group and nitrogen containing bases. How this structure became the written language of the genetic code is discussed in Chapter 1. Understanding the chemistry and thermodynamics of interaction of nucleic acid is critical to realizing the importance of the genetic code leading to every body function. DNA, RNA, codons, transcription, translation are all parts of the sequences that lead to the supply of essential proteins. The statistical odds of such simple molecules with no more than five options of nitrogen groups producing proteins are astronomical; and more surprising are the odds of a translated chain of amino acids turning into a three-dimensional protein. But all of these observations are now well-understood and form the basis of new drug discoveries.

Chapter 3: RNA Therapeutics: RNA therapeutics is a wide field, including therapies and prevention of infection and autoimmune disorders. The role of RNA and its dozens of types are now well recognized, and a few applications have been introduced. The consistency with which RNA operates at all levels of its operation, from translation to its limited lifecycle, makes it an ideal modality for treating, preventing, and treating diseases. Unlike chemical drugs, its toxicity is limited to a localized distribution site. Unlike DNA therapies, it does not enter the nucleus, reducing the risk of any damage to the genes in the nucleus. It is anticipated that RNA therapeutics will be the most forthcoming branch of new drug discovery; and for this reason, a contemporary understanding of RNA developments is essential for developers.

Chapter 4: Nucleoside Vaccines: More lives have been saved by vaccinations than any other modality in the history of humanity; however, the arrival of nucleoside vaccines has transformed the future of disease prevention and expanded it to a level never possible before. Now we can be confident that every immune disorder can be prevented with a proper RNA vaccine; we are also entering the era where instead of expressing antibodies ex vivo, we will have RNA to produce these therapeutic entities. While the RNA vaccines are still produced using a DNA template, they will no longer be needed, as PCR techniques become more efficient. The chemical nature of RNA also makes it possible to create copies of these vaccines. This effort will boost the availability of vaccines across the globe and at a cost that would be readily affordable. The technology for RNA vaccine manufacturing is relatively cheaper than any other vaccine, and the speed of development brings us the possibility of managing future pandemics with greater efficiency and fewer deaths.

Chapter 5: cGMP mRNA Vaccine Manufacturing: The cGMP manufacturing of mRNA vaccines is a complex process; however, the process is validated, and it should result in consistent product. Therefore, of great importance are the in-process control QC checks.

Chapter 6: Regulatory Guidance: In the post-COVID-19 age, it is expected that the experience of the COVID-19 pandemic will also allow a better response to future pandemics. The regulatory approval of RNA products took years, and the traditional vaccines even decades; all of that has changed as the regulatory agencies are now providing guidelines that will allow faster development of RNA products. While the EU and US still have many differences, and these are closing fast, the core requirements remain unchanged. Therefore, as presented in this chapter, developers are advised to plan their development programs in close collaboration with the regulatory agencies and be prepared for what is considered essential and non-negotiable.

Appendix 1: COVID-19 mRNA Vaccine Manufacturing Feasibility: Financial and scientific projections of establishing COVID-19 vaccine manufacturing as an example for all types of mRNA vaccines.

Appendix 2: Pharmacopeial Testing: The development of RNA products requires extensive quality testing for safety and efficacy. The testing methods used for biological drugs, traditional vaccines, and gene therapy are widely available and applicable to the development of mRNA products. Recently, the USP has proposed quality control methods that should soon evolve into specific chapters in the USP. Several books on this subject are available, and so is a vast volume of data in the patent applications and publications to establish optimal testing protocol.

Appendix 3: Suggested Readings: With over 100,000 literature references that arose over the past decade, a selection of comprehensive reviews of RNA technology are provided.

Acknowledgments

I am thankful to many of my scientific and professional colleagues, particularly those I came to know through the landmark literature in the field but never met. I may have quoted their work thinking that this is all in the public domain subconsciously; I hope they would excuse me for taking this liberty as it would be impossible to recognize them well. An elaborate bibliography does not necessarily replace this obligation that I have to acknowledge their work correctly.

Finally, I would like to admit my mistakes. I couldn't find a better statement than that which appeared in the first edition of Encyclopedia Britannica (1786):

"WITH regard to errors, in general, whether falling under the denomination of mental, typographical, or accidental, we are conscious of being able to point out a greater number than any critic whatever. Men *(and women)* who are acquainted with the innumerable difficulties attending the execution of a work of such an extensive nature will make proper allowances. To these, we appeal and shall rest satisfied with the judgment they pronounce."

I will appreciate receiving your comments to improve this treatise in the future, and most kindly, if you find any mistakes.

Disclaimer: The author does not accept responsibility for any technical or legal suggestions or advice provided in this book; all views expressed in this book are those of the authors in their personal capacity and not as the Patent Agent of the US Patent and Trademark Office, as an officer of any company or in any academic positions held, or in any capacity as advisors to regulatory agencies.

Sarfaraz K. Niazi, Ph.D., Deerfield, Illinois, USA, June 2022

Author

Sarfaraz K. Niazi, Ph.D., is an Adjunct Professor at the University of Illinois and the University of Houston; he has authored 60+ major books, 100+ research papers, and 100+ patents, mainly in the field of bioprocessing, drug discovery, drug formulations, thermodynamic systems, alcohol aging, nutraceuticals, and treatment of autoimmune diseases. He has hands-on experience establishing biotechnology projects from concept to market, including FDA approvals. In addition, he has firsthand experience in establishing RNA therapeutic product development and manufacturing, including the mRNA vaccine for COVID-19. He also serves as an advisor to major pharmaceutical and biopharmaceutical companies, regulatory agencies, and many heads of state. He is also a patent law practitioner. Email: niazi@niazi.com

Background

Evolution does nothing in vain. There are four times the strips of nucleotides watching over the translating ones to ensure there is no mistake made. We have just begun to understand, and someday, we will find a resolution for every disease. This is going back to Nature that helped us survive for millions of years.

The Author

RNA discovery dates to 1953, when Alfred Day Hershey reported RNA formation in Escherichia coli RNA after infection with bacteriophage T2. In 1961, Brenner, Jacob, and Watson isolated mRNA. In the 2000s, it was understood how the in vitro transcription leads to instant translation in the cytoplasm, and thus began the field of RNA therapeutics. However, the mRNA is only transiently active and is wholly degraded via physiological and metabolic pathways, requiring a delivery system to protect the naked or complexed RNA. The first mRNA vaccine was reported in mice in 1993 by using liposome-encapsulated in vitro transcription (IVT) mRNA to encode the nucleoprotein of influenza to induce virus-specific T cells. The IVT mRNA was then combined with synthetic lipid nanoparticles, which resulted in protective antibody responses in mice against the respiratory syncytial virus (RSV), and the influenza virus.

Robert Conry demonstrated in 1995 that injecting naked RNA encoding carcinoembryonic antigen into the muscle produced antigen-specific antibody responses. It was then expanded upon by showing that dendritic cells (DCs) injected into tumor-bearing mice and exposed to mRNA coding for specific antigens or total mRNA isolated from tumor cells triggered T cell immune responses and decreased tumor growth. T cell responses were induced by direct injection of naked IVT mRNA into lymph nodes, which led to the first in-human testing of naked IVT mRNA encoding cancer antigens to treat melanoma (NCT01684241; BioNTech).

Nucleic acids, DNA, and RNA are genetic materials that are the most powerful tools today for gene therapy, curing or preventing hundreds of diseases. The history of exploring the use of DNA and RNA as therapeutic modalities goes back to 1947, correcting the phenotypic abnormalities in rats; the subsequent, most crucial discoveries were gene transfer into mouse muscle without a vector in 1990, and in 2001 to show that RNAi works in mammalian cells in vitro. However, naked DNA and RNA in the 1990s did not go much farther because of their instability until the past decade, when techniques were developed to protect the nucleic acids during their entry and reach into the cells (Figure B.1).

One application of nucleosides that has brought much attention is gene therapy, first proposed about half a century ago. Since both DNA and mRNA serve as a model for protein synthesis, it allows the cell to produce missing or defective proteins instead of introducing exogenous proteins. This is a faster and cheaper treatment

DOI: 10.1201/9781003248156-1

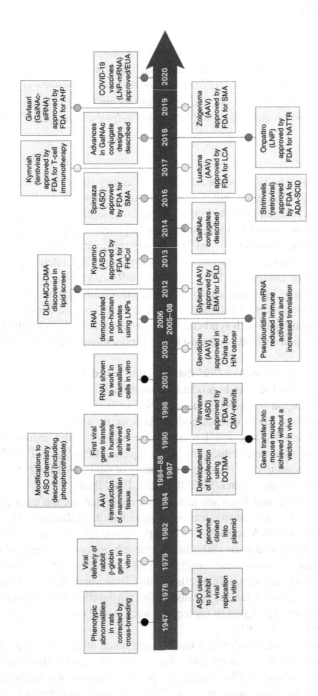

FIGURE B.1 Timeline of key discoveries and events during the development of nucleic acid therapeutics.

with no protein size restrictions or the complexity of producing proteins in vitro. Additionally, the nucleic acid allows protein post-translational modifications that are difficult to gain in heterologous systems. Also, in vivo delivery of protein helps protect it chemically upon reaching the target. The production cost is also a factor in delivering exogenous mRNA into cells to manipulate protein expression.

Most of the human genome is transcribed, though only less than 2% of the transcriptome is protein-coding, leaving vast possibilities of finding new therapies for hundreds of untreatable diseases—essentially every disease.

The mRNA therapeutic mechanisms of action are through immune stimulation and protein replacement. Other mechanisms in the decreasing order of use frequency include agonist (protein replacement), gene silencing, gene activation, increasing translation, agonist (immune stimulation), gene knockout, splice modulation, and antagonist (inhibition). What had prevented the use of RNA therapeutic products in the past was the high chemical instability of RNA. This is now addressed through modifications to RNA and improved delivery systems, like liposomes and LNPs, all resulting in a longer half-life and reduced immunogenicity. DNA-based therapeutics have been popular approaches to treat inherited diseases due to missing or dysfunctional proteins. However, unlike RNA therapeutics, DNA therapeutic elements must enter the nucleus to enable transcribing into mRNA. Nuclear delivery is a crucial barrier to DNA-based therapy since most differentiated cells are post-mitotic cells that do not divide frequently. There is also a risk of unwanted modifications being made to the genes.

The nucleic acid-based therapies are preferred, as they directly supply an absent or replace a faulty protein; they are also easier to design and have fewer size limits. Furthermore, some proteins, such as membrane proteins, are difficult or impossible to generate properly in vitro. Another advantage of employing nucleic acids as biotherapeutics is that it avoids manufacturing difficulties, particularly post-translational modifications, which are required in proteins but extremely difficult to achieve in heterologous systems. The difficulties with post-translational modifications may result in considerable variations between endogenous and exogenous (in vitro) proteins, resulting in likely higher immunogenicity. These disadvantages of creating a protein of larger size and achieving the in vivo concentrations necessary to generate a therapeutic effect, and the lower cost advantage make nucleic acid biotherapeutics the most desirable modus of therapy, without the risk of integration into the genome.

A major push for RNA therapies and vaccines came with the approval of mRNA vaccines to prevent SARS-CoV-2 infections recently. The rise of mRNA is a model for the study of how our understanding shifts when facing a crisis. A model for this change is presented in Figure B.2.

The paradigm shift brought by SARS-CoV-2 was made possible by the multitude of developments over the past couple of decades; the key problem of assuring mRNA stability and choosing a proper vector was resolved by the liquid nanoparticle (LNP) technology that provided the protection. In addition, the science of RNA nucleoside modification was also validated, as an mRNA vaccine that did not modify the nucleosides failed.

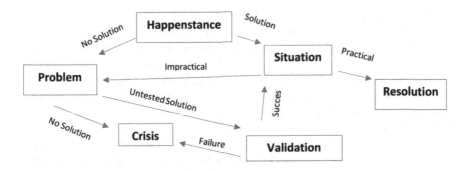

FIGURE B.2   Shifting understanding in a crisis. An event that upsets everyday life, or happenstance, is first evaluated if there is a solution available or not; if there are solutions, then it is termed a situation or a problem. If a solution exists, it is evaluated to see if it is practical or not; if it is practical, the solution is reached and resolved. If it is impractical, it is labeled as a problem. However, if there is no solution, the happenstance also goes into the problem category. If there are untested solutions, then a validation step determines whether it is a success; if yes, the happenstance becomes a situation; otherwise, it goes into crisis. In 1918, the Spanish Flu could not be resolved and ended up as a crisis since we did not have any solutions to try then. The COVID-19 in 2019 came a hundred years later, but we had many possible solutions, such as using an mRNA vaccine to prevent infection by this time. It had never been tried, but there was little choice left not to try. The trial was successful because of the rapid spread of the infection, proving it to be the best vaccine ever for safety and efficacy.

Table B.1 lists the major events in the life of the discoveries of RNA.

How significant these discoveries are demonstrated by the 30 Nobel Prizes awarded, the highest for any single technology. (Table B.2). The most prominent name Johannes Friedrich Miescher is missing, as he died long before the Nobel Prize was established. A Swiss physician and biologist, he isolated nucleic acid in 1869, identified protamine, and made a number of other discoveries. He isolated various phosphate-rich chemicals (which he called nuclein, now nucleic acids) from the nuclei of white blood cells, paving the way for the identification of DNA as the carrier of inheritance.

B.1   THE RNA LEAD

Until recently, DNA-based therapy techniques were the preferred option to suggest treating hereditary disorders caused by missing or malfunctioning proteins. However, realizing that DNA must be transcribed into mRNA before the therapeutic protein molecule can be generated, therapeutic use of DNA necessitates rapid transport of DNA to the cytoplasm and efficient entry into the nucleus. Furthermore, because most differentiated cells are post-mitotic cells that do not divide frequently, nuclear delivery is a significant barrier to DNA-based therapy. In contrast, as soon as mRNA enters the cytoplasm, the translation process can begin without the need for it to be sent to the nucleus.

TABLE B.1

Major Events in the History of RNA

1930–1950

The chemical characteristics of RNA and DNA are different.

The chemical and biological differences between RNA and DNA were not apparent when they were initially investigated in the early 1900s, so they were given names based on the materials from which they were isolated: RNA was called "yeast nucleic acid," and DNA was called "thymus nucleic acid." Carbohydrate chemists used diagnostic chemical tests to prove that the two nucleic acids contained distinct sugars, and the popular name for RNA was changed to "ribose nucleic acid." Other early biochemical investigations revealed that RNA was easily degraded at high pH, whereas DNA remained stable (although denatured) in alkali. A nucleoside composition study revealed that RNA had nucleobases that were comparable to DNA but had uracil instead of thymine and a variety of minor nucleobase components, such as modest amounts of pseudo uridine and dimethyl guanine.

Cellular localization and morphogenetic function

Jean Brachet proposed that DNA is contained in the cell nucleus, and RNA is only found in the cytoplasm while investigating virgin sea urchin eggs in 1933. "Yeast nucleic acid" (RNA) was supposed to be found only in plants at the time, while "thymus nucleic acid" (DNA) was thought to be found only in animals. The latter was considered to be a tetramer that buffered the pH of the cell. Joachim Hämmerling began to separate the contributions of the nucleus and cytoplasm substances (later known to be DNA and mRNA, respectively) to cell morphogenesis and development during research on Acetabularia in the 1930s.

1951–1965

The genetic information that drives protein synthesis is carried by messenger RNA (mRNA).

The term "messenger RNA" was used by Francis Crick in the late 1950s to describe his "Central Dogma of Molecular Biology," which said that DNA led to the production of RNA, which led to the synthesis of proteins. The nature of messenger RNA and the genetic code were defined in the early 1960s by an advanced genetic study of mutations in the lac operon of E. coli and the rII locus of bacteriophage T4. The biochemical isolation of mRNA was difficult due to the short half-life of bacterial RNAs and the highly complicated nature of the cellular mRNA population. The utilization of reticulocytes in vertebrates, which produce huge amounts of mRNA that is substantially enriched in RNA encoding alpha- and beta-globin (the two major protein chains of hemoglobin), solved this problem in the 1960s. A hemoglobin-producing machine gave the first direct experimental evidence for the existence of mRNA.

Ribosomes make proteins.

Radioactive amino acids were associated with "microsomes" (later described as ribosomes) relatively quickly after injection and before they were broadly integrated into cellular proteins, according to labeling experiments in rat liver in the 1950s. Ribosomes were originally observed using electron microscopy. Their ribonucleoprotein components were discovered using biophysical approaches, most notably sedimentation studies in ultracentrifuges capable of producing extremely high accelerations (equivalent to hundreds of thousands times that of gravity). Polysomes (many ribosomes traveling along a single mRNA molecule) were discovered in the early 1960s. Their investigation led to a better understanding of how ribosomes read mRNA in a 5′ to 3′ direction, creating proteins in the process.

The physical link between RNA and protein is transfer RNA (tRNA).

(Continued)

TABLE B.1 (CONTINUED)

Major Events in the History of RNA

According to biochemical fractionation experiments, radioactive amino acids were promptly integrated into small RNA molecules that remained soluble under conditions where bigger RNA-containing particles would precipitate. These molecules were initially known as soluble (sRNA) and then renamed transfer RNA (tRNA). Following research, it was discovered that (i) every cell has multiple species of tRNA, each of which is associated with a single specific amino acid, (ii) a matching set of enzymes is responsible for linking tRNAs to the correct amino acids, and (iii) tRNA anticodon sequences form a specific decoding interaction with mRNA codons.

The genetic code has been cracked.

The genetic code consists of particular nucleotide sequences in mRNA that are translated into specific amino acid sequences in proteins (polypeptides). The ability to decipher the genetic code resulted from the convergence of three areas of research: (i) new methods for creating synthetic RNA molecules of defined composition to serve as artificial mRNAs, (ii) development of in vitro translation systems that could be used to convert the synthetic mRNAs into protein, and (iii) experimental and theoretical genetic work that established that the code was written in three-letter "words" (codons). The amino acid sequence of the protein products of the tens of thousands of genes whose sequences are being discovered in genome research can now be predicted thanks to our grasp of the genetic code.

The RNA polymerase is purified.

The biochemical separation and characterization of RNA polymerase from the bacteria Escherichia coli allowed researchers to better understand the methods by which RNA polymerase initiates and terminates transcription and how these activities are regulated to control gene expression (i.e, turn genes on and off). Following the discovery of E. coli RNA polymerase, the three RNA polymerases found in the eukaryotic nucleus and those found in viruses and organelles were identified. Many protein factors that control transcription, including repressors, activators, and enhancers, have been discovered due to transcription studies. The availability of purified RNA polymerase allowed researchers to develop a wide range of new methods for investigating RNA in the test tube, which led to many later significant RNA biology findings.

1966–1975

A biological nucleic acid molecule's first complete nucleotide sequence.

Although it was becoming more common to determine the sequence of proteins, technologies for sequencing nucleic acids were not available until the mid-1960s. This seminal study isolated a specific tRNA in large amounts and then sliced it into overlapping fragments using several ribonucleases. The information needed to derive the tRNA sequence came from analyzing the nucleotide composition of each fragment in detail. Studying considerably larger nucleic acid molecules is now highly automated and significantly faster.

Folding patterns are revealed by the evolutionary diversity of homologous RNA sequences.

The first comparative sequencing study revealed that the sequences evolved so that all of the tRNAs could fold into extremely similar secondary structures (two-dimensional structures) and had identical sequences in many places (for example, CCA at the 3′ end). The radial four-arm structure of tRNA molecules is known as the "cloverleaf structure." It evolved from sequences with shared ancestry and biological purpose. Since the discovery of the tRNA cloverleaf, researchers have been able to identify shared sequences and folding patterns in a variety of related RNA molecules.

(Continued)

TABLE B.1 (CONTINUED)

Major Events in the History of RNA

The first entire genomic nucleotide sequence is discovered.

A massive team of researchers spent several years determining the 3569-nucleotide sequence of all of the genes of the RNA bacteriophage MS2, which was published in a series of scientific papers. These findings allowed scientists to examine the first entire genome, albeit modest by today's standards. In addition, several surprise traits were discovered, including genes that partially overlapped and the first indications that different organisms may use codons in slightly different ways.

RNA can be copied into DNA by reverse transcriptase.

Retroviruses contain a single-stranded RNA genome and replicate via a DNA intermediary, the opposite of the normal DNA-to-RNA transcription route. This procedure requires an RNA-dependent DNA polymerase (reverse transcriptase), which they encode. Some retroviruses, such as those linked to cancer and the HIV-1 virus that causes AIDS, can cause sickness. In the laboratory, reverse transcriptase has been widely employed to analyze RNA molecules, particularly the conversion of RNA molecules to DNA before molecular cloning and polymerase chain reaction (PCR).

RNA replicons are constantly changing.

The enzyme systems that replicate viral RNA molecules (reverse transcriptases and RNA replicases) lack molecular proofreading (3′ to 5′ exonuclease) activity, and RNA sequences do not benefit from extensive repair systems similar to those that exist in maintaining and repairing DNA sequences, according to biochemical and genetic analyses. As a result, RNA genomes experience much higher mutation rates than DNA genomes. For example, HIV-1 mutations that result in the generation of viral variants resistant to antiviral medicines are prevalent and provide a significant therapeutic issue.

All life forms' ribosomal RNA (rRNA) sequences serve as a record of their evolutionary past.

The study of ribosomal RNA sequences from a wide range of organisms revealed that all extant forms of life on Earth share structural and sequence properties of the ribosomal RNA, indicating a common ancestor. Mapping the similarities and differences across rRNA molecules from various sources yields quantitative and obvious information about the links between organisms' phylogenetics (i.e., evolution). In addition to the prokaryotes and eukaryotes, rRNA molecules were used to identify a third major kingdom of creatures, the archaea.

RNA molecules have non-encoded nucleotides appended to their ends.

Following transcription, according to molecular analysis, non-DNA-encoded nucleotides are added to both the 5′ and 3′ ends of mRNA molecules (guanosine caps and poly-A, respectively). Enzymes that add and maintain the ubiquitous CCA sequence on the 3′ end of tRNA molecules have also been discovered. These are some of the first examples of RNA processing, a complicated set of activities required to turn RNA primary transcripts into physiologically active RNA molecules.

1976–1985

Small RNA molecules abound in the nucleus of eukaryotes.

Immunological experiments with autoimmune antibodies, which bind to small nuclear ribonucleoprotein complexes, were used to identify small nuclear RNA molecules (snRNAs) in the eukaryotic nucleus (snRNPs; complexes of the snRNA and protein). Many of these molecules have critical roles in essential RNA processing events within the nucleus and nucleolus, including RNA splicing, polyadenylation, and the maturation of ribosomal RNAs, according to subsequent biochemical, genetic, and phylogenetic investigations.

(Continued)

TABLE B.1 (CONTINUED)

Major Events in the History of RNA

RNA molecules need a specialized, complex three-dimensional structure for them to function.

X-ray crystallography was used to identify the detailed three-dimensional structure of tRNA molecules, revealing highly complicated, compact three-dimensional structures with tertiary interactions built on top of the fundamental cloverleaf secondary structure. The coaxial stacking of neighboring helices and non-Watson–Crick interactions among nucleotides within the apical loops are important aspects of tRNA tertiary structure. Additional crystallographic investigations revealed that a variety of RNA molecules (including ribozymes, riboswitches, and ribosomal RNA) fold into particular structures with various 3D structural patterns. The single-stranded nature of RNA makes it possible for RNA molecules to adopt specific tertiary structures, which is critical for their biological function. RNA folding is more closely related to protein folding than the highly repetitive folded structure of the DNA double helix in many aspects.

Introns, which must be eliminated by RNA splicing, frequently interrupt genes.

According to research, the size of mature eukaryotic messenger RNA molecules is generally significantly less than the DNA sequences that encode them. The genes were discovered to be discontinuous, with introns (sequences not present in the final mature RNA) positioned between sequences kept in the mature RNA (exons). After transcription, introns were eliminated through a process known as RNA splicing. Splicing of RNA transcripts necessitates a very precise and coordinated sequence of molecular events, which includes (a) the defining of exon and intron boundaries, (b) RNA strand cleavage at those specific points, and (c) the covalent joining (ligation) of the RNA exons in the correct order. The discovery of discontinuous genes and RNA splicing shocked the RNA biology community, and it remains one of the most surprising discoveries in molecular biology research.

Multiple proteins are produced from a single gene through alternative pre-mRNA splicing.

Multiple introns are found in most protein-coding genes encoded in the nucleus of metazoan cells. In several cases, these introns were shown to be processed in multiple ways, resulting in a family of related mRNAs that differed, for example, by the presence or absence of specific exons. As a result of alternative splicing, a single gene can encode a range of distinct protein isoforms, each of which can perform a different (typically related) biological function. Alternative splicing produces the majority of the proteins encoded by the human genome.

Catalytic RNA is discovered (ribozymes).

An experimental setup was constructed to splice an intron-containing rRNA precursor from the nucleus of the ciliated protozoan Tetrahymena in vitro. Following biochemical research, it was discovered that this group I intron was self-splicing, meaning that the precursor RNA can carry out the entire splicing reaction without proteins. Furthermore, the RNA component of the bacterial enzyme ribonuclease P (a ribonucleoprotein complex) catalyzed the tRNA-processing reaction in the absence of proteins in a separate study. These findings were watershed moments in RNA biology because they proved that RNA could catalyze certain biochemical events and hence play a role in cellular processes. Prior to these discoveries, biological catalysis was thought to be limited to protein enzymes.

(Continued)

TABLE B.1 (CONTINUED)

Major Events in the History of RNA

Prebiotic evolution was most likely aided by RNA.

Catalytic RNA (ribozymes) was discovered to be able to both encode genetic information (like DNA) and catalyze certain metabolic reactions (like protein enzymes). The RNA World Hypothesis was born out of this realization: RNA may have played a vital role in prebiotic development before more specialized molecules (DNA and proteins) dominated biological information coding and catalysis. Furthermore, functioning RNA molecules with shared ancestry in all modern-day life forms is a strong indication that RNA was extensively extant at the time of the last common ancestor, even though we cannot know the course of prebiotic evolution with any confidence.

Introns are genomic components that can move around.

Some self-splicing introns can spread throughout an organism's population by "homing," or inserting copies of themselves into genes where there was previously no intron. These sequences indicate transposons that are genetically quiet—i.e., they do not interfere with the expression of the gene into which they have inserted because they are self-splicing (that is, they remove themselves at the RNA level from genes into which they have been inserted). These introns can be thought of as self-serving DNA. Some mobile introns code for homing endonucleases, which start the homing process by cleaving double-stranded DNA at or near the intron-insertion site of alleles lacking an intron. Self-splitting introns belonging to the group I or group II families is typically found in mobile introns.

Spliceosomes mediate nuclear pre-mRNA splicing.

Spliceosomes, huge ribonucleoprotein complexes made up of snRNA and protein molecules whose composition and molecular connections fluctuate throughout RNA splicing events, remove introns from nuclear pre-mRNAs. Spliceosomes assemble on and around splice sites in mRNA precursors, using RNA-RNA interactions to identify key nucleotide sequences and, most likely, catalyze the splicing events. Self-splicing group II introns are similar to nuclear pre-mRNA introns and spliceosome-associated snRNAs. Furthermore, the splicing pathways of nuclear pre-mRNA introns and group II introns are very similar. These resemblances have led to speculation that these molecules may have shared a common ancestor.

1986 to 2000.

RNA sequences can be altered within cells.

Before being translated into protein, messenger RNA precursors from various organisms can be altered. Non-encoded nucleotides can be introduced into specified locations in the RNA, while encoded nucleotides can be deleted or changed during this process. The earliest evidence of RNA editing was found in the mitochondria of kinetoplastid protozoans, where it was widespread. Some protein-coding genes, for example, encode less than half of the nucleotides seen in mature, translated mRNA. In addition, mammals, plants, microbes, and viruses all have RNA editing events. Although there are fewer nucleotide changes, insertions, and deletions in these editing events than in kinetoplast DNA, they nonetheless have a significant physiologic impact on gene expression and regulation.

Telomerase maintains chromosomal ends by using a built-in RNA template.

(Continued)

TABLE B.1 (CONTINUED)
Major Events in the History of RNA

Telomerase is an enzyme found in all eukaryotic nuclei that helps maintain the ends of linear DNA in the eukaryotic nucleus' linear chromosomes by adding terminal sequences lost after each cycle of DNA replication. Before telomerase was discovered, its activity was predicted based on a basic knowledge of DNA replication, which showed that existing DNA polymerases could not replicate the 3' end of a linear chromosome due to the lack of a template strand. Instead, telomerase was discovered to be a ribonucleoprotein enzyme with an RNA template strand and a protein component that has reverse transcriptase activity and adds nucleotides to the chromosome ends using the internal RNA template.

Peptide bond formation is catalyzed by ribosomal RNA.

Because the covalent bonding of amino acids is one of the most fundamental chemical events in biology, scientists have spent years figuring out which protein(s) within the ribosome were responsible for peptidyl transferase function during translation. According to careful biochemical tests, extensive deproteinized big ribosomal subunits might catalyze peptide bond formation, hinting that the sought-after activity might be found in ribosomal RNA rather than ribosomal proteins. Using X-ray crystallography, structural biologists were able to pinpoint the peptidyl transferase center of the ribosome to a highly conserved region of the large subunit ribosomal RNA (rRNA), which is located at the point within the ribosome where the amino-acid-bearing ends of tRNA bind but no proteins are present. The ribosome was discovered to be a ribozyme due to these experiments. Moreover, the rRNA sequences that make up the ribosomal active site are the most conserved in biology. These findings suggest that RNA-catalyzed peptide bond production was a trait of the last common ancestor of all known forms of life.

In vitro evolution is enabled via a combinatorial selection of RNA molecules.

In vitro molecular experiments that used powerful selective replication strategies used by geneticists and amounted to evolution in the test, tubes were invented, allowing investigators to use large, diverse populations of RNA molecules to carry out in vitro molecular experiments that used powerful selective replication strategies used by geneticists. Different names have been given to these trials, the most common of which are "combinatorial selection," "in vitro selection," and systematic evolution of ligands by exponential enrichment (SELEX). These methods have been used to isolate RNA molecules with various features, including the ability to bind to certain proteins, catalyze specific processes, and bind low molecular weight chemical ligands. They can be used to elucidate relationships and mechanisms known as attributes of naturally occurring RNA molecules and isolate RNA molecules with unknown biological properties. Laboratory systems for synthesizing complex populations of RNA molecules were established as part of the development of in vitro selection technology for RNA. They were used in conjunction with the selection of molecules with user-specified biochemical activities and in vitro replication schemes. (a) Mutation, (b) Selection, and (c) Replication are the three phases. These three steps, when combined, enable in vitro molecular evolution.

(Continued)

TABLE B.1 (CONTINUED)

Major Events in the History of RNA

2001–present

Several mobile DNA elements use an RNA intermediate.

Transposons are transposable genetic elements that can replicate through transcription into an RNA intermediate, then transformed into DNA by reverse transcriptase. Many of these sequences, presumably connected to retroviruses, make up a large portion of the DNA in eukaryotic nuclei, particularly in plants. For example, retrotransposons make up 36% of the human genome and more than half of the genomes of crucial cereal crops, according to genomic sequencing (wheat and maize).

Riboswitches are proteins that attach to cellular metabolites and regulate gene expression.

RNA segments, which are often found in the 5′-untranslated region of many bacterial mRNA molecules, have a significant impact on gene expression via a previously unknown method that does not involve proteins. In many circumstances, environmental variables (such as ambient temperature or concentrations of certain metabolites) cause riboswitches to modify their folded form, which regulates the translation or stability of the mRNA in which the riboswitch is embedded. Gene expression can be substantially controlled at the post-transcriptional level in this way.

Post-transcriptional gene silencing is how small RNA molecules control gene expression.

In the 1990s, another previously unknown mechanism of RNA molecules' involvement in genetic regulation was found. In eukaryotic cells, small RNA molecules called microRNA (miRNA), and small interfering RNA (siRNA) exert post-transcriptional regulation over mRNA expression. They work by binding to specific locations within the mRNA and causing mRNA breakage via a silencing-associated RNA degradation process.

Non-coding RNA regulates epigenetic changes.

Non-coding RNA (ncRNA) families have recently been discovered to play functions in genome defense and chromosome inactivation and their well-known involvement in translation and splicing. For example, piwi-interacting RNAs (piRNAs) protect germline cells from genomic instability, while X-inactive-specific-transcript (Xist) is required for X-chromosome inactivation in mammals.

TABLE B.2
Nobel Prizes Awarded for Discoveries in RNA

Name	Born-Died	Field	Award Year
Alexander Todd	1907–1977	Chemistry	1957
Severo Ochoa	1905–1993	Physiology or Medicine	1959
Francis Crick	1916–2004	Physiology or Medicine	1962
James Watson	1928	Physiology or Medicine	1962
Maurice Wilkins	1916–2004	Physiology or Medicine	1962
François Jacob	1920–2013	Physiology or Medicine	1965
Jacques Monod	1910–1976	Physiology or Medicine	1965
Robert W. Holley	1922–1993	Physiology or Medicine	1968
H. Gobind Khorana	1922–2011	Physiology or Medicine	1968
Marshall Nirenberg	1927–2010	Physiology or Medicine	1968
David Baltimore	1938	Physiology or Medicine	1975
Renato Dulbecco	1914–2012	Physiology or Medicine	1975
Howard Temin	1934–1994	Physiology or Medicine	1975
Walter Gilbert	1932	Chemistry	1980
Aaron Klug	1926–2018	Chemistry	1982
Sidney Altman	1939–2022	Chemistry	1989
Thomas Cech	1947	Chemistry	1989
Richard Roberts	1943	Physiology or Medicine	1993
Philip.	1944	Physiology or Medicine	1993
Sydney Brenner	1927–2019	Physiology or Medicine	2002
Andrew Fire	1959	Physiology or Medicine	2006
Roger Kornberg	1947	Chemistry	2006
Craig Mello	1960	Physiology or Medicine	2006
Françoise Barré-Sinoussi	1947	Physiology or Medicine	2008
Luc Montagnier	1932–2022	Physiology or Medicine	2008
Elizabeth Blackburn	1948	Physiology or Medicine	2009
Carol Greider	1961	Physiology or Medicine	2009
Venkatraman Ramakrishnan	1952	Chemistry	2009
Thomas Steitz	1940–2018	Chemistry	2009
Jack Szostak	1952	Physiology or Medicine	2009
Ada Yonath	1939	Chemistry	2009
Emmanuelle Charpentier	1968	Chemistry	2020
Jennifer Doudna	1964	Chemistry	2020

Because of its instability and immunogenicity, mRNA was thought to be unsuitable for gene therapy. With the advancement of understanding of mRNA, the finding of stabilizing changes, and the development of new nucleic acid delivery systems, the disadvantages of the use of mRNA have been removed. Improvements in mRNA translation, half-life, and better transfection efficiency have resulted in a dramatic reduction in immunogenicity of the therapy. mRNA has been studied as a potential therapeutic replacement for DNA or recombinant proteins as a temporary carrier of genetic information capable of influencing protein expression. Because of its temporary nature, mRNA has greater flexibility and therapeutic value than almost all other kinds of known medicines. This heightened interest in mRNA's potential to change many health fields, including immunization, cell reprogramming, protein replacement therapies, and the treatment of genetic illnesses in a safer manner than conventional gene therapy approaches. mRNA has now progressed from a fragile molecule to a therapeutic drug in clinical trials. Overall, this biomolecule outperforms DNA vectors in terms of inactive cell transfection efficiency and lacks the risk of insertional mutagenesis in the genome, making mRNA a more appealing molecule for protein replenishment therapy.

Furthermore, mRNA allows for faster protein creation, greater control over expression levels, and the absence of exogenous sequences, such as antibiotic resistance or virus-derived promoters, demonstrating mRNA's safety and efficacy. The structure of mRNA can be used to predict its degradation, allowing improved, controlled, and transient pharmacokinetics. Another important element is the ability to synthesize mRNA using various ways, such as chemical synthesis or in vitro transcription. In vivo production, based on recombinant technology, is one option being explored.

To obtain the desired therapeutic results, one strategy that can assist in overcoming this challenge is to use a drug delivery system (DDS) capable of preserving mRNA against nucleases and inhibiting immune system detection. mRNA, as previously said, has a transitory therapeutic impact. Although the temporary nature of mRNA is advantageous in some situations, it also proves to be a drawback. Repeated delivery of this biomolecule is required to maintain therapeutic levels of a protein in hereditary and/or metabolic illnesses that require long-term treatment, which can be impractical.

The therapeutic use of mRNAs has shown significant promise in recent years, both for prophylaxis (for example, antiviral vaccinations) and for treating a wide range of illnesses, including myocardial infarction, HIV infection and several types of cancer. RNA as the nucleic acid for a genetic vehicle has numerous advantages over DNA, including:

1. The mRNA therapeutic mechanisms of action are mainly through immune stimulation and protein replacement. Other mechanisms in the decreasing order of use frequency include agonist (protein replacement), gene silencing, gene activation, increasing translation, agonist (immune stimulation), gene knockout, splice modulation, and antagonist (inhibition).
2. The RNA that is injected into the cell does not become part of the genome; whereas DNA does integrate into the genome, to a certain degree, and can also be inserted into an intact gene of the genome of the host cell, causing a mutation of this gene, and leading to a partial or total loss of the genetic information or misinformation).
3. For successful RNA transcription, viral sequences such as promoters are unnecessary; whereas a strong promoter (e.g., the viral CMV promoter) is

required to express DNA injected into the cell. The integration of such promoters into the host cell's genome can result in unfavorable modifications in gene expression regulation.

4. The RNA degradation that has been introduced occurs over a short period, allowing for transitory gene expression that can be stopped when the required treatment period has passed. This does not happen in the case of DNA that has been integrated into the genome.

5. The production of harmful anti-RNA antibodies in the patient is not caused by RNA; whereas the induction of anti-DNA antibodies is known to cause an undesirable immune response.

6. RNA has a wide range of applications; any desired RNA for any desired protein of interest can be made quickly for therapeutic purposes, including customized medicine.

B.2   DEVELOPMENT PERSPECTIVE

Currently, there are less than a dozen FDA-approved RNA therapeutics, the bulk of which are antisense oligonucleotides (ASO) and small interfering RNA (siRNA) candidates for genetic disorders. However, following the success of the COVID-19 mRNA vaccine technology, the mRNA space is expanding a wide range of disease indications. As of April 2022, there were 402 mRNA-based therapies under development (https://beacon-intelligence.com/); 123 of these therapies are clinically active, and 238 are still in preclinical development; 60 of the programs are targeting SARS-CoV-2, with the overall space being dominated by mRNA-based vaccines (52%). Nanoparticle development is the largest effort involving 80% of projects. Figure B.3 shows the active programs.

The routes of administration are compared in Figure B.4.

The indications for these projects are given in Figure B.5.

A major hurdle to new drug discovery is drug target selection. Not more than 1% of all approved drugs do not bind to proteins, whereas more than 80% of all drugs target only two protein classes: enzymes or receptors. Furthermore, the number of

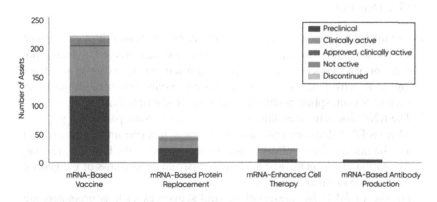

FIGURE B.3   Distribution of current mRNA projects.

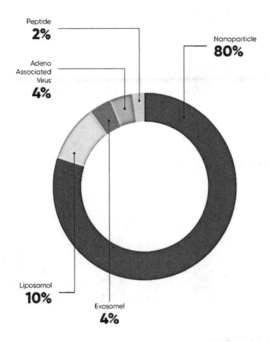

FIGURE B.4 Routes of administration of RNA therapies and vaccines.

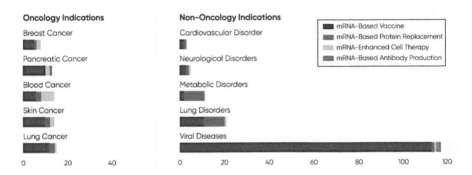

FIGURE B.5 Indications of currently developed RNA therapies and vaccines.

proteins as drug targets is limited, even though the human genome encodes more than 25,000 genes, while only 600 disease-modifying protein drug targets have been identified.

B.3 INTELLECTUAL PROPERTY PERSPECTIVE

A significant hurdle in the deployment of RNA technology is the vast patent landscape. Figures B.6– B.10 list the distribution of patents that present RNA as its mode of the invention.

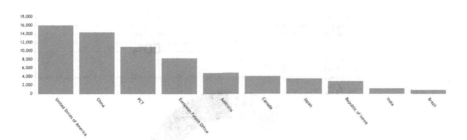

FIGURE B.6   Patent holding jurisdictions.

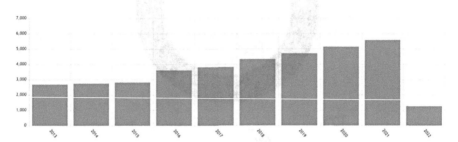

FIGURE B.7   Yearly issuances.

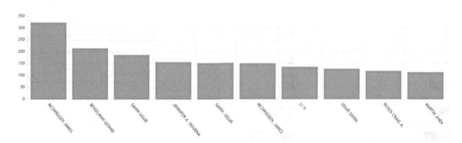

FIGURE B.8   Inventors.

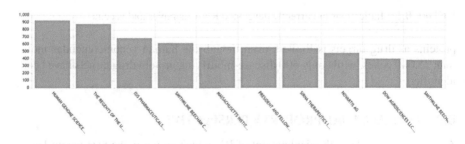

FIGURE B.9   Companies holding the patents.

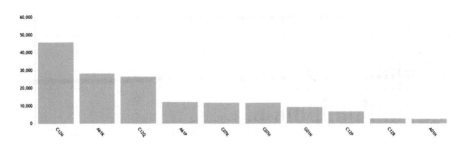

FIGURE B.10   IPC Codes of issued patents.

The complexity of the intellectual property goes further as many chemical suppliers have patents that are not included in the figure. These hurdles have prevented developing countries from taking advantage of the low-cost and fast development of mRNA vaccine production to protect their citizens. The US, the European Union (EU), India, and South Africa agreed on a proposed "TRIPS" patent waiver for Coronavirus Disease 2019 (COVID-19) vaccines on March 15, 2022. This permits an "eligible" World Trade Organization member to temporarily authorize the use of patented inventions necessary for COVID-19 vaccine production and supply without the right holder's consent. This agreement has drawn concerns from waiver opponents, claiming it threatens medical innovation and US competitiveness.

B.4   PUBLICATIONS

One way to judge the progress of science is to examine the peer review publications that arrive; Figure B.11 shows the mRNA vaccine-related publications. Figure B.12 show the papers published on the topic of RNA Therapeutics.

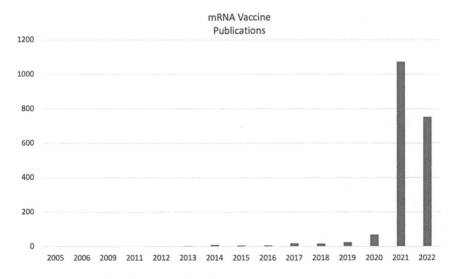

FIGURE B.11   mRNA Vaccine publications.

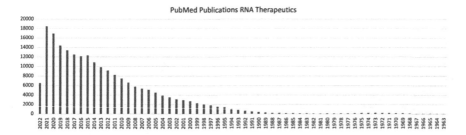

FIGURE B.12 RNA Therapeutics publications.

1 The Genome Machine

1.1 BACKGROUND

Around 14 billion years ago, it was a nightmare—an entropy explosion. "It" was so compressed that it had no alternative but to expand, as the second law of thermodynamics teaches us. It was the "Big Bang." There was just one glitch, however: entropy change requires producing more chaos, and at that moment, there was no matter present to push the expansion to increase entropy. At first, it was just energy, with no space or time or spacetime. Still, within a billionth of a second, the spreading of energy reduced the intensity of energy, causing the formation of fundamental particles. As the heat dissipated, matter was formed: first hydrogen, then helium, and later, the rest of the elements that can be found in the Periodic Table. When a bond of any type is formed, energy is released but first an increase in energy is required to bring the components together. It was the energy of the Big Bang that resulted in the formation of all elements we now know and may discover in the future. Particle physics describes what the universe (matter, energy, and forces) is made of. Forces are defined by the interaction of particle–particle or particle–energy. Scientists have created a standard model that defines the properties of the particles and forces (Figure 1.1).

To understand the arrival of RNA, let us go back to the Big Bang. We know how things worked out after that one-billionth of a second after the Big Bang, when energy was converted into particles, forces, time, and space. The laws of physics were formed, and a bit later, the fundamental particles converged into the hydrogen and helium that still light up trillions of stars. Some day in the future, we may know more about what happened during that one-trillionth of a second, but then we may not; for many, this inquiry is essential—what was there before the Big Bang? But to humble realists, it is not necessary to know.

Time as we experience it is a measure of distance. Everything around and within us is in motion, and the fundamental elements are moving at the speed of light. For this reason, time slows down as our speed increases and comes to half if we reach the speed of light. The fundamental particles can no longer move because their path is moving at the same speed. Time comes to a halt. Everything was condensed into a tiny entity blocking any movement at the point (not time) of the Big Bang. Thus, there was no time; as the expansion began and the fundamental particles could cover a certain distance, time came into existence.

The word "element" refers to a component of a whole. Philosophers of earlier centuries believed and tried to experiment with alchemy to analyze elements observed in nature. Even Sir Isaac Newton practiced it; much of Newton's writing on alchemy was lost in a fire in his laboratory. The concept of alchemy went against the term elements; if an element is viewed as a building block, then it should not be able to create

DOI: 10.1201/9781003248156-2

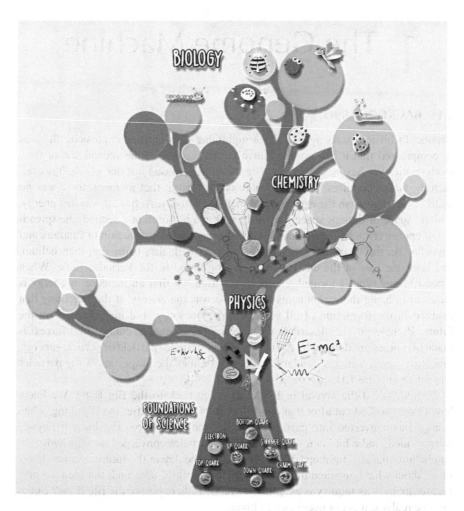

FIGURE 1.1 Family tree of elementary particles leading to biology.

another building block. For example, mercury cannot be an element if its chemical combination with other elements can produce the element gold. At best, they can be used to make alloys. Before the twentieth century, there were no means to break open complex objects into smaller parts. The principal elements required for life are hydrogen, oxygen, nitrogen, carbon, phosphorus, sulfur, and iron. As already mentioned, at the present state of our knowledge, the universe was formed about 13.7 billion years ago, the result of the Big Bang. Hydrogen formed within 10 seconds after the creation of the universe, but the rest of the elements were created inside the stars.

The first group of stars formed 200 million years after the Big Bang. The oldest star died 10 billion years ago. As most stars die, they explode in an incredible death spasm, called a nova; this process spews out the heavier elements required for life. Once the required elements come together, organic compounds form—they are found throughout the universe. The required elements for life formed 10 billion years ago, i.e., after the death of the first star. Earthlike planets formed at the same time as their corresponding stars were formed. Earth, as per current estimation, was formed about 4.54 billion years ago.

About 400 million years ago, the current form of carbon-based life emerged. Out of all the elements in the periodic table, only one element, carbon, is small enough (six protons in the nucleus, two electrons in the inner orbit, and four in the outer, called the valence electrons) to combine with itself and other elements in an incredible number of ways. These combinations gave rise to more than ten million organic compounds, which continue to increase further. Carbon-based chemistry is called "organic chemistry" because all the molecules that make up any known life-form are organic, but the reverse is not true. The small size of carbon enables it to combine with another carbon, and the C–C-bond energy (83 kcal/mol) is very close to its bonding capability with other atoms. For example, the bonding energy of the C–H-bond is 97 kcal/mol. However, we do not know yet how the sheer complexity and interconnection of different organic compounds ultimately creates an externally complex behavior—life, which contemplates, writes, and reads about itself and is *aware* of itself.

Now comes $E=mc^2$. Breaking an atom releases massive energy; only 15 g of uranium was squeezed to fuse the bombs dropped on Hiroshima and Nagasaki, weighing around 8 kg. The reason uranium was used had to do with its unstable atomic structure that requires less energy to break; once it breaks, the energy created breaks others, and a chain reaction follows. If all 8 kg were consumed, the blast would have been so large as to annilihate the entire country.

This book is not about theoretical physics, so why I am bringing this topic up? I intend to connect this concept to the creation of life thanks to ribonucleic acid.

Four billion years ago or so on our planet, basic chemical building blocks gave rise to longer polymers that could self-replicate and perform essential functions: storing information and catalyzing chemical reactions. My argument is straightforward: if different environmental conditions could form other elements, then it is entirely possible that these chemical building blocks are capable of self-replication. Three things were needed for life-forms to arrive: RNA, protein, and lipids (the last one to form a holding pouch). How these chemicals were formed is no longer a mystery. Neither is there any mystery about how some molecules began self-replicating; it is all chemistry, and so is the chemistry of death, all driven by the laws of thermodynamics.

Let us see how the complex chemicals came to be that gave birth to life on Earth. One of the most important chicken-or-the-egg questions for scientists exploring the origins of life is: which came first, proteins or nucleic acids (like DNA and RNA)?

1.2 MOLECULAR CLOCK

Molecular biology began with James Watson and Francis Crick's announcement of the structure of deoxyribose nucleic acid (DNA) in 1953. Ten years later, in a groundbreaking publication by Émile Zuckerkandl and Linus Pauling, the "molecular clock" was named. By 1963, numerous proteins had already been sequenced, including hemoglobin. But the new breed of molecular biologists noticed something unusual. Proteins from different animal species were not identical, and the architectures of proteins from distantly related species diverged even more. In other words, human and chimp hemoglobin molecules were similar, while shark hemoglobin was quite different. According to Zuckerkandl and Pauling, the degree of difference was proportional to time. Human and chimp hemoglobin had minimal difference, indicating that these two species separated very recently geologically, whereas human and shark hemoglobin had a 79 percent difference, indicating a divergence 400 million years ago or more.

Protein sequencing was a time-consuming operation in the 1960s, and new information was slow to arrive. Still, by 1967, the hemoglobin of the great apes was well-known enough that the first attempt at creating an evolutionary tree was made. As a result, the field of molecular phylogenetics came into being. In a three-page report published in the American magazine *Science*, Vincent Sarich and Allan Wilson charted the links between humans and apes, revealing that the chimp was our closest relative, followed by the gorilla, and then the orangutan. This was not entirely unexpected, and it corresponded to the pattern of links revealed by anatomical research.

The molecular clock determined that humans and chimps separated about 5 million years ago, rather than the 15–20 million years predicted by early humanlike fossils from Africa's Miocene. More animals were added to the tree as the protein data sets developed, and the branching dates for most other taxa seemed credible. However, an examination of the fossils reveals that the ostensibly "human" qualities of the Proconsul and his relatives were everything but human. Because this fossil was linked to the shared ancestors of humans and African apes, it could not be used to determine the exact time of divergence. Nevertheless, discoveries in Africa since the 1970s have revealed that humans and chimps diverged at least 6–7 million years ago.

DNA sequences are being used by molecular biologists interested in the tree of life, the vast pattern of links that connects all species. But protein sequencing is time-consuming, and evidence is scarce. DNA, or genetic code, contains more information, and new techniques developed in the 1980s have made sequencing nearly automatic. Sequencers are delighted to run long portions of the genetic code, consisting of many genes and many species, to establish patterns of relationships for specific groups or huge sectors of life because computers can now crunch enormous amounts of data. For example, it is possible to analyze the genomes of 20 different lizard species and create a tree that shows the evolution over 10 million years. Similarly, the analyst can choose 20 genomes from diverse species—a person, shark, mollusk, tree, fern, and bacteria—and create a tree of relationships that stretches back through time.

1.3 EVOLUTION

Evolution is the process of a living species going through billions of reproductions. Aristotle (384–322 BC) focused on *spontaneous generation*. He believed that all marine shellfish originated spontaneously on the seabed and among the coastal rocks from mud, sand, and slime. He made similar assumptions about other life-forms: moths arose from woolen garments, garden insects appeared from the spring dew or decaying wood, and many fishes emerged from froth on the ocean's surface. Until the nineteenth century, such viewpoints were prevalent. Louis Pasteur (1822–95) famously and decisively demonstrated, by sterilizing utensils and heating water, that life does not begin spontaneously.

Earth was first supposed to be something akin to a massive iron ball—iron is one of the most abundant metals—that had been molten and was cooling down. Based on this premise and his understanding of thermodynamics, Lord Kelvin (1824–1907) speculated that the Earth formed only 20–40 million years ago. Charles Darwin thought it had to be hundreds or thousands of millions of years old, although he never speculated more closely. Nonetheless, he could observe how the oceans may have gathered and what it took for the oceans to split from the molten rock and turn salty.

By the 1950s, the age of the Earth was estimated at 4.5 billion years, the currently accepted figure based on radiocarbon studies. However, it is still hard to date the exact origin of the Earth because rocks were presumably molten then, so there are no solidified crystals that may be dated.

Most geologists suggest that the Earth became habitable about 600 million years ago. After all, any organic components would have been burned off if the initially molten surface had not cooled to below 100°C. Carbon, hydrogen, and oxygen are the building blocks of life, and they all stay gaseous at high temperatures. But, of course, water boils at 100°C, and life is essentially water (H_2O) with carbon.

The gas into which earlier generations of stars expelled hydrogen and helium and minuscule amounts of carbon, oxygen and other elements produced in their cores formed the Sun and its companion planets 4.6 billion years ago. The Earth used to be a molten mass. Lighter components like silicon ascended to the surface, whereas heavier iron sunk to the core. The separation took 50 million years, and during that period, the Moon may have spun off, potentially resulting from a collision with a colossal planetoid. Massive volcanic eruptions at the Earth's surface emitted significant gases such as carbon dioxide, nitrogen, water vapor, and hydrogen sulfide from semi-molten silicon-rich rocks.

Temperatures on the earth's surface were too high, and the crust was too unstable for any form of carbon-based life to exist. At this time, the record of craters on the Moon suggests a few huge impacts on Earth, impacts from large comets or asteroids that would have provided enough energy to turn the ocean into steam. Thus, if life had started before 4 billion years ago, it would probably have been wiped out, only to start afresh.

The oldest sedimentary rocks have been discovered in Greenland's Isua Group, dating back 3.7–3.8 billion years. There is no doubt that there was water on the Earth at this time and that part of the Isua Group rocks is made up of accumulated sand that was put down underwater and derived from older rock sources. It has also been suggested that these ancient sedimentary rocks contain indications of life, but this is still a hot topic of controversy.

1.4 LIFE

There are numerous ideas about the beginning of life, all of which are based on our understanding of how today's tiniest living organisms function. The earliest modern hypothesis for the origin of life was established in the 1920s by two outstanding scientists, Russian biochemist A. I. Oparin (1894–1980) and British evolutionary biologist J. B. S. Haldane (1892–1964). Oparin and Haldane founded the biochemical hypothesis for the origin of life. Accordingly, life arose through organic chemical reactions that resulted in progressively complex biochemical structures. In early Earth's atmosphere, common gases interacted to produce simple organic compounds, which eventually joined to build more complex molecules. The complex molecules were then separated from the surrounding media and began to resemble living organisms. They learned to absorb nutrients, grow, divide (reproduce), and perform other duties. However, the Oparin–Haldane model was not tested until the 1950s.

In 1953, Stanley Miller (1920–2007), then a University of Chicago student studying under Harold Urey (1893–1981), produced a laboratory glass jar duplicate of the Precambrian atmosphere and oceans. After exposing a mixture of water, nitrogen, carbon monoxide, and nitrogen to electrical sparks to simulate lightning, he noticed a brownish sludge in the container after a few days. However, nucleotides, sugars, and amino acids were all present. Miller had thus recreated the first two steps of the Oparin–Haldane model, mixing the fundamental components to produce simple organic molecules and then combining them to generate proteins and nucleic acids.

Further research in the 1950s and 1960s observed the next stage in the suggested sequence: the production of polypeptides, polysaccharides, and other bigger organic molecules. In 2001, Euan Nisbet (University of London) and Norman Sleep (Stanford University) published the hydrothermal model for the origins of life, a modern twist on the classic Oparin–Haldane biochemical model. According to this theory, the ancestor of all living things was a hyperthermophile, an important organism that flourished in excessively hot settings. It is possible that the transition from isolated amino acids to DNA occurred in a hot-water system related to active volcanoes rather than in some primordial soup at sea level. There are two types of hot-water systems on Earth today: "black smokers," located in deep waters above mid-ocean ridges where magma meets seawater, and hot pools and fumaroles, which are found around active volcanoes and are fed by rainwater.

Let us examine the nature of three major forces dominating the molecular interaction.

- Van der Waal's force. This type of force arises from the induced dipole, and the interaction is weaker than the dipole–dipole interaction. In general, the heavier the molecule, the stronger is the van der Waal's force of interaction. Each interaction has a characteristic optimal distance of twice the atomic radius. Van der Wall's sphere is related to the atomic radius. Although, individually, it is a weak force, they collectively play an important role in determining biomolecular structure and interactions. This force is significant in molecular dynamic modeling.

- Hydrogen bond. Hydrogen bonds affect the molecular structure of organic compounds such as alcohols, acids, amines (an amino acid chain of proteins), and nucleotide chains of DNA, RNA, etc. Hydrogen bonding is the most dominant and important force in biological science. The hydrogen bond is an attractive force between a hydrogen atom from a molecule or a molecular fragment Z–H in which Z is more electronegative than H. Hydrogen bonding is easily found in liquid water, it is the reason for its higher boiling point. The hydrogen atom in a water molecule is attracted towards the oxygen atom of the neighboring water molecule, as the oxygen atom is partially negatively charged, and the hydrogen atom is partially positively charged. It is also described as an electrostatic dipole–dipole interaction.
- Covalent bonding. Covalency of an atom refers to the number of electrons it shares with other atoms. It is an intramolecular force between a pair of atoms rather than an intermolecular force like an H-bond. It shapes the molecule itself rather than affecting the shape of a polypeptide chain.

In addition to the above three, other electrostatic interactions lead to sulfur bonds, salt bridges, and hydrophobic core due to hydrophobic forces.

The objects in nature are made out of simple building blocks; each block has properties expressed in numbers. The numbers dictate how they self-organize or interact with other blocks; a set of rules guides this processing of data/information contained in the object. This happens with subatomic particles, the building blocks of everything in the universe.

At a certain level of complexity, the blocks are formed of organic entities based on carbon and a few other elements. They can store, modify information, and self-replicate. The behavior of these known macro-blocks of life is modeled using Cellular Automata (CA).

If matter, energy, and space are informatics in origin, so are the molecules of life. As first demonstrated by Gregor Mendel, genetic information is passed through generation by discrete means, though he did not know about DNA. We have seen the discreteness of life as established through DNA. The earliest cells built from fragile organic materials developed along a path of planned obsolescence. Born perfect are cells, molecules, and organisms; they live for a minute, a year, or a century before reproducing to generate a new molecule, cell, or organism and then dying. Within this cycle of birth, life, and death, one strand of immortality survives the millennia: the information about one's genetics as it is passed down from generation to generation. But that too changes as it mutates and alters with time, resulting in the diversity of life that we currently enjoy. If necessary, all of our cells are preprogrammed with a means to die on command. When a cell enters programmed cell death, it safely and methodically disassembles its molecular machinery. A cytotoxic T-cell sends the signal for another cell to die. The death process begins when death receptors identify proteins on the T-cell surface. The BID (BH3 Interacting Domain Death Agonist) protein creates a pore in the surface of mitochondria, allowing cytochrome c to escape into the cytoplasm. This is the signal for forming an apoptosome (a big quaternary protein), which then triggers the activation of initiator caspases. More caspases are activated; as a result, unleashing an ordered attack on critical proteins throughout the cell. Caspases, for example, cut the protein gelsolin and convert it into an active form capable of disassembling actin filaments. This account of death should teach us a lot about how the genome in our bodies functions so well—it is guided by thermodynamic rules.

But there's more to get rid of in our bodies. For example, proteins are produced to perform a particular activity, and they are promptly destroyed once that work is completed. In a typical cell, 20–40% of freshly synthesized proteins are eliminated within an hour. Some proteins with time-critical functions, such as transcription regulators or cell division regulators, are only present for minutes. This kind of planned obsolescence may appear wasteful, yet it has a significant benefit: it enables the cell to react swiftly to changes in its surroundings.

This, of course, presents a problem for the cell. You can't just make protein-degrading enzymes and release them into the cytoplasm at random. They would kill everything in sight, just like the digestive enzymes in our gut. Proteasomes, on the other hand, are created by the cell. Proteasomes are voracious protein shredders, yet the equipment for shredding proteins is carefully contained inside a barrel-shaped structure. As a result, the proteasome is free to roam within the cell, and only the appropriate proteins are fed into its hungry maw.

Cells must be able to regulate protein breakdown, ensuring that only obsolete or degraded proteins are delivered into the proteasome. Ubiquitin, a tiny protein, plays a crucial function in this process. It binds to aged proteins, alerting the cell that they are ready to be dismantled and recycled. Ensuring that ubiquitin is only bound to suitable proteins is the most challenging component of this process. A group of enzymes known as ubiquitin ligases is responsible for this. They detect short-lived proteins and attach ubiquitin to them with the help of two additional enzymes. A protein is targeted for destruction by a string of four or more ubiquitin molecules. The ubiquitin string is recognized by caps on either end of the proteasome, which feed the associated protein into the destruction chamber, where it is snipped into little pieces and recycled.

Environmental enemies are continually attacking our molecular machinery. They are eroded by reactive chemicals, unfolded and denatured by heat, and broken by ultraviolet light. These molecules are frequently damaged and unable to execute their jobs. Damaged proteins can be discarded by the cell, but this is not the case with DNA. It must be kept in excellent condition since it contains crucial genetic information that governs the cell's life and must be handed down to progeny. To keep this information from being lost, the cell uses various methods to protect the DNA from being destroyed, and if damage does occur, repairs it.

Several significant abnormalities can occur at the ends of DNA strands. For starters, they are susceptible to damage due to unwinding. Also, because DNA polymerase has problems copying DNA to the end, the DNA gets shorter and shorter after numerous rounds of replication. Many bacteria overcome this challenge by completely removing the ends of their DNA and forming a large circle. On the other hand, our cells are made up of 46 linear strands, each with two ends that must be protected.

Our DNA strands feature a specific nucleotide sequence called a telomere at either end to tackle this problem. The telomere is made up of the pattern GGGTTA, repeated a thousand times in a row. A group of proteins binds to the telomere and forms a loop around it, sealing the end and protecting it from DNA-cutting enzymes. The telomere also addresses the issue of telomere shortening. The telomeres lose 50–100 bases from each end when the cell divides, and the DNA is copied. The enzyme telomerase then latches to the telomere and extends it with new copies of the repeating sequence, using its internal RNA template. It does not matter how much it adds because it is a recurring sequence; all that matters is that it adds enough to keep up with the losses.

Embryonic and stem cells, such as those that make blood cells continuously throughout our lifetimes, include active telomerase, which protects their DNA throughout replication. However, most of our cells have switched off their ability to prolong telomeres. Adult human fibroblasts, for example, can divide 60 times before irreversible damage occurs and the cells die. This could help protect us from cancer by putting a stop to the proliferation of cells. As cells grow out of control, their telomeres shorten, and they all die off after a few generations.

Gravely wounded cells leave a mess when they die. They enlarge and burst, spilling the cell's contents into uncomfortable locations. Damage to lysosomes (small compartments inside cells that undertake digestion) might release damaging enzymes. The body reacts by inflaming the region with immune cells that try to clean up the debris without causing too much damage to the healthy tissue in the surrounding area.

Our cells have been programmed to commit suicide rapidly and painlessly to avoid this nasty situation. This mechanism, known as programmed cell death or apoptosis, permits the cell to break down in a controlled manner and signals the immune system that it is ready to be recycled. Apoptosis is triggered by cells for a variety of causes. They may enter programmed cell death if damaged, such as if the DNA is disrupted in multiple places or if the cell is infected with a virus. It is also crucial in the development of cancer. Our toes, for example, were produced by programmed cell death while we were still embryos. A flat flipper-like appendage split into toes, then small regions of cells died neatly. Tadpole tails go through a similar transformation as they develop into frogs. Because cells that demonstrate unusual growth are usually pushed to die, programmed cell death plays a crucial role in cancer prevention.

One myth has held on tenaciously: every few years, herds of lemmings commit mass suicide by jumping off seaside cliffs. Instinct, it is said, drives them to kill themselves whenever their population becomes unsustainably large.

Of course, this lethal system needs checks and balances. Apoptosis must be initiated only when essential to cells. The Bcl-2 family of proteins regulates apoptosis. They analyze the advantages and disadvantages of cell death every time. Some of these proteins are survival-enhancing. When a cell is healthy and useful, these proteins take over and inhibit apoptosis-inducing signals. However, the second group of proteins sentences the cell to death if DNA damage or infection is detected or cells become detached from their neighbors.

The ultimate executors of planned cell death are caspases. They are protein-cutting enzymes, like those that help us digest our food. They are, however, significantly more discriminating than our digestive enzymes, and the caspases' targets are deliberately picked to allow piecewise cell death. First, the breakdown of essential regulatory proteins and polymerases stops the cell from dividing and preventing the creation of new nucleic acids. Next, cleavage and disassembly of structural proteins, such as the lamins that support the membrane around the nucleus, occurs. Next, the cell's adhesion proteins are broken to allow for quicker processing, which frees the cell from its neighbors. Finally, the cell membrane is altered gradually, indicating that the cell is ready to be absorbed and regenerated into the surrounding tissue.

1.4.1 AGING

When we are born, our cells are brand new, and they function according to the genomic plan. Our molecules, cells, and bodies, on the other hand, steadily age as we become older, becoming less efficient and eventually failing and dying. Aging has been the focus of many scientific and medical studies as we try to find ways to slow down the aging process that remains mysterious with so many unknown variables. However, a few crucial discoveries have identified some of the most critical aspects. When we look at a range of species, we can see that the maximum lifetime is linked to body size and metabolism. Small animals have a faster metabolism than giant creatures; therefore, they age and die younger. The slow but persistent accumulation of damage from reactive forms of oxygen, according to research, is a primary underlying cause of this aging.

In respiration, our cells rely on oxygen as the last acceptor of electrons, allowing us to extract significantly more energy from food than we could without it. However, highly reactive forms of oxygen, such as superoxide and hydroxyl radicals, are generated during these processes. These hazardous compounds occasionally escape the respiratory enzymes before being entirely transformed into water. They next go after proteins and DNA, producing damage or mutations. They also assault the lipids in our membranes, converting them into reactive forms that can subsequently attack other molecules. The formation of liver spots on aged skin is a noticeable indicator. Lipofuscin, a brownish peroxidized version of our regular lipids, makes them up.

Oxidation is a severe issue. One of our most active molecular systems is our respiratory system, and these reactive forms of oxygen move through the cell as a by-product. But we have a mechanism in place to safeguard us from this ever-present threat. A sequence of enzymes that seek out and detoxify reactive forms of oxygen serves as our first line of defense. Superoxide dismutase, which eliminates superoxide (oxygen with an extra electron), and two enzymes that remove peroxides are among these enzymes. Several tiny antioxidant compounds aid this task. Glutathione and vitamin C fight oxygen species in the cell's water-filled compartments, detoxifying them if they discover one. However, reactive oxygen forms are significantly more soluble inside membranes, so we need membrane-bound vitamins A and E to detoxify them. Because vitamin E's role is important, there may only be 100 lipid molecules for every cell.

However, infusing with extra antioxidants, such as vitamins A, C, and E, does not slow down the aging process. The typical level of antioxidants has been fine-tuned by evolution to give us the best possible protection, so antioxidant supplements do not appear to have much impact. However, restrictive diets do increase lifespan. The animal's diet still contains all of the nutrients required for normal growth and maintenance, but the calories consumed are reduced to extend survival. The diet's success is related to damage caused by reactive oxygen. The metabolism slows down on a calorie-restricted diet, which means less oxygen is utilized and fewer molecules of reactive oxygen leak from the respiratory enzymes.

1.4.2   Humans

The peculiarly human characteristics stem from two features. First, the large brain permitted or enabled language, socialization, extended care of children, adaptability to challenging environments, and technology. Second, bipedalism freed the hands for gathering food, tool-making, pot-making, scratching, and writing. It seemed clear that humans acquired their large brains first and then bipedalism.

So far as we know, human evolution occurred only in Africa. But the following species, *Homo erectus*, escaped from Africa. The oldest examples are indeed known from Africa in rocks dated about 1.9 million years ago, and similar dates have been suggested for *H. erectus* specimens from Georgia and China. *H. erectus* had a brain size of 830–1,100 cc in a body up to 1.6 meters tall.

Indeed, modern humans, *Homo sapiens*, may have arisen as long as 400,000 years ago, and certainly by 150,000 years ago, in Africa, having evolved from *H. erectus*. It seems that all modern humans arose from a single African ancestor and that the *H. erectus* stocks in Asia and Europe died out. *H. sapiens* spread to the Middle East and Europe 90,000 years ago.

The Neanderthals disappeared as the ice withdrew to the north, and more modern humans advanced across Europe from the Middle East. This new wave of colonization coincided with the spread of *Homo sapiens* over the rest of the world, crossing Asia to Australasia before 40,000 years ago and reaching the Americas 11,500 years ago, if not earlier, by crossing from Siberia to Alaska. With brain sizes averaging 1,360 cc, these modern humans brought more refined tools than those of the Neanderthals, art in cave paintings and carvings, and religion. In addition, the nomadic way of life began to give way to settlements and agriculture about 10,000 years ago.

And here we are making a synthetic RNA to force ribosomes to translate the proteins of our choice to bring immunity to our body—a giant leap for humanity!

1.4.3   Biological Cell

The cell is the basic structural, functional unit of all known living organisms. A cell can replicate independently. Cells are the building blocks of life. Organisms consisting of a single cell are called unicellular, for example, bacteria. Higher organisms, such as plants, contain multiple cells. Humans contain more than 10 trillion cells. Cell dimension varies from 1 to 100 micrometers.

Cells consist of a membrane enclosing a disordered colloidal solution called cytoplasm. The material properties of the cytoplasm remain an ongoing investigation. Recent measurements reveal that the cytoplasm can be likened to an elastic solid rather than a viscoelastic fluid (Figure 1.2).

The simplest cell does not have a nucleus inside the cell membrane; these are called prokaryotic cells and were the first form of life on earth which emerged at least 3.5 billion years ago. The DNA of the prokaryotic cell consists of a single chromosome that is in direct contact with the cytoplasm. The dimension of a prokaryotic cell ranges from 0.5 to 2.0 um in diameter. Bacteria fall in the domain of prokaryotic cellular organisms.

Enclosing the cell is the plasma membrane covered by a cell wall, but the cell wall is absent in some microorganisms. The cell wall gives rigidity to the cell and serves as a protective filter. Inside the cell is the cytoplasmic region that contains DNA, ribosome, etc. There are variations in the internal elements of a cell depending on different unicellular life-forms. This shows the diversity and evolutionary dynamics that even the simplest cell goes through.

Plants, animals, fungi, slime molds, protozoa, and algae belong to the eukaryotic group. Eukaryotic cells are 15 times larger than prokaryotic cells (and hence a

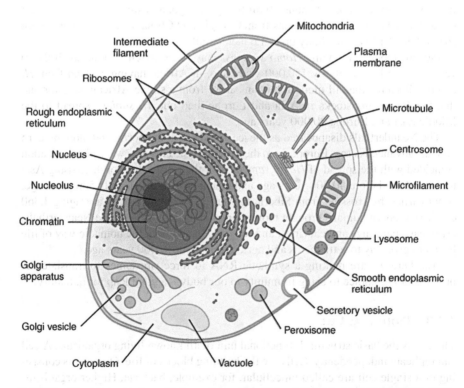

FIGURE 1.2 Anatomy of a cell. (https://cnx.org/contents/FPtK1zmh@8.25:fEI3C8Ot@10/ Preface Licensed under the Creative Commons Attribution 4.0 International)

thousand times more in volume). The various organelles that perform specific metabolic functions are categorized inside the cell membrane. The most important is
the cell nucleus, an organelle that houses the cell's DNA. The plasma membrane
resembles prokaryotes, i.e., physical communication with the environment for nour-
ishment and waste disposal.

The eukaryotic DNA is organized in one or more linear molecules called chromosomes. The cell nucleus stores all chromosomal DNA, isolated from the cytoplasm
by a membrane. DNA can also be found in some eukaryotic organelles, such as
mitochondria.

Cells use DNA for their long-term information storage. The biological information contained in an organism is in its DNA sequence. RNA that is used for communication is called messenger RNA (mRNA). Transfer RNA (tRNA) adds amino
acids during protein translation. The organelle "ribosome" is the organic body that
connects genomics to proteomics.

A human cells have genetic material contained in the cell nucleus and the mitochondria. In humans, the nuclear genome is divided into 46 linear DNA molecules
called chromosomes, including 22 homologous chromosome pairs and a pair of sex
chromosomes. The first 22 pairs are called autosomes. The chromosomes of the 23rd
pair are called allosomes (sex chromosomes), consisting of two X chromosomes in
women, and a Y chromosome in men.

The X chromosome is always present as the 23rd chromosome in the ovum, while
either an X or Y chromosome can be present in individual sperm. Early in female
embryonic development, in cells other than egg cells, one of the X chromosomes is
randomly and partially deactivated; in some cells, the X chromosome inherited from
the mother is deactivated. In others, the X chromosome from the father is deactivated. This ensures that both sexes always have exactly one functional copy of the X
chromosome in each cell.

The mitochondrial genome differs from nuclear DNA in that it is a circular DNA
molecule. As a result, it is tiny compared to nuclear chromosomes, and it codes
for 13 proteins involved in mitochondrial energy production and specific tRNAs. In
humans, mitochondrial DNA (mtDNA) is inherited solely from the mother.

Foreign genetic material (most commonly DNA) can also be artificially introduced
into the cell by transfection. Transfection is transient if the DNA is not inserted into the
cell's genome. Transfection is stable if it is inserted. Certain viruses also insert their
genetic material into the genome. There are various methods of introducing foreign
DNA into a eukaryotic cell, including electroporation, cell squeezing, and nanoparticles. Several chemical materials and biological particles (viruses) are used as carriers.

The anatomy of a cell structure in Figure 1.2 describes various organelles.
Analogous to the different functions of organs in a human body, organelles are parts
of the cell that are adapted and specialized for carrying out one or more vital cell
functions. Both eukaryotic and prokaryotic cells have organelles; prokaryotic organelles are generally more straightforward and are not membrane-bound.

There are several types of organelles in a cell. A few, such as the nucleus and
Golgi apparatus, are typically solitary in number. Others such as mitochondria and
lysosomes exist in large numbers.

Mitochondria are self-replicating organelles that occur in various numbers, shapes, and sizes in the cytoplasm of all eukaryotic cells. The biological processes are often called "respiration" that occurs in the mitochondria and generate the cell's energy, using oxygen to release energy stored in cellular nutrients. Mitochondria multiply through binary fission like prokaryotic cells. They are known as the cell's powerhouses, organelles that function as a digestive system, absorbing nutrients, breaking them down, and converting them into energy-rich molecules for the cell. Cellular respiration refers to the cell's metabolic processes.

In contrast to molecules that float freely in the cytoplasm, the endoplasmic reticulum (ER) is a transport network for molecules targeted for specific modifications and destinations. The rough ER, which has ribosomes on its surface that secrete proteins into the ER, and the smooth ER, which does not have ribosomes, are the two types of ER. The smooth ER controls calcium sequestration and release. The Golgi apparatus' principal purpose is to process and package proteins and lipids produced by the cell.

Lysosomes contain enzymes that digest excess or worn-out organelles, food particles, viruses, or bacteria. Peroxisomes secrete enzymes to get rid of toxic peroxides in the cell. The centrosomes produce the microtubules of a cell. It directs the transport through the ER and the Golgi apparatus. Centrosomes are two centrioles, which separate during cell division and help form the mitotic spindle. A single centrosome is present in the human cell. Vacuoles provide structural support and service functions such as storage, waste disposal, protection, and growth.

Cell division involves a single cell (called a *mother cell*) dividing into two daughter cells. Such procreation of cells results in the growth of the multicellular organism. Prokaryotic cells divide by binary fission, while eukaryotic cells usually undergo a process of nuclear division, called mitosis, followed by division of the cell, called cytokinesis. A diploid cell (cells that have two homologous copies of each chromosome) may also undergo meiosis (a specialized type of cell division that reduces the chromosome by half) to produce haploid cells (usually four). Haploid cells serve as gametes in multicellular organisms, fusing to form new diploid cells.

In mitosis, DNA replication always happens when a cell divides into two. In meiosis, the DNA is replicated only once, while the cell divides twice. DNA replication only occurs before meiosis I. DNA replication does not occur when the cells divide in meiosis II. Cell division is a highly complex and essential process.

In complex multicellular organisms, cells specialize in in that they are adapted to execute specific functions. In mammals, major cell types include skin cells, muscle cells, neurons, blood cells, and others. Cell types differ in appearance and function, yet they are genetically identical. Cells can be of the same genotype, but different cell types, due to the differential expression of the genes they contain.

Cells emerged at least 3.5 billion years ago. The early cell membranes were probably simpler and more permeable than modern ones, with only a single fatty acid chain per lipid. Lipids are known to spontaneously form bi-layered vesicles in water and could have preceded RNA. Still, the first cell membrane could have been produced by catalytic RNA or even required structural proteins before they could form.

Prokaryotes are single-celled organisms with no nucleus, membrane, or other specialized organelles. Bacteria and archaea are examples of prokaryotes. Prokaryote life appears to have begun over 4 billion years ago, feeding on the early atmosphere's carbon dioxide, carbon monoxide, steam, nitrogen, hydrogen, and ammonia.

Archaea and bacteria are the two domains of prokaryotes. All internal water-soluble components, proteins, DNA, and metabolites are found in the cytoplasm of prokaryotes rather than in discrete cellular compartments in the cytoplasm and contained by the cell membrane. Bacteria have protein-based bacterial micro-compartments that operate as primitive organelles encased in protein shells. Cyanobacteria and other prokaryotes can create huge colonies. Myxobacteria, for example, exhibit multicellular stages in their life cycles.

Figure 1.3 depicts the evolution of prokaryotes from a primitive carbon dioxide, carbon monoxide, steam, nitrogen, hydrogen, and ammonia atmosphere to the present day, starting 4.3–4.4 billion years ago and extending from a primitive carbon dioxide, carbon monoxide, steam, nitrogen, hydrogen, and ammonia atmosphere to an oxygen–nitrogen atmosphere. Despite billions of years of development or progress, prokaryotic life is a very primitive life-form.

The cytoskeleton of prokaryotes is substantially more rudimentary than that of eukaryotes. Flagellin, the helically structured building block of the flagellum, is a significant cytoskeletal protein in bacteria, providing structural backdrops for the basic physiological response of chemotaxis bacterium. Some prokaryotes have internal structures that are similar to rudimentary organelles. Some prokaryotes have membrane organelles or intracellular membranes, such as vacuoles or membrane systems dedicated to specific metabolic features, such as photosynthesis.

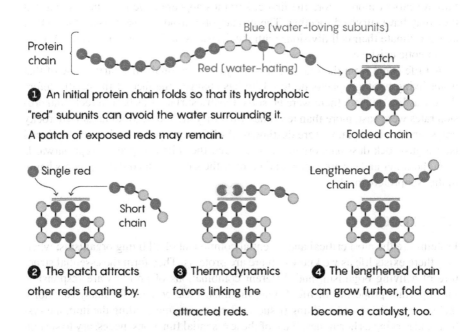

FIGURE 1.3 Folding of the chain leads to complex proteins.

Protein-enclosed micro-compartments with specific physiological functions are also seen in some animals.

A five-kingdom classification of life was popular for a while, with plants and animals supplemented by fungi among the larger forms and two major groups of microscopic organisms, the eukaryotic protoctists and the prokaryotic monerans. The five-kingdom model was demolished after 1977 in a remarkable series of papers by Carl Woese and colleagues from the University of Illinois (my alma mater). Their molecular trees showed a deep split into three fundamental divisions, the domains Bacteria (or Eubacteria), Archaea (or Archaebacteria), and Eucarya (or Eukaryota). So, the prokaryotes are no more, forming the domains Bacteria and Archaea, and it is still unclear whether Archaea and Bacteria split first, or Archaea and Eucarya. Despite this uncertainty at the root, Woese had produced the first universal tree of life.

So, all living things fall into these three great domains. The Domain Bacteria includes Cyanobacteria and most groups commonly called bacteria. The Domain Archaea ("ancient ones") comprises the Halobacteria (salt-digesters), Methanobacteria (methane-producers), Eocytes (heat-loving, sulfur-metabolizing bacteria), and others. Finally, the Domain Eucarya includes an array of single-celled forms often lumped together as "algae" and multicellular organisms. Perhaps the most startling observation is that, within Eucarya, the fungi are more closely related to the animals than the plants, which has been confirmed in several analyses. This may pose a moral dilemma for vegetarians: should they eat mushrooms or not?

While it had long been assumed that prokaryotes had dominated the Earth for a billion years or more before the first eukaryotes appeared, we now understand that they may have survived together. The prokaryotic invaders that possess their DNA and coordinate their cell divisions with the divisions of the larger host cells allowed a symbiotic existence.

All life came from the sea, and it is not just the animals that carry some of that water-living heritage: plants do too. Life has changed the face of the earth. Before there was life on land, there were no soils. Earth's surface was barren rock, and erosion rates were vast, more than ten times what they are today. Mountains were rocky crags, and lowland plains were dustbowls. As life moved onto land, soils developed (soil is just rock dust plus organic matter), and the soils and plants crept outwards from the water and covered more and more of the surface. But did this process begin in the Neoproterozoic?

1.5   PROTEINS

Proteins are the most critical and essential component of all living organisms; wherever there exists life as we know it, there are proteins. They form the essential structure of a living organism, and different combinations of proteins are responsible for important properties of life. Living organisms use proteins for many functions, including repairing and building tissues, acting as enzymes, aiding the immune system, and serving as hormones. Each of these essential functions, necessary to sustain life, requires different classes of proteins. Despite their differences in structure, all proteins contain the same basic sub-components (micro-molecules). Proteins communicate, acquire and store energy, modify themselves, and do many more things. The polymeric macromolecules are assembled from nucleotides.

Protein chains spontaneously grew to support life about 4 billion years ago by catalyzing one another's growth. They were produced by nucleic acids, DNA and RNA, constituting the eternal pair. The instructions for creating proteins are carried by DNA and RNA, which proteins extract and copy as DNA or RNA. So, which one could have done both roles on its own at first? For decades, RNA has been the preferred contender, especially after the revelation in the 1980s that RNA can fold up and catalyze processes in the same way that proteins do. Life arose from RNA with the ability to catalyze the synthesis of additional RNA. However, RNA is very sophisticated and delicate, raising questions about its prebiotic origins. To conduct their catalytic activity, both RNA molecules and proteins must assume the form of long, folded chains. The early environment prevented nucleic acid or amino acid chains from becoming long enough. Lengthy polymers likely folded into protein forms initially, leading to RNA synthesis (Figure 1.3).

The "protein-folding problem" is concerned with how a protein's amino acid sequence determines its folded structure. The hydrophobic-polar (HP) protein-folding model treats the 20 amino acids as merely two types of subunits, hydrophobic and hydrophilic, with the hydrophobic ends' ability to cluster together to avoid water as the only difference. Foldable polymers, also known as foldamers, serve as a sticky platform for elongating polymers. The majority of those elongated polymers just keep going. However, a few fold, some even have their hydrophobic patch, just like the original catalyst. When this happens, the folded molecules with landing pads continue to build lengthy polymers in increasing numbers. Still, they can also form an autocatalytic set, in which foldamers catalyze the development of copies of themselves either directly or indirectly. Two or more foldamers can sometimes engage in reciprocal catalysis by promoting processes that form one another. Despite the rarity of such pairings, the number of these molecules would expand exponentially and eventually take over the prebiotic soup—a modest event's potential to leverage itself to far more significant events. This productive, information-rich environment may have grown more conducive to RNA's emergence. Natural selection would have favored RNA in the long run since it is stronger at autocatalysis.

Whether any sticky strands existed before RNA or not becomes a moot point since they cannot translate proteins, giving the RNA an upper single hand or strand.

Proteins are large molecules composed of one or more long chains of amino acids. It is a single class of macromolecule consisting of amino acid residues joined by peptide bonds. The building blocks of an amino acid are the atoms—carbon, hydrogen, nitrogen, oxygen, sulfur, and occasionally phosphorus—the most abundant elements in the universe.

Amino acids are organic compounds containing two functional groups, amine and carboxyl, and an R group (an alkyl group or hydrogen). Amines (derivative of ammonia) are compounds and functional groups composed of a basic (opposite to acidic) nitrogen atom with a two valence electron (lone pair). There are four classes of amines—primary, secondary, tertiary, and cyclic. Morphine and heroin are tertiary amines, while antidepressants like amoxapine are secondary amines. The breakdown of amino acids releases amines. The smell of decaying fish is due to the breakdown of amino acids; it is of trimethylamine, another tertiary amine.

The amino acid molecules are not rigid like a ball and stick; they are vibrating, dynamic, and influenced by the medium they are in which, in the present case, is water. The dynamism gives rise to the redistribution of charges over the surface of the molecules. For example, when two glycines join together, they must get rid of one water molecule thus forming glycine residue. We can now envisage the behavior of linkages between amino acids that result in complex properties.

Some amino acid residues are polar, meaning they have an electric charge difference across themselves. These polar amino acid residues happily interact with water and are called hydrophilic. Other amino acids are non-polar, without a charge—they are called hydrophobic.

There are about 500 amino acids—proteinogenic and non-proteinogenic. Interestingly, only 20 common ones are synthesized from the genetic code during translation. These are called proteinogenic amino acids, each having a common backbone linked to a side chain that differs for each one. One end of the backbone covers an N–H group, while the other end covers a C=O group of atoms with an alpha carbon. Peptide bonds link a chain of amino acids. The formation of a peptide bond linking a pair of amino acids releases two hydrogens and one oxygen atom; the resulting amino acid is referred to as amino acid residue. The specific sequence of residues in a polypeptide chain imparts a unique property to a protein concerning its structure and function. One particular amino acid, cysteine, has a sulfur atom. Sulfur atoms on two separate cysteine residues can bond, forming a disulfide bridge; disulfide bonds (Figure 1.4) are essential in determining the quaternary structure of some proteins.

The amino acid residue chain making up the long strand is the main determining factor that decides what shape a particular protein will fold into. The sequence of amino acids behaves like a string of instructions, and their properties depend on their physical and chemical characteristics and their neighbor's. The 3D structure of the proteins is derived from a uniquely encoded primary structure (the amino acid sequence).

Proteins fold into unique three-dimensional structures during protein folding. They fold through the interaction of the different amino acids in the medium. Before settling down to its quaternary structural conformation, the intermediate conformations of a protein structure are summarized below and illustrated in Figure 1.5.

- The primary structure of the protein is made of amino acid residue sequence.
- The secondary structure of the protein is composed of regularly repeating local structures. It is stabilized by hydrogen bonds that get formed. The most common examples are the alpha-helix, beta-sheet, and turns.
- The tertiary structure of the protein is the overall shape that the single protein molecule folds into. It essentially characterizes the spatial relationship of the secondary structures to one another. The tertiary structure of the protein essentially dictates the basic function of the protein.

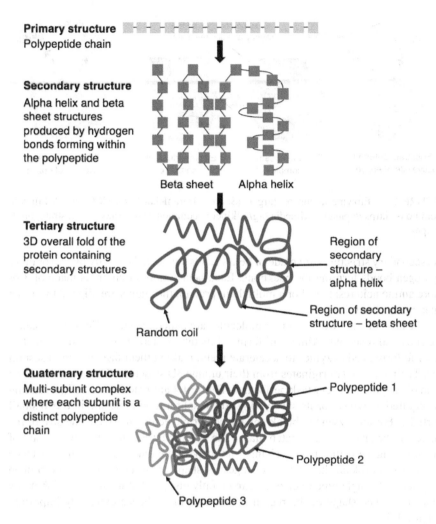

FIGURE 1.4 Structures of protein. (Kep17, CC BY-SA 4.0 <https://creativecommons.org/licenses/by-sa/4.0>, via Wikimedia Commons)

- The quaternary structure of the protein is formed by several chains of multichain protein that combine to function as a single protein complex.

The protein's primary structure is the sequence of amino acid residues in the polypeptide chain. The primary structure is held together by covalent bonds, mostly the peptide bonds. The primary structure then evolves into the secondary structure. Given different electrostatic forces, the secondary structure is formed out of the primary structure linear chain. By convention, common structural blocks are referred to as "motifs." For example, the alpha-helix is a common motif formed in the secondary structure of proteins. It is a right-handed coil-like formation. Beta sheets in

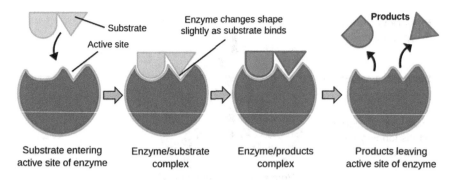

FIGURE 1.5   Enzyme action on target. (Source: ImranKhan1992, CC0, via Wikimedia Commons. https://upload.wikimedia.org/wikipedia/commons/4/40/Enzyme-substrate_binding.png)

the secondary structures are made of beta strands connected laterally by two or more hydrogen bonds forming the backbone. Each beta-strand, or chain, is made of 3 or more amino acid residues. For a multichain protein, the chains are aligned to form a quaternary structure.

The proteins that work on other molecules are called enzymes. Enzymes accelerate chemical reactions. Almost all forms of metabolic activities in the living cell of any life-form need enzymes to accelerate them, making them fast enough to sustain life. Their *specificity* originates from their unique 3D structure. There is at least one kind of enzyme for every task performed. Figure 1.4 animates how a cell (consisting of required enzymes for its survival) needs to split a food molecule into two small particles. For an enzyme to break any particular molecule, the shape and size of the "hole" in the enzyme must match that of the specific target molecule. As a result of the target entering, the enzyme changes its shape and breaks the target in two. Once the target is broken, the enzyme changes its shape again and releases the broken fragments. A single type of enzyme can do only one job, but it can do the job many times over. The shape of the region in this enzyme is hence extremely important (Figure 1.5).

It might be easier to predict how a protein would fold if they were all very structured; unfortunately, they are not. There are unstructured regions that current methods cannot capture. The oldest method of finding the structure of a protein is protein crystallography. However, many large protein regions could not be assigned in X-ray data sets. This happens because they occupy multiple positions. This suggests that regions are disordered. New microbiological imaging methods, such as Nuclear Magnetic Resonance (NMR), demonstrated the presence of large flexible linkers that terminates in many structural ensembles. In the present state of the art, it is accepted that proteins exist as motifs, which are an ensemble of similar structures, and some regions are more structurally constrained than others. At this stage, we must mention that Intrinsically Unstructured Proteins (IUP)s occupy the end of structural flexibility. Intrinsically, unstructured proteins are highly abundant among disease-related proteins.

Although presented as solid rigid bodies, proteins are highly dynamic and impart an essential feature in their function and regulation. When in a solution, fragments of proteins and the entire protein do not have a well-defined structure. When in a specific functional state, they assume such a structure. Nevertheless, the presence of unstructured regions in a protein is a reality, which probably explains why the prediction of protein structure has not achieved the desired success even after strenuous effort over the last few decades.

Databases of 3D structures of proteins obtained from X-ray crystallography, NMR spectroscopy, and cryo-electron microscopy are in the Protein Data Bank (PDB); this is freely available through the Internet. Predicting structure through different means, mainly through computer-based modeling, is a continuous endeavor through the Critical Assessment of protein Structure Prediction (CASP) competition. The large-scale study of proteins is called Proteomics. It is one of the most difficult branches of study in biological systems. The proteome is the entire set of proteins produced or modified by an organism or system.

The flexibility and variety of protein molecules depend on how they fold and function. Proteins working as a team perform complex functions depending on a sequence of amino acids (the information). The study of Proteomics provokes us to think that proteins are alive—without the capability or mechanism to reproduce themselves.

Proteins are regularly destroyed or broken down; therefore, a mechanism must exist that can make proteins. To achieve this goal, different amino acid sequence data must be stored in encrypted form, and a physical process must exist in a biological system to construct the required protein chain out of that form.

RNA-binding proteins are a large and varied group of proteins associated with posttranscriptional gene regulation. They bind to various regions either upstream or downstream from the coding region of the RNA to control five major processes in mRNA metabolism—splicing, polyadenylation, export, translation, and decay. A small domain of around 80 amino acids of retinol-binding protein (RBP) displays a motif referred to as RRM (RNA Recognition Motif) with four beta strands and two alpha-helixes. The RRM mainly controls various biological functions. An RBP also binds either to the double-stranded siRNA or single-stranded miRNA to derive a multi-protein complex RISC (RNA-Induced Silencing Complex). The single strand of miRNA/siRNA acts as a template for RISC to recognize the specific region of mRNA transcript to initiate gene silencing and defense against viral infection.

1.6   CONCLUSION

The genome machine is a creation of the evolution of the universe. Starting from what we do not know, the fundamental particles and the rules of physics have formed that lead to chemistry and then to biology. Life, as we feel, is merely a set of chemical and physical reactions, all governed by physics; the formation of life is best described as a cellular automaton that depends on the charge and size of the molecule. Carbon being the smallest and with the least charge, led the trail. Self-replication, driven by the charge interactions as demonstrated in the famous Game of Life, also known simply as Life, is a cellular automaton devised by the British mathematician John Horton Conway in 1970. It is a zero-player game, meaning that its evolution is determined by its initial state, requiring no further input. One interacts with the Game of Life by creating an initial configuration and observing how it evolves. It is Turing complete and can simulate a universal constructor or any other Turing machine. Any live cell with two or three live neighbors survives; any dead cell with three live neighbors becomes a live cell. All other live cells die in the next generation. Similarly, all other dead cells stay dead. The initial pattern constitutes the seed of the system. The first generation is created by applying the above rules simultaneously to every cell in the seed, live or dead; births and deaths co-occur, and the discrete moment at which this happens is sometimes called a "tick." Each generation is a pure function of the preceding one. The rules continue to be applied repeatedly to create further generations. [https://playgameoflife.com/]. This game teaches us how cells replicate, how a polypeptide chain turns into a three-dimensional protein, and how genes are mutated.

DESPITE ITS INSTABILITY, the RNA started life as it got tagged with other molecules. Now, after the incident that happened almost four billion years ago, we are returning to finding the solutions to all ailments of life through RNA, as it formed life so long ago.

2 Understanding Nucleic Acids

2.1 BACKGROUND

The human body produces thousands of proteins in the trillions of body cells continuously (Figure 2.1).

These proteins are needed for our survival. So, each cell has a nucleus within which lies 21 chromosomes that are a long-twisted chain of DNA (deoxyribonucleic acid) made up of nucleotides.

The nucleotides are the monomers of nucleic acids (Figure 2.2).

Nucleotides contain either a purine or a pyrimidine—two significant groups of bases. The three building blocks of nucleic acid are:

1. A five-carbon sugar
2. A phosphate group
3. Nitrogen-containing base. The nitrogen-containing bases (or just base) come in five types—Adenine (A), Uracil (U), Guanine (G), Thymine (T), and Cytosine (C). The base U in RNA gets replaced with T in DNA.

A and G are purines, while U, T, and C belong to the pyrimidine group. Purines and pyrimidine are the nitrogen-containing bases found in the nucleotides of DNA and RNA. They have been artificially synthesized. All the bases (Figure 2.2) are nearly two-dimensional flattish rings and, therefore, stackable; due to these shapes, they can form hydrogen bonds only on the plane of this paper. G and A are larger than T and the other base—uracil. Thymine (T) of DNA is replaced with Uracil (U) (Figure 2.1) in the RNA base sequence. Uracil misses a methyl group (CH_3) present in thymine (Figure 2.3).

In a living organism, nucleotides function to create, encode, and store information. The encoded information is contained and conveyed via the nucleic acid sequence. Strings of nucleotides are linked to form the sugar-phosphate backbone of a nucleic acid. The backbone of DNA covers two chains forming a stable helical structure. On the other hand, the RNA backbone is formed out of a single chain, and its structure displays a set of structural motifs (loop, turn, etc.). The deoxyribonucleic acid (DNA) has deoxy sugars in its molecule, meaning that it is derived from the sugar ribose by losing an oxygen atom. This shape shows how the bases stick out and occupy the same plane.

DNA, or deoxyribonucleic acid, is a code that living organisms follow to stay alive. The RNA, or ribonucleic acid, helps carry out the instructions embedded in the DNA code, making it more versatile. RNA, a single-stranded, linear molecule, is

DOI: 10.1201/9781003248156-3

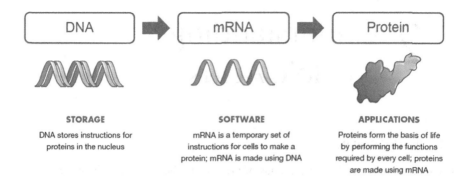

FIGURE 2.1   Genetic coding to manufacture proteins in the body.

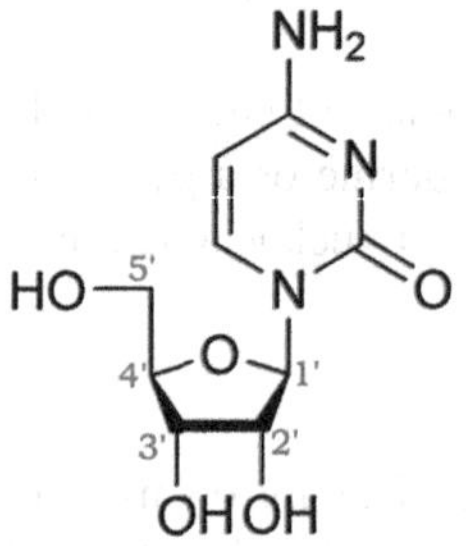

FIGURE 2.2   Nucleic acid structure.

generated during transcription. It works in tandem with DNA, assisting it in completing the duties that DNA has assigned to it (Figure 2.4).

The nucleobases are connected to their sugar-phosphate backbone in both molecules. Adenine ties to thymine, cytosine links to guanine, and each nucleobase on a nucleotide strand of DNA joins its companion nucleobase on a second strand. The two strands of DNA twist and spiral around each other, generating various shapes such as the iconic double helix (DNA's "relaxed" form), circles, and supercoils resulting from this joining (Figure 2.5).

2.2   THE DNA

The structure of DNA is a double helix (Figure 2.6). Two antiparallel strands contain a sugar-phosphate backbone to the exterior with interior-facing nitrogenous bases that form hydrogen bonds to the nitrogenous bases on the other strand to hold the two strands together.

They can store information long term (as DNA) as a sequence of multiple nucleic acids, use that information to duplicate a cell (when DNA splits), and use that information through a messenger (mRNA) to create proteins that are produced inside the cell but in the cytoplasm, not the nucleus where the DNA resides. This process protects the DNA (the genetic code).

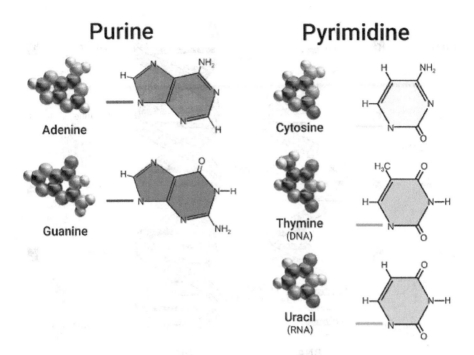

FIGURE 2.3 Structure of nucleic acids purine and pyrimidine.

The DNA or RNA strands grow as new nucleotides are added to the existing nucleotide at the 3' hydroxyl (OH) group through dehydration synthesis regardless of whether it is DNA or RNA. This is because an unbounded 5' phosphate group always remains on one end of the strand, and an unbounded 3' hydroxyl group is found on the opposite end of the strand. Therefore, building new nucleic acids always occurs from a 5' to 3' direction.

The complementary base pairs (C–G and A–T) are linked in two strands with H-bonds in the DNA. The two strands of DNA have redundant information, and reading the sequence of one strand is good enough. However, in genetics, they are differentiated; the segment that runs from 5' to 3' is called the sense strand or coding strand, while the other strand runs from 3' to 5' and is called the antisense strand. The sense strand is the strand of DNA taken as the template for the generation of the mRNA string, as depicted in Figure 2.2. In the process, the mRNA becomes complementary to the sense strand, and so it becomes identical to the antisense strand. RNA is later translated to protein. The pairing of A–T and C–G in DNA is realized through hydrogen bonds. A hydrogen bond is a weak bond between two molecules created because of an electrostatic attraction between a proton in one of the molecules and a negatively charged atom.

The DNA double helix is a very long, fragile thread occasionally wrapped around a series of 8 histone proteins. The area where the DNA is wrapped around the histones is called a nucleosome. The area between nucleosomes where only the DNA thread is called linker DNA (Figure 2.6).

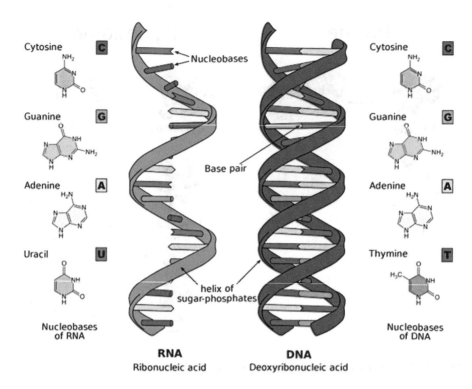

FIGURE 2.4 Structural differences between DNA and RNA. [By Users Antilived, Fabiolib, Turnstep, Westcairo, Creative Commons Attribution]

The linker DNA and nucleosomes fold back on one another to form a thicker thread or a rope called chromatin. The chromatin folds back on itself to form one of two types of chromosomes: euchromatin (true) or heterochromatin. Euchromatin is loosely packed, so it is not seen under the microscope. (Figure 2.7)

Heterochromatin is the tightly condensed chromosomes that can be seen in a cell when cell division occurs, or in females, one of their X chromosomes is heterochromatin (Barr Body). Heterochromatin is chromosomes that have either been deactivated entirely or are not used at that very minute to conduct cellular metabolism. Because their DNA is circular, the DNA in prokaryotic cells is supercoiled. Therefore, instead of histones, they use histone-like proteins because they are similar but not the same.

Human DNA consists of approximately 3 billion bases. More than 99% of DNA bases are common in all humans, but only 55% of human DNA is common in the potato. The sequence of these DNA bases determines the genetic information available for building and maintaining a life-form. The common analogy is how letters of the alphabet appear in a specific order and sequence to form meaningful words and sentences.

An essential trait of DNA is that it can replicate, i.e., make copies of itself. Each strand of DNA in the double helix can serve as a pattern for duplicating the sequence

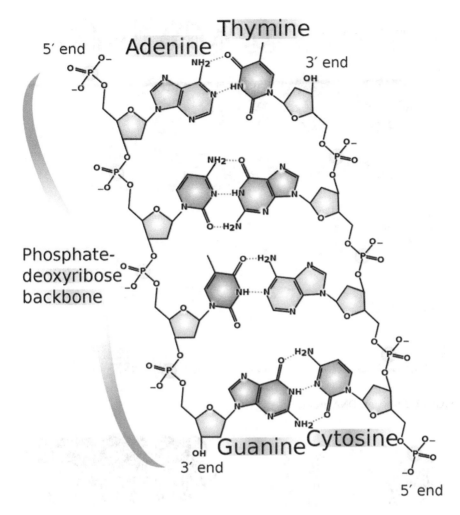

FIGURE 2.5 Structure of nucleotides. (Source: https://upload.wikimedia.org/wikipedia/commons/e/e4/DNA_chemical_structure.svg)

of bases when required. This is DNA's most critical ability. When cells divide, each new cell now has a replica of the DNA from the old cell.

DNA sequences that encode protein sequences are referred to as "coding DNA." There exists non-coding DNA that does not encode protein. DNA has a complex structure; its double helix structure gives it the structural rigidity required to store the information for inheritance. They have an inherent redundancy—if one strand breaks, it could be recreated from the complementary strand. However, such a stable structure triggers the question—are there precursors of DNA in a primitive life-form that got replaced with the current form of life? Though there is no conclusive proof, it is plausible that the two basic nucleotide groups, purine and pyrimidine, were the starting point from which the five bases evolved—A and G from purine and U, T,

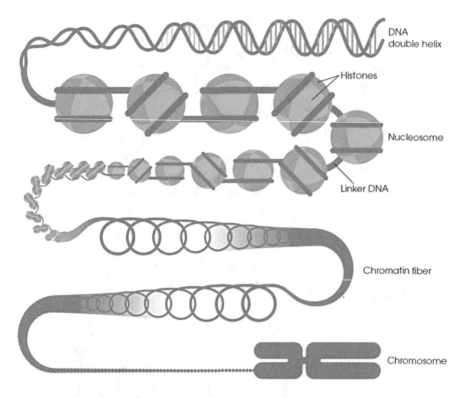

FIGURE 2.6   How DNA grows.

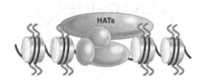

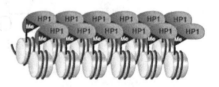

Euchromatin

Heterochromatin

- less condensed
- chromosome arms
- unique sequences
- gene rich
- replicated throughout S phase
- recombination during meiosis

- highly condensed
- centromeres and telomeres
- repetitious sequences
- gene poor
- replicated in late S phase
- no meiotic recombination

 Transcriptional activators

 Heterochromatin Protein 1 complex

SS Hyper-acetylated histone tail

Hypo-acetylated histone tail;
methylated H3K9

FIGURE 2.7   Threading of DNA.

and C from pyrimidine. As a result, single-strand RNA with two bases was replaced with a more complex RNA string with four bases, A, U, G, and C, similar to the current life-form. The big problem is—to sustain primitive life-forms of RNA, from where can we get the protein enzymes? For current life-forms, these enzymes are transcribed from DNA.

Sustaining life requires that molecules have a crucial property: the fundamental ability to catalyze reactions that lead to the production of more molecules similar to themselves. The first biological molecules may have been created by metal-based catalysis on crystalline surfaces of minerals. It has been proposed that an elaborate system of molecular synthesis and breakdown could have persisted on these surfaces long before the first living cell came into existence. These catalysts have special self-promoting properties which could ideally use raw materials to reproduce and replenish themselves and thus divert these same materials from the production of other substances. In living cells, the most flexible catalysts are polypeptides, composed of different amino acids with versatile and chemically diverse side chains. Hence, they can take on various three-dimensional structures that rise with reactive chemical groups. But, although polypeptides are versatile as catalysts, there is no recognized way in which they can reproduce themselves.

Polynucleotides have one unique property that contrasts with those of polypeptides. Polynucleotides can direct the formation of exact copies of their sequence. This unique capability is because of complementary base pairing that enables one polynucleotide to act as a template for creating another.

The "gene" is a part of DNA. Human genes vary in size from a few hundred DNA bases and may go up to more than two million bases. A gene is a section of DNA responsible for coding a specific protein. Thus protein, as explained earlier, is the final product of a gene of a DNA molecule. For example, in the case of humans, one gene will code for the protein insulin, which has the important role of controlling sugar in our blood.

If we take the DNA from all the cells in the human body and line it up, end to end, it would form a fragile (order of 10^{-4} mm) 5000 million miles long. To store such a large volume of information in chromosomes, DNA molecules are tightly packed around proteins called histones. Nature has achieved some efficient packing mechanisms to store voluminous information coded in DNA.

2.3 THE RNA

The RNA is made up of a single polynucleotide strand. However, some small sections within the RNA molecule can be complementary and create secondary structures (hairpins and loops, for example) (Table 2.1). The secondary structure of the RNA is determined by the base sequence of the nucleotide chain so that different RNA molecules can assume other structures. Moreover, as RNA structure determines its function, this diversity is also responsible for RNA engagement in multiple cellular roles.

RNA polymerase synthesizes RNA from template DNA, and mRNA acts as a bridge between DNA expression and protein translation. Both coding and non-coding

TABLE 2.1

Comparison of DNA and RNA

	DNA	RNA
Stands For	Deoxyribonucleic Acid.	Ribonucleic Acid.
Definition	A nucleic acid is a molecule that provides the genetic instructions that all modern living creatures must follow to grow and function properly. DNA nucleotides generate proteins that express or manifest DNA genes with the help of RNA.	DNA includes information determining whether features are created, activated, or deactivated, whereas RNA has the same function.
Function	The living thing must follow the existing genetic information storage and transmission code. The notion of evolution is defined by the slow, constant changes found in DNA through time. Mutations can be harmful, neutral, or advantageous to an organism. Humans have roughly 19,000 genes found in tiny portions of long DNA strands. The distinctions between various living organisms and similar living organisms are caused by the specific instructions present in genes, which are dictated by how nucleobases in DNA are arranged.	RNA causes the execution of DNA blueprint instructions. Transfers genetic code from the nucleus to the ribosome, required for protein production. Messenger RNA (mRNA) transcribes genetic information from a cell nucleus' DNA and transports it to the cytoplasm and ribosome. Transfer RNA (tRNA) is located in the cytoplasm of a cell and functions as a helper for mRNA. For example, a ribosome's tRNA transports amino acids, the building blocks of proteins, to the mRNA. The cytoplasm of a cell contains ribosomal RNA (rRNA). The ribosome accepts the information provided by mRNA and tRNA, and translates it. This data "learns" whether a polypeptide or protein should be created or synthesized.
Structure	Double-stranded. Four nitrogen-containing nucleobases and five-carbon sugar (the stable 2-deoxyribose) make up two nucleotide strands (adenine, thymine, cytosine, and guanine) and the phosphate group.	Single-stranded. Phosphate, a five-carbon sugar (ribose), and four nitrogen-containing nucleobases: adenine, uracil (not thymine), guanine, and cytosine, are all found in RNA.
Base Pairing	The pairing of Bases Cytosine connects to guanine (C-G), while adenine connects to thymine (A-T) (C-G). In addition, adenine binds to uracil (A-U), while cytosine binds to guanine (C-G).	Adenine connects to uracil (A-U), while cytosine connects to guanine (C-G) (C-G).

(Continued)

TABLE 2.1 (CONTINUED)

Comparison of DNA and RNA

	DNA	RNA
Location	The nucleus of a cell and mitochondria contain DNA	This molecule can be located in the nucleus, cytoplasm, or ribosome, depending on the type of RNA.
Stability	Because of C-H linkages, deoxyribose sugar in DNA is less reactive. In alkaline circumstances, it is stable. Enzymes have a tougher time "attacking" DNA because the grooves are smaller.	The C-OH (hydroxyl) bonds in ribose sugar make it particularly reactive. It is not stable in alkaline environments. Because of its larger grooves, enzymes can "attack" RNA more easily.
Propagation	Self-replicating.	It is synthesized from DNA when needed.
Unique Features	The DNA helix has a B-form helix geometry. Because DNA is tightly packed in the nucleus, it is safeguarded. UV rays can cause DNA damage.	This molecule can be found in the nucleus, cytoplasm, or ribosome, depending on the kind of RNA.

Ribose sugar is highly reactive due to the C–OH (hydroxyl) bonds. It is not stable under alkaline conditions. Enzymes can more easily "attack" RNA because of their broader grooves.

When RNA is needed, DNA is used to make it.

The A-Form helix geometry is apparent in RNA. RNA strands are constantly created, degraded, and reused. Therefore, ultraviolet photons are less likely to harm RNA. |

RNA share characteristics such as being single-stranded, having a 2′ OH group, and the ability to adopt a variety of secondary and tertiary structures.

mRNA, a single-stranded molecule, is complementary to one of a gene's DNA strands that transports a piece of the DNA code to other cell areas so that proteins can be made. To be translated into RNA, DNA therapies require access to the nucleus, and their effectiveness is dependent on nuclear envelope collapse during cell division. mRNA therapies do not need to enter the nucleus to act because they are quickly translated as they reach the cytoplasm. Furthermore, unlike plasmids and viral vectors, mRNA do not integrate into the genome and do not cause insertional mutagenesis, making them ideal for cancer vaccines, tumor immunotherapy, and infectious disease prevention.

As RNA cannot integrate into the genome, it does not present the risk of insertional mutagenesis, an inherent risk in therapies based on DNA modifications.

Two RNA sensors have been discovered: toll-like receptors (TLRs) and the RIG-I-like receptor family. TLRs are found in the endosomal compartment of macrophages and dendritic cells (DCs), among other cells. A pattern recognition receptor (PRR) belongs to the RIG-I-like family of receptors. However, the immune response mechanisms and processes of cellular sensors that recognize mRNA vaccines and the mechanism of sensor activation are unknown.

Adenine and uracil (rather than thymine) constitute the connection in RNA, as cytosine remains connected to guanine. Linking to its nucleobases, RNA folds in on itself as a single-stranded molecule, but not all of them pair up. The hairpin loop is the most common of these three-dimensional forms, and it aids in determining if the RNA molecule is messenger RNA (mRNA), transfer RNA (tRNA), or ribosomal RNA (rRNA). A comparison of the two nucleic acids can be seen in Table 2.1.

rRNA, tRNA, mRNA, and various additional non-coding RNAs are found in all living creatures. However, there are significant differences between eukaryotes and prokaryotes in the kinds and frequency of various forms of RNA. The ribosome, which contains ribosomal RNA, converts mRNA into protein after transcription. A riboswitch that changes conformation (dotted segment) upon binding a signal molecule may control mRNA expression (green hexagon). Small RNA (sRNA) binding, in most cases, regulates mRNA expression by encouraging RNA breakdown.

RNA is also the catalyst for the peptidyl transferase reaction that takes place inside the ribosome.

Different forms of RNA act as the template for the translation of genes into proteins, transfer amino acids to the *ribosome* (the cell organelle where protein synthesis takes place) to form proteins, and translate the transcript into proteins. RNA that acts like an enzyme is called a *ribozyme*.

This minimum requirement that two RNA molecules should interact requires that one acts as the enzyme, to bring together the components, and the other acts as the gene template. Together the template and the enzyme RNA combine as an *RNA replicase*. But these components have to be kept together inside some form of compartment or cell, or they would only occasionally come into contact to work together. This is the second pre-life structure, a self-replicating vesicle, a membrane-bound structure made primarily of lipids (organic molecules not soluble in water, such as fats) that develop and divide over time. The RNA replicase, at some point, entered a self-replicating vesicle, which allowed the RNA replicase to function efficiently. However, it is a protocell, and it is not yet living. It is just a self-replicating membrane bag with an independent self-replicating molecule inside. To make the protocell function, both components have to interact, the vesicle protecting the RNA replicase, and the RNA replicase perhaps producing lipids for the vesicle. If the interaction works, the protocell has become a living cell. The cell is alive because it has the ability to feed itself, grow, and replicate. Evolution can happen because the cells show differential survival ("survival of the fittest"), and the genetic information for replication is coded in the RNA.

The mRNA carries the message from the DNA, which controls and coordinates the cellular activities within a cell. For example, if a cell requires a particular protein to be synthesized, the corresponding gene is "turned on," and then the mRNA is synthesized through transcription. In the subsequent translation process, the mRNA interacts with the ribosome and other mechanisms within the cell to direct the synthesis of the protein that it encodes. Compared to double-stranded DNA, single-stranded mRNA, in general, are relatively unstable and short-lived in the cell to ensure that the proteins are only made when needed, especially in prokaryotic cells.

Ribosomal RNA (rRNA) and protein make up a ribosome. As its name suggests, it is a key component of ribosomes, accounting for around 60% of the ribosomal mass and defining the binding site for mRNA. The rRNA ensures that the mRNA, tRNA (transfer RNA), and ribosomes are properly aligned. Furthermore, the rRNA catalyzes the creation of peptide bonds between two aligned amino acids during elongation of the peptide chain for protein synthesis by an enzymatic activity (peptidyl transferase).

tRNA (transfer RNA) is the third main type of RNA and one of the smallest, usually only 70–90 nucleotide bases long. It is responsible for carrying the correct amino acid to the site of protein synthesis in the ribosome. Nature has designed a fail-safe design of base pairing between the tRNA and mRNA that allows the correct insertion of amino acid in the polypeptide chain being synthesized. Consequently, a mutation in the tRNA or rRNA can result in severe problems for the cell. Hence, both the molecules are necessary for ensuring proper protein synthesis as the proteins control the functions of living cells.

siRNA (small interfering RNA) have a well-defined structure—a short, usually 20–24-bp (base pair) derived out of a longer RNA molecule is called double-stranded RNA (dsRNA). A dsRNA has a phosphorylated 5 prime (5′) end and hydroxylated 3 prime (3′) end with two overhanging nucleotides. An enzyme referred to as a dicer catalyzes the production of siRNA and Small Hairpin Loop (HPL) RNA from long dsRNA. For wet-lab experiments, siRNA may be introduced into cells by transfection. In principle, though, any gene could be knocked down by a synthetic siRNA with a complementary sequence. Consequently, siRNA have become a principal tool for validating gene function and drug targeting in the postgenomic era.

Similar to siRNA, miRNA (micro-RNA) resemble other small RNA in the RNA interference (RNAi) pathway. However, while miRNA are derived from regions of RNA transcripts that fold back onto themselves to form short hairpins, the siRNA are usually derived out of longer regions of double-stranded RNA. The human genome may encode over 1000 different miRNA. They are abundant in many mammalian cell types and target more than 60% of the genes of mammals including humans.

Self-amplifying RNA (saRNA) is similar to mRNA. It comprises a 5′ cap, a poly(A) tail, and 5′ protein and 3′ untranslated regions. Still, it also encodes non-structural proteins that form a replicase to aid intracellular amplification. When mRNA and saRNA vaccines are compared in the same formulation, saRNA can be hundreds to thousands of times more potent, lowering the dose and consequently the cost of RNA vaccines. This will also allow for smaller, less expensive manufacturing plants.

Self-replicating RNA produced from the genomes of positive-strand RNA viruses is a valuable tool for both molecular research of virus biology and the development of new, safe, and effective vaccinations. For successful self-replicating RNA recovery, the 3′ end of viral RNA is crucial. A poly(A) tail is found on the 3′ end of many viruses, which matches the structure of eukaryotic mRNA and ensures effective translation. The poly(A) tail should be critical for viral RNA replication because it is the section where transcription must commence during minus-strand production. Other viral genomes lack poly-A, but they contain secondary structures that act as translation and RNA replication cis-acting factors. Therefore, any virus with a poly(A) tail in its genome should have one in its infectious cDNA construct. In contrast, viruses without a poly(A) tail will be susceptible to changes in the sequence at their genomic 3' end, necessitating steps to ensure the correct genomic end is generated during transcription.

2.3.1 REPLICATION

Replication begins with one double-helix DNA and ends with two double-helices DNA (Figure 2.8).

While it occurs in the nucleoid area of prokaryotes (cytoplasm), the replication takes place in the eukaryote nucleus, making DNA from DNA, using each strand of DNA as a template to build new DNA to reduce the number of errors produced when making DNA. Replication only occurs when the cell is about to divide to make daughter cells. Replication or DNA duplication occurs in the S or synthesis phase in the cell cycle (Figure 2.9).

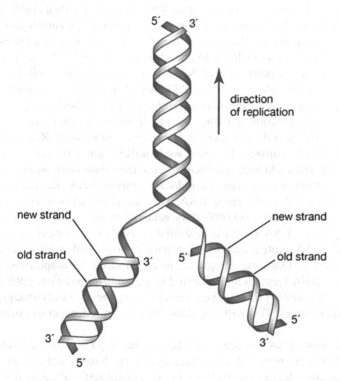

FIGURE 2.8 DNA replication and transcription.

CELL CYCLE

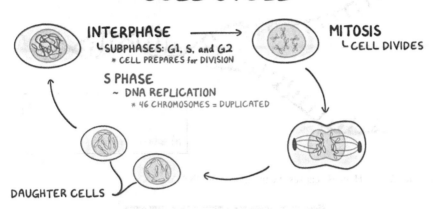

FIGURE 2.9   Synthesis phase cell division.

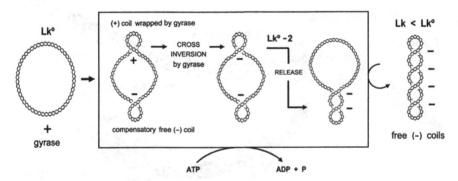

FIGURE 2.10   Relaxation of twisting of DNA by gyrase.

Replication only happens in "stem" cells that can produce new cells. For example, stem cells would include the fibroblasts of connective tissue, blood-producing cells in the bone marrow, select cells in regenerative tissues of the skin, and mucous membranes. The liver also has this ability.

DNA is twisted, and as replication proceeds, it becomes even more twisted. DNA gyrase relieves the twists ahead of the replication area so that the DNA does not become too compact to unzip. Gyrase will nick the DNA, allow it to untwist, and then attach it back (Figure 2.10)

Helicase unzips the DNA, which means that it breaks the hydrogen bonds between the nitrogenous bases of each strand to allow for enzymes to bond to the individual strands (Figure 2.11).

Stabilizing proteins keep the replication fork open and prevent the DNA from reforming its original hydrogen bonds while replication occurs (Figure 2.12).

Complementary base pairing involves guanine that can form 3 hydrogen bonds with another nucleotide. So does cytosine. Adenine and thymine only can form 2

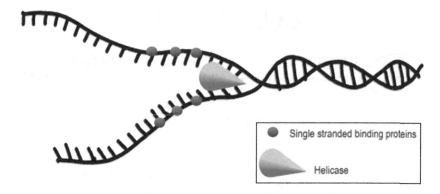

FIGURE 2.11   Helicase causes the unzipping of DNA.

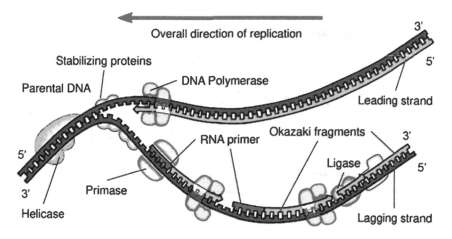

FIGURE 2.12   Stabilizing proteins in DNA replication.

hydrogen bonds with another nucleotide. Therefore, guanine usually bonds to cytosine (G≡C), and adenine usually always bonds to thymine (A=T). This allows the use of one strand of the DNA as a template to build a new strand.

DNA melts at different temperatures depending on A, T, C, and G's relative numbers. The temperature required to melt the two strands apart is higher in DNA with a heavy G≡C content than the lower melting temperature of DNA with mostly A=Ts. This is due to the extra hydrogen bond between G and C. If there is 30% cytosine in the DNA, the other nucleotides' amounts can be calculated. If cytosine is 30%, and always bonded to guanine, then guanine is also 30%. That leaves 40% so, if adenine is always bonded to thymine, they must be equal at 20% each.

2.3.2   TRANSCRIPTION

The entire DNA is not transcribed—just a piece of it is. An area is called a gene (a gene usually codes for a specific product, and there are many genes throughout the entire DNA for various products). The sense strand is normally transcribed to make mRNA; the antisense strand is usually used to make rRNA and tRNA.

RNA will also be built in a 5′ →3′ direction. So, the RNA polymerase sets down on what will be the 5′ end of the mRNA and then inserts RNA nucleotides (A, U, C, G) based on the complement of the template DNA.

    5′ CTACAAATTTGGGCCCAAATTTGGGCCCATC   3′
    3′ GAUGUUUAAACCCGGGUUUAAACCCGGGUAG   5′

The pre-mRNA is built using one strand of the DNA as a template.

    3′   GATGTTTAAACCCGGGTTTAAACCCGGGTAG 5′

New nucleotides are added to the growing mRNA strand one at a time by RNA polymerase. After the pre-mRNA is made, it detaches from the DNA template—the two strands of the DNA reform hydrogen bonds and reform an unchanged helix. For bacteria, the pre-mRNA is the mRNA ready to be used to make proteins. However, for eukaryotic cells, like humans, some modification is required before the pre-mRNA can be used to make protein.

    3′ GAUGUUUAAACCCGGGUUUAAACCCGGGUAG   5′

Once the mRNA is built, it needs modification; three things happen: first, extra nucleotides (introns) must be removed, and the essential nucleotides (exons) must be joined together. This occurs by a spliceosome. Second, a modified (methylated) guanine is added to the 5′ end, called a 5′ cap. Third, a string of adenine nucleotides is added to the 3′ end called the 3′ poly(A) tail.

    3′ AAAGAUGUUUAAACCCGGGUUUAAACCCGGGUAGG   5′

Let's rewrite the above to go from 5′ to 3′ and doing the three steps again. Let us also say that Cs are introns for this exercise to give the eventual product.

    5′ GGAUGGGCCCAAAUUUGGGCCCAAAUUUGUAGAAA   3′

And after the introns are removed:

    5′ GGAUGGGAAAUUUGGGAAAUUUGUAGAAA   3′

Now mRNA is ready for translation. The transcription takes place in the nucleus of the cell in eukaryotes. So, our little mRNA will have to leave the nucleus to be used to build protein in the cytoplasm.

During the transcription process, a portion of the cell's DNA serves as a template for creating an RNA molecule. The newly created RNA molecule produced out of the non-coding DNA may become a finished product; this is referred to as non-coding RNA that performs important functions within the cell. Typical examples are messenger RNA (mRNA), tRNA (transfer RNA), ribosomal RNA (rRNA), and a set of regulatory RNAs. While the first three types of RNAs are associated with protein synthesis, the fourth group performs different regulatory functions within a cell. If one can see that DNA is working as a code memory, the various other types of RNA are putting the code into action (Figure 2.13).

mRNA is produced out of the coding region of the DNA sequence; it carries the messages from the DNA to other parts of the cell for processing. This information is used to manufacture proteins. The first step in the transcription process is the mechanism of unzipping the two strands of a DNA gene apart and then using one strand (sense strand) as a template to make a copy of the sequence information of nucleotides. A set of proteins called polymerases does this process of transcription. The polymerases transcribe a gene (non-coding and coding DNA) to produce an RNA (ribo nucleic acid) molecule. It is called "ribo" because the sugars in RNA are different from the sugars in DNA; "deoxy" infers that deoxyribose has lost an oxygen atom—ribose has not.

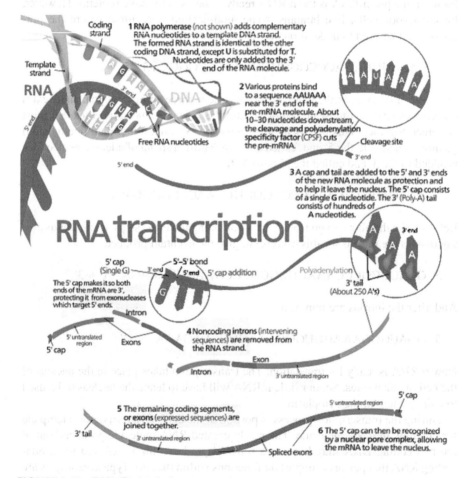

FIGURE 2.13   RNA Transcription.

The copy of the coding DNA sequence is called messenger ribonucleic acid, mRNA if we consider an mRNA strand transcripted from the DNA sequence A-A-T-T-A-A-C-G-T-T-A-C-T-A. The two ends, 5′ and 3′ (called 5 prime and 3 prime), become important at this stage. The 5′ and 3′ indicate the specific carbon numbers in the DNA's sugar backbone. A phosphate group is attached to the 5′ carbon, and the 3′ carbon has a hydroxyl (–OH) group attached. This asymmetry provides the DNA strand a direction. The transcription process itself can be divided into sub-processes to describe each process for clarity. First, the RNA polymerase binds onto the DNA template strand. This first step is called "initiation."

In the initiation phase, the RNA polymerase and its associated transcription factors bind to the DNA strand at a specific site that facilitates the transcription process. This area of binding is called the promoter region. Sometimes, it includes a specialized nucleotide sequence, TATAAA, referred to as the "TATA box." Approximately 23% of human genes contain this TATA box within the core promoter.

Once the RNA polymerase and its related transcription factors are in position, the single-stranded DNA is exposed and is ready for transcription. The RNA polymerase now begins moving down the DNA template strand in the 3′ to 5′ direction, stringing together complementary nucleotides as it does so. The very process of complementary base pairing creates a new strand of mRNA organized in the 5′ to 3′ direction. As the RNA polymerase continues down the DNA strand, more nucleotides are progressively added to the mRNA, leading to a long chain of nucleotides. This process is aptly named "elongation." thus, the process of elongation follows the initiation process.

All of the bases of DNA are present in RNA, except thymine, which is replaced with the base uracil. The presence of thiamine in the DNA template strand instructs RNA polymerase to bind uracil to the matching region of the developing RNA strand during the elongation phase.

A new mRNA molecule is produced from a single template strand of DNA during the elongation phase of transcription. The mRNA peels away from the template as it elongates. This mRNA molecule conveys information to the ribosome, a type of organelle.

After elongation, the mRNA can only execute its given function before it separates from the DNA template. This is the "termination" phase of the process. In some circumstances, the polymerase is terminated as soon as it reaches a specific sequence of nucleotides along with the DNA template. Also in some situations, the presence of a protein known as the termination factor is essential for termination.

The mRNA molecule falls off the DNA template at the end of the termination phase. Non-coding nucleotide sequences, known as introns, are cut out of the mRNA strand by the newly generated mRNA, referred to as precursor mRNA. This "splicing" procedure cleans up the molecule by removing nucleotides that are not needed for protein synthesis. The splicing process necessitates using a complex molecule known as a spliceosome.

On the 5′ and 3′ ends of a normal mRNA, there are two untranslated regions (UTRs): 5′ UTR and 3′ UTR. In addition, a sequence of adenine nucleotides is added to the 3′ end of the mRNA before it is exported to the cytoplasm for translation, and a

5′ cap is added to the 5′ end. A poly-specific sequence of nucleotide bases is covered by the UTRs and caps. The attachment of the poly(A) tail sequence to the mRNA molecule informs the cell that it is now ready to depart the nucleus and reach the cytoplasm for translation.

2.3.3 Codons

A "codon" is a triplet of nucleotides in an mRNA string that can be thought of as the information unit for information transfer from DNA to RNA.

The message of the mRNA codon string encodes a sequence of amino acids. The codon-amino acid Table 2.2 displays the amino acids encoded by different codons. There are 64 combinations of 4 nucleotides taken three at a time (referred to as codon) and only 20 amino acids. As a result, there is more than one codon per amino acid in most cases. This phenomenon is referred to as "codon degeneracy." This is because, for example, the simplest amino acid glycine (gly) is encoded by codons GGU, GGC, GGA, and GGG (Table 2.2).

A degenerate code points to several code words having the same meaning. The genetic code is degenerate because there are multiple instances in which different codons specify the same amino acid; the simplest amino acid glycine (gly) is encoded with four codons GGU, GGC, GGA, and GGG with first two bases as GG followed by any one of the four bases in the third base location. It has been suggested that the degeneracy makes the DNA more tolerant of pointing mutations—replacing

TABLE 2.2
Mapping of 64 Codons to 20 Amino Acids

First Letter	Second Letter U	C	A	G	Third Letter
U	phenylalanine	serine	tyrosine	cysteine	U
	phenylalanine	serine	tyrosine	cysteine	C
	leucine	serine	stop	stop	A
	leucine	serine	stop	tryptophan	G
C	leucine	proline	histidine	arginine	U
	leucine	proline	histidine	arginine	C
	leucine	proline	glutamine	arginine	A
	leucine	proline	glutamine	arginine	G
A	isoleucine	threonine	asparagine	serine	U
	isoleucine	threonine	asparagine	serine	C
	isoleucine	threonine	lysine	arginine	A
	methionine (start)	threonine	lysine	arginine	G
G	valine	alanine	aspartate	glycine	U
	valine	alanine	aspartate	glycine	C
	valine	alanine	glutamate	glycine	A
	valine	alanine	glutamate	glycine	G

the third base with another in the base triplet of a codon. Degeneracy is associated with translating an mRNA codon to an amino acid in a protein chain. To present the underlying principle of the CA model for degeneracy is used (Table 2.3).

A position of a codon is said to be an n-fold degenerate site if only $n(n = 4, 3, 2)$ of four possible nucleotides (A, C, G, and U) at this position specify the same amino acid. A nucleotide substitution at an n-fold degenerate site is a synonymous mutation. On the other hand, substitutions resulting in the amino acid change are denoted as non-synonymous mutations.

There are three base locations in a codon triplet: left, center, and right. If any mutation at a codon location results in amino acid substitution, it is referred to as a non-degenerate site. There is only one triple degenerate location where altering three of the four nucleotides has no effect on the amino acid but results in an amino acid substitution when changing to the fourth nucleotide. This is the third position of iso-leucine (ile) codons: AUU, AUC, and AUA all encode isoleucine, but AUG encodes Methionine (Met). Hence, this condition is often treated as a twofold degenerate site for computation. An inverted genetic code in Table 2.3 shows each of the 20 amino acids and their associated codons.

2.3.4 TRANSLATION PROCESS

The function of translation is to translate mRNA to protein using the mRNA made in transcription. For example, if it reads a base triplet, say GGU in mRNA string, the amino acid glycine gets attached to the growing peptide chain. The ribosome is a highly specialized molecule of great importance because it is the biological entity that acts as a bridge between Proteomics and Genomics (Figure 2.14).

The ribosome is a central entity to the process of life. Ribosomes occur both as free particles within cells and as particles attached to the membranes inside the cells. A ribosome is made of about 4 nucleic acid molecules and 70 different types of

TABLE 2.3
Codon Degeneracy for 20 Amino Acids and Start/Stop Codons

Amino acid	Codons	Amino acid	Codons
Ala/A	GCU, GCC, GCA, GCG	Leu/L	UUA, UUG, CUU, CUC, CUA, CUG
Arg/R	CGU, CGC, CGA, CGG, AGA, AGG	Lys/K	AAA, AAG
Asn/N	AAU, AAC	Met/M	AUG
Asp/D	GAU, GAC	Phe/F	UUU, UUC
Cys/C	UGU, UGC	Pro/P	CCU, CCC, CCA, CCG
Glu/E	GAA, GAG	Thr/T	ACU, ACC, ACA, ACG
Gly/G	GGU, GGC, GGA, GGG	Trp/W	UGG
His/H	CAU, CAC	UAU, UAC	UAU, UAC
Ile/I	AUU, AUC, AUA	Val/V	GUU, GUC, GUA, GUG
START	AUG	STOP	UAA, UGA, UAG

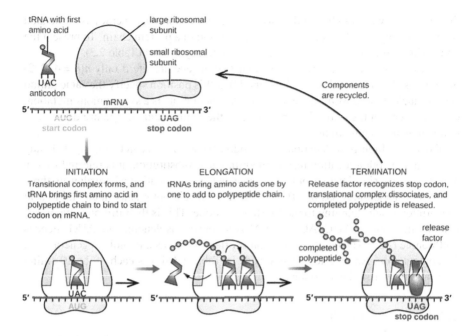

FIGURE 2.14   Process of translation. (Source: Author, based on: http://publications.nigms .nih.gov/insidethecell/images/ch2_ribosome_proteinbig.jpg, http://fig.cox)

proteins. Ribosomes are several numbers within a cell and account for a large proportion of its total nucleic acid. There are so many ribosomes because the translation process is prolonged. In an animal cell, around 1 million amino acids are added to growing proteins every second. However, each ribosome can add only 3–5 amino acids to the growing peptide-protein chain each second.

The RNA and proteins that make ribosomes in bacteria are different from that of eukaryotes. Also, these vary between different species of eukaryotes. However, their basic structure and function are always the same.

The amino acids for protein synthesis in the ribosome come from the Transfer RNA (tRNA) molecules that transport amino acids to the ribosome. The A, P, and E sites are the three tRNA slots on the ribosome. As tRNA supply amino acids during translation, they pass through these sites (A to P to E) (Figure 2.15).

The small and large subunits of ribosomes come together to provide three locations for tRNA to bind (the A site, P site, and E site). The sites appear in A-PE order from right to left in the diagram. After the initial binding of the first tRNA at the P site, an incoming charged tRNA would bind at the A site. Peptide bond formation transfers the amino acid of the first tRNA, and methionine to the amino acid of the second tRNA (in this case, Tryptophan). This chain of two amino acids would be attached to the tRNA in the A-site. The ribosome would then move along the mRNA template by one codon. The tRNA in the A site (with the polypeptide chain) would shift to the P site (Figure 2.15), and the empty tRNA previously in the P site would

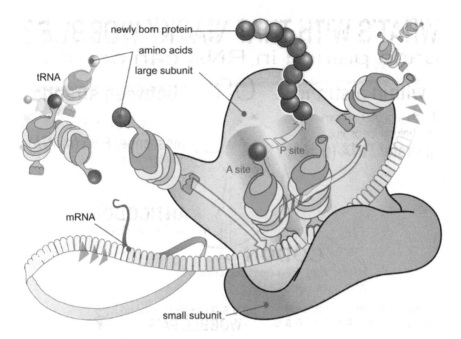

FIGURE 2.15 Translation process.

exit the ribosome. A new tRNA, in this case, one bearing phenylaniline (Phe), would bind to the newly exposed codon in the A site, and the process then repeats.

A transfer RNA (tRNA) molecule is a unique type of RNA molecule. Its job is to match the amino acid that an mRNA codon codes for with the amino acid that the codon codes for. An anticodon is a set of three nucleotides found in each tRNA molecule (Figure 1.16). A particular tRNA's anticodon can bind to one or a few specific mRNA codons. The amino acid encoded by the codons that the tRNA binds to is also carried by the tRNA molecule. Because the two ends of a strand of DNA or RNA are different, information flow has a direction, and the nucleotide chain in DNA and RNA has a direction. Many biological activities, such as DNA replication and transcription, can only occur in one direction of a DNA or RNA strand. For example, Figure 2.15 shows a tRNA loaded with the amino acid "Met" for the codon AUG.

A tRNA acts as an adaptor, connecting an mRNA codon to an amino acid in Figure 2.15. The anticodon of 3'-UAC-5' on one end of the tRNA binds to a codon in an mRNA with a sequence of 5'-AUG-3' by complementary base pairing of the first two bases and wobble pairing for the third base. The amino acid methionine (Met), which is specified by the mRNA codon AUG, is carried on the other end of the tRNA.

There are many different types of tRNA in a cell, each with its anticodon and corresponding amino acid. In addition, as explained below, certain tRNA bind to several codons via "wobble" pairing (Figure 2.16).

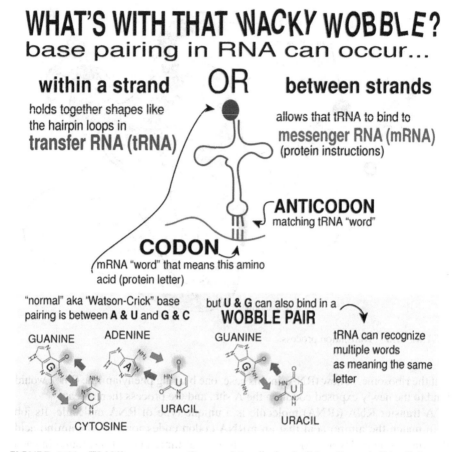

WHAT'S WITH THAT WACKY WOBBLE?
base pairing in RNA can occur...

within a strand OR between strands

holds together shapes like the hairpin loops in
transfer RNA (tRNA)

allows that tRNA to bind to
messenger RNA (mRNA)
(protein instructions)

ANTICODON
matching tRNA "word"

CODON
mRNA "word" that means this amino acid (protein letter)

"normal" aka "Watson-Crick" base pairing is between **A & U** and **G & C**

but **U & G** can also bind in a
WOBBLE PAIR

tRNA can recognize multiple words as meaning the same letter

GUANINE   ADENINE

GUANINE

URACIL

CYTOSINE

URACIL

FIGURE 2.16 Wobbling process. (Source: https://upload.wikimedia.org/wikipedia/commons/0/0e/Wobble_base_pairing.svg)

Some tRNAs can create base pairs with several codons. Wobble occurs when a typical base-pair involving nucleotides other than A–U and G–C forms at the codon's third position (Figure 2.16). Although it has their own laws, normal regulations do not apply to wobble pairing. For example, a G in the anticodon might pair with a C or U (but not an A or G) at the codon's third position. Wobble pairing allows a single tRNA to identify several codons for the amino acid it transports, as seen in Figure 1.16 with the tRNA for the amino acid "Phe." The anticodon of phenylalanine (Phe) tRNA is 3'-AAG-5'. It can couple with either the 5'-UUC-3' or 5'-UUU-3' mRNA codons (both of which specify Phe). Because it can form a normal base pair with the third codon position (5'-UUC-3' codon with 3'-AAG-5' anticodon) and an atypical base pair with the third codon position (5'-UUU-3' codon with 3'-AAG-5' anticodon) with the third codon position (5'-UUU-3' codon with 3'-AAG-5' anticodon), tRNA can bind to both codons (Figure 2.16).

Wobble pairing rules ensure that a tRNA does not bind to the incorrect codon. For example, the anticodon of phenylalanine tRNA is 3'-AAG-5', which can mate with two phenylalanine codons but not with the 5'-UUA-3' or 5'-UUG-3' codons (Figure 2.16).

Because these codons indicate leucine rather than phenylalanine, the laws of wobble pairing allow a single tRNA to cover numerous codons for the same amino acid while removing any confusion about which amino acid will be delivered to each codon. Wobble pairing permits fewer tRNAs to cover all of the genetic code's codons while still ensuring that the code is correctly read. This is a computational mechanism used by nature to improve the accuracy and efficiency of data translation.

The L-shaped structure of a tRNA molecule is held together by hydrogen interactions between bases in different portions of the mRNA sequence. The anticodon is on one end of the L shape, while the amino acid attachment site is on the other. Various tRNAs have slightly different shapes, which is critical for ensuring that the correct amino acid is loaded into them.

The right amino acid gets linked to the right tRNA to ensure that codons are read correctly. Enzymes called aminoacyl-tRNA synthetases perform this very important job. Each amino acid has its own synthetase enzyme, which recognizes only that amino acid and its associated tRNAs (and no others). Once the amino acid and its tRNA have linked to the enzyme, the enzyme binds them together in a reaction powered by the molecule adenosine triphosphate, which acts as an "energy currency" (ATP). Each aminoacyl-tRNA synthetase's active site fits an associated tRNA and a specific amino acid like a "lock and key." The amino acid is subsequently attached to the tRNA using ATP.

An aminoacyl-tRNA synthetase may occasionally make a mistake and bind to the erroneous amino acid (one that resembles its intended target). The threonine synthetase, for example, can accidentally capture serine and bind it to the threonine tRNA. Fortunately, the threonine synthetase possesses a proofreading site that removes the erroneous amino acid from the tRNA.

The ribosome acts as an enzyme to align the tRNA to the mRNA properly. It also catalyzes the dehydration synthesis reaction between the amino acid of one tRNA (in the P site) to the amino acid of another tRNA (in the A site). Finally, the ribosome also catalyzes the decomposition reaction between the amino acid of the tRNA in the P site and the tRNA itself.

The mRNA is aligned in the ribosome such that the initial AUG lies within the P site of the ribosome. The sequence AUG is a signal to a ribosome to start translation here. mRNA is read in a series of 3 nucleotides called a codon. There are 64 different combinations of nucleotides that make a codon. tRNA reads the mRNA codons by having a complementary sequence of RNA (called the anticodon, located at the base of its structure).

tRNA is t-shaped with the anticodon at the bottom that reads the mRNA, and an amino acid at the top, added to the growing polypeptide chain. In this way, the mRNA is the message which codes for the next amino acid to be added to the chain.

An anticodon should be complementary to the codon of the mRNA. Each tRNA carries a different sequence of nucleotides in the anticodon. There are 64 different combinations of nucleotides that make up a codon, but a tRNA has only 20 other amino acids; some of the codons must be redundant. The start codon initiates translations. It is AUG. It codes for Methionine which begins each protein. Thus, there are 3 codons that stop translation. They are UAA, UGA, and UAG. So, of the 64 possible combinations, there are 60 left to code for 20 different amino acids. This leads us to the "wobble" hypothesis. The first nucleotide of the codon is required, and the second is needed most of the time. But the third nucleotide may not matter to get the same amino acid inserted into the protein. When the mRNA is read, it first opens a pocket for tRNA to bind complementarily to the mRNA. Second, it catalyzes a dehydration synthesis process between the amino acid in the P site of the tRNA, and the amino acid in the A site of the tRNA. Third, it catalyzes the hydrolysis (decomposition reaction) between the tRNA in the P site, and its amino acid. Fourth, it slides by one codon (3 nucleotides) to eliminate the tRNA with no amino acid attached, and opens the A site.

- The E site begins to empty of tRNA, and the P site would contain a tRNA with the anticodon of UAC, and the tRNA in the A site would contain the anticodon CCU. AUG codes for the amino acid Methionine (Met), GGA codes for the amino acid Glycine (Gly).
- First, the ribosome catalyzes a dehydration synthesis between Met and Gly. Second, the ribosome catalyzes a decomposition reaction between Met and its tRNA. Third, the ribosome shifts to the right by one codon.
- The UAC tRNA is now in the E site and is let go, the CCU tRNA is in the P site, and the A site with the mRNA sequence AAU is empty of tRNAs. Finally, the tRNA enters the A site with the anticodon UUA. AAU codes for Asparagine (Asn).
- After that, first a dehydration synthesis reaction is catalyzed between Gly and Asn. Second, a decomposition reaction occurs between Gly and its tRNA. Third, the ribosome shifts to the right by one codon.
- The tRNA containing the CCU anticodon is now in the E site and is let go, the P site now includes the tRNA with the anticodon UUA, and the A site is empty of tRNA containing the UUG mRNA sequence. Finally, the tRNA with the AAC anticodon enters the A site. UUG codes for Leucine (Leu).
- Translation continues until the UAG appears; The E site contains the UUA anticodon with its tRNA let go. The P site contains the tRNA with the AAC anticodon. The A site is empty, containing only the GGA mRNA. Finally, the tRNA with the CCU anticodon and the amino acid Glycine (Gly) enters the A site.
- Dehydration synthesis between Leu and Gly is catalyzed. Decomposition between Leu and its tRNA is catalyzed. The ribosome moves to the right by one codon.
- The E site contains the tRNA with the anticodon AAC and is let go. The P site contains the tRNA with the CCU anticodon. The A site with the mRNA AAU does not contain a tRNA. Instead, a tRNA with the anticodon UUA and the amino acid Asparagine (Asp) enter the A site.

- Dehydration synthesis between Gly and Asp is catalyzed. Decomposition between the Gly and its tRNA is catalyzed. The ribosome shifts to the right by one codon.
- The E site contains the tRNA with the CCU anticodon and is let go. The P site contains the tRNA with the UUA anticodon. The A site contains the mRNA with the UUG codon and does not contain a tRNA. A tRNA with the anticodon AAC and the amino acid Leucine (Leu) enters the A site. Dehydration synthesis between the Asp and the Leu. Decomposition between the Asp and its tRNA ribosome shifts to the right by one codon.
- The E site contains the tRNA with the UUA anticodon and is let go. The P site contains the tRNA with the ACC anticodon. The A site with the UAG mRNA does not contain a tRNA. The tRNA with the AUC anticodon enters the A site.
- The UAG codon is a stop codon. Three mRNA codons stop translation (UAA, UAG, UGA). The tRNAs with the AUU, AUC, and ACU anticodons do not contain an amino acid. Therefore, the ribosome cannot catalyze a reaction between the amino acid held by the P-site tRNA and the A-site tRNA. This serves as a signal to stop translation. The decomposition reaction between the Leu and the P-site tRNA occurs, releasing the polypeptide. The ribosomal subunits dissociate and release the mRNA, ending translation.

All pieces are now free to do other things. The ribosome can go on to repeat translation with another mRNA. The mRNA can be translated again and even by multiple ribosomes before being degraded. The protein will undergo folding to assume its final 3-D shape, and the tRNA will be recycled to regain its amino acid. But, at this point, translation of this one mRNA has been completed.

2.4 LEVENTHAL PARADOX

Of significance to note is the Levinthal paradox, according to which a polypeptide chain comes out of a ribosome.

In 1969, Cyrus Levinthal noted that the molecule has an astronomical number of possible conformations because of the very large number of degrees of freedom in an unfolded polypeptide chain. An estimate of 10^{300} was made; for example, a polypeptide of 100 residues will have 99 peptide bonds and 198 different phi and psi bond angles. If these bond angles can be in one of three stable conformations, the protein may misfold into a maximum of 3^{198} different conformations (including any possible folding redundancy). Therefore, if a protein were to attain its correctly folded configuration by sequentially sampling all the possible conformations, it would require a time longer than the universe's age to arrive at its correct native conformation. This is true even if conformations are sampled at rapid (nanosecond or picosecond) rates. The "paradox" is that most small proteins fold spontaneously on a millisecond or microsecond time scale. Computational approaches have established the solution to this paradox to protein structure prediction. Levinthal suggested that the paradox can be resolved if

> " protein folding is sped up and guided by the rapid formation of local interactions which then determine the further folding of the peptide; this suggests local amino acid sequences which form stable interactions and serve as nucleation points in the folding process."
> **(https://web.archive.org/web/20090902211239/http://www.biochem.wisc.edu/ courses/biochem704/Reading/Levinthal1968.pdf)**

Indeed, the protein folding intermediates and the partially folded transition states were experimentally detected, explaining the fast protein folding. Levinthal also suggested that the native structure might have higher energy, if the lowest energy was not kinetically accessible. An analogy is a rock tumbling down a hillside that lodges in a gully rather than reaching the base.

The Leventhal solution is akin to an algorithm that is a finite sequence of well-defined instructions, typically used to solve a class of specific problems or to perform a computation. By using artificial intelligence, algorithms can perform automated deductions (referred to as automated reasoning) and use mathematical and logical tests to divert the code through various routes (referred to as automated decision-making). Using human characteristics as descriptors of machines in metaphorical ways was already practiced by Alan Turing with terms such as "memory," "search," and "stimulus."

2.5 CONCLUSION

Nucleic acid is a five-carbon sugar, with a phosphate group and nitrogen-containing bases. How this structure became the written language of genetic code was discussed in Chapter 1. Understanding the chemistry and thermodynamics of interaction of nucleic acid is important to realize the importance of the genetic code leading to every bodily function. DNA, RNA, Codons, Transcription, Translation are all parts of the sequences that lead to a supply of essential proteins. The statistical odds of such simple molecules with no more than five options of nitrogen groups producing proteins are astronomical. And more surprising are the odds of a translated chain of amino acids turning into a three-dimensional protein. But all of these observations are now well-understood and form the basis of new drug discoveries.

3 RNA Therapeutics

3.1 BACKGROUND

RNA Therapeutics is a new, rapidly growing field of biotherapeutics, that treats diseases with biological products. It is set to revolutionize the standard of care for many diseases, as the number of RNA medications being developed and tested in clinical trials increases. The development of RNA-based treatments for a wide range of uses has been made possible by technical and scientific advances in the production, purification, and cellular delivery systems for RNA. As a result, RNA therapies are the fastest growing class of drugs, revolutionizing the treatment of many as yet "undruggable" diseases and enabling personalized therapy. In addition, RNA medications are inexpensive, motivating many small companies to lead this field.

Small molecule medications that can target active regions of proteins to block or change their function are central to traditional drug strategy. However, given that only 10–14% of proteins have active binding sites that can be "drugged" by tiny compounds and that only around a quarter of the human genome is thought to code for proteins, it creates a constraint that is now partially resolved by the recombinant protein technology that originated in the Silicon Valley in the late 1970s. The development of genetic engineering by Stanford University's Stanley Cohen and UCSF's Herb Boyer created the foundation for the production of recombinant proteins. The University of California earned billions of dollars; now, all of Boyers patents have expired. The FDA has approved 140+ recombinant products as of 2022, and there are over 180 such products worldwide. However, recombinant proteins have limitations in molecular size, stability, and folding—requiring post-translational changes and complicating the manufacturing process. In contrast, the nucleic acid-based techniques bypass many drawbacks by utilizing the mammalian cell's translational machinery.

RNA therapeutics are a class of drugs based on ribonucleic acid (RNA): RNA aptamers, messenger RNA (mRNA), RNA interference (RNAi), and antisense RNA (asRNA). The mRNA-based therapy triggers the synthesis of proteins within cells, making it particularly useful in vaccine development, as demonstrated by the recent success of vaccines against the SARS-CoV-2 viral pandemic. The asRNA is complementary to coding mRNA. Therefore, it triggers mRNA inactivation to prevent it from being used in protein translation; RNAi-based systems use a similar mechanism involving small interfering RNA (siRNA) and micro-RNA (miRNA). RNA aptamers are short, single-stranded RNA molecules that bind to biomolecular targets altering their in vivo activity.

While the focus of this book is on RNA therapeutics, we need to review DNA therapeutics, which pre-dated RNA therapeutics, for essential purposes.

3.2 DNA THERAPEUTICS

DNA therapies are advantageous over RNA therapies, including gene therapy, as mRNAs are not sufficiently stable for long-term gene therapy applications. DNA can be inserted into an intact gene in the host cell's genome, generating a mutation resulting in a partial or complete loss of genetic information or misinformation. Likewise, the RNA that enters the cell does not integrate into the genome (whereas DNA does to some extent) and can potentially be inserted into an intact gene in the host cell's genome, resulting in a mutation and a partial or complete loss of genetic information or misinformation.

When DNA medications are transported to the nuclei of the patient's cells, either incorporated into a viral vector or transmitted as plasmids, they produce therapeutic proteins. However, all DNA-based medications must pass through two membranes, the cytoplasmic and nuclear membranes, to have an effect. In addition, DNA medicines create safety issues since they enter the nucleus and may integrate into the host genome. RNA therapies can solve these restrictions, which just need to reach the cell cytoplasm and pose no risk of chromosomal integration.

3.2.1 DNA PLASMIDS

DNA plasmids are circular molecules with a high molecular weight that encodes therapeutic proteins. These proteins could be used to replace missing or faulty proteins in patients. DNA plasmids can be utilized in gene therapy, immunization, and cell therapy, among other applications. Plasmid DNA (pDNA) must pass through the cytoplasmic and nuclear membranes to access the nucleus. The pDNA is transcribed into mRNA in the nucleus, encoding the desired protein in the patient's body. Gene treatment using pDNA, for example, VM202 is a plasmid DNA gene therapy with 7377 base pairs that encode both isoforms of human hepatocyte growth factor.

3.2.2 VIRAL VECTORS

DNA-based therapeutics replace missing or faulty proteins. However, concerns about foreign DNA integrating into host chromosomes and disrupting normal gene activity have prompted a search for non-integrating techniques. Adeno-Associated Virus (AAV) is a typical viral vector for delivering therapeutic protein-coding DNA with little integration risk. The AAV is a tiny (25 nm) icosahedral human parvovirus with single-stranded linear DNA (4.7 kb). After critical AAV viral genes are deleted, the desired gene is introduced into the AAV DNA for expression. To restore normal protein function, the AAV vector delivers the desired gene to the target cell. In addition, the AAV vector is used to deliver interference RNA to suppress the expression of a certain gene. The AAV, for example, is employed to express hairpin siRNA in HeLa S3 cells to suppress caspase 8 and p53 expression.

In 2003, the Chinese Food and Medication Administration approved Gendicine, the first DNA therapy drug, to treat head and neck squamous carcinoma. Gendicine is an adenoviral vector encoding the wild type (wt) p53 gene that is used to treat cancer by restoring the tumor suppressor gene's expression; a p53 deficiency is found in 60–80% of all cancers.

Glybera was the first DNA therapy to be approved in Europe in 2012. It is a serotype 1 adeno-associated virus that encoded the lipoprotein lipase (LPL) gene and was used to treat LPL deficiency; it is a rare hereditary disorder causing pancreatitis by increasing fat levels in the blood. Unfortunately, Glybera did not work well, and it is no longer available.

Luxturna is an AAV (serotype 2) treatment that encodes the RPE65 gene; it improves eyesight by restoring RPE65 protein levels in RPE65-mediated hereditary retinal degeneration patients. In addition, Zolgensma targets motor neuron cells and delivers a fully functioning copy of the human SMN gene to express SMN protein in a child's motor neurons after a single intravenous injection, improving muscle mobility, function, and survival in children with spinal muscular atrophy, or SMA.

Antigen(s) encoded in DNA-based vaccinations induce a protective immune response. For example, Imlygic is a genetically engineered medication removing the ICP34.5 gene to reduce the natural herpes simplex virus type 1 (HSV-1) infection of normal tissues while increasing tumor-killing preference. It acts by entering tumor cells and replicates and expresses a protein that causes the cancer cells to become cytotoxic.

Infectious pathogens are targeted by DNA-based vaccinations such as Innovio, which encode the SARS-CoV-2 spike protein to provide virus protection. This was the first DNA vaccine to enter clinical testing. However, this product has not received approval and is unlikely to be approved since the mRNA-based vaccines against SARS-CoV-2 have proven useful.

New cell treatments can be created using DNA vectors. Therapeutic DNA is usually transfected into the cells ex vivo to change their phenotypic or function, and then the cells are expanded and supplied to the patient. For example, Kymriah is a single-dose CAR T cell immunotherapy that targets CD19 to treat leukemia, lymphoma, and pediatric cancer. Lentiviral vectors express a chimeric antigen receptor (CAR) targeting CD19 and are transduced into enriched T cells from a patient's peripheral blood mononuclear cells. The transduced T cells are then grown, formed into a suspension, and frozen for future delivery.

Yescarta is another CAR immunotherapy that targets CD19 in treating large B cell lymphoma. First, it inserts the CD19-specific CAR into T cells via a retroviral vector. Then the anti-CD19 CAR T cells are reintroduced into the patient's body and employed to attack CD19-expressing target cells.

Strimvelis is a personalized DNA-based drug to treat patients with Severe Combined Immunodeficiency caused by a lack of Adenosine Deaminase (ADA-SCID). Strimvelis employs CD34+ cells derived from the patient's hematopoietic stem cells (HSCs). The CD34+ cells are then reinfused into the patient after being transduced with a gamma-retrovirus vector containing the human adenosine deaminase (ADA) gene. As a result, CD34+ cells proliferate and produce normal ADA protein in the patient's bone marrow, correcting the deficit.

Zyntelgo for the treatment of beta-thalassemia is a lentiviral vector that, ex vivo, introduces the beta-globin gene into autologous blood-derived CD34+ cells. The genetically modified cells are subsequently reinfused into the patient's bone marrow, resulting in normal hemoglobin levels in red blood cells. A similar method treats severe combined immunodeficiency (SCID), often known as "bubble boy" disease. Mutations in the gene encoding the common chain (IL2RG), shared by several cytokine receptors, cause this rare, life-threatening illness. Children with this condition have impaired immune function because this protein is required for lymphocyte formation and function.

3.3   TYPES OF RNAs

For successful RNA transcription, no viral sequences, such as promoters, are required; whereas, for the expression of DNA carried into the cell, a strong promoter (e.g., the viral cytomegalovirus (CMV) promoter) is necessary. Therefore, integrating such promoters into the host cell's genome can result in unfavorable gene expression regulation alterations.

Because the inserted RNA degrades quickly, transitory gene expression can be achieved that can be switched off after the treatment period (which is not possible with DNA that has been incorporated into the genome).

Dangerous anti-RNA antibodies due to RNA are not created in the patient, although it is widely known that anti-DNA antibodies produce an adverse immunological response.

RNA has several applications: for example, in a short time, any required RNA for any desired protein of interest can be synthesized for therapeutic purposes, even for a single patient, and labeled as personalized medicine.

RNA comes in various forms, the most common being the mRNA that codes the proteins. But many of these RNAs are also crucial in creating new therapies (Table 3.1).

3.4   APPROVED THERAPIES

The approved nucleic acid (DNA/RNA) therapeutics (Table 3.1) treat diseases by targeting their genetic blueprints in vivo, unlike targeting proteins which is a conventional transient approach. The long-term curative effects of nucleic acid therapies are driven by gene inhibition, addition, replacement, or editing. Unlike other treatment techniques, nucleic acid therapies' efficacy and applicability depend on delivery technologies that have enhanced stability, facilitated internalization, and boosted target affinity over the last few decades. The nucleic acid therapeutics include antisense oligonucleotides (ASOs), ligand-modified small interfering RNA conjugates, lipid nanoparticles (LNPs), and adeno-associated virus vectors (AAVs) (Figure 3.1).

Fomivirsen, the first-ever FDA-approved RNA therapy, is used to treat cytomegalovirus retinitis, a symptom of DNA herpes cytomegalovirus (CMV), which is frequent in advanced acquired immunodeficiency syndrome (AIDS). Table 3.2 lists the approved nucleoside therapeutic products.

TABLE 3.1

Types of RNAs

Designation	Type
5.8S rRNA	5.8S ribosomal RNA
5S rRNA	5S ribosomal RNA
6S RNA	6S RNA
aRNA	antisense RNA
asmiRNA	antisense micro RNA
asRNA	antisense RNA
cfRNA	cell-free RNA
circRNA	circular RNA
cis-NAT	cis-natural antisense transcript
CRISPR RNA	CRISPR-Cas RNA
crRNA	CRISPR RNA
DD RNA	DNA damage response RNA
diRNA	DSB-induced small RNAs
dsRNA	double-stranded RNA
endo-siRNA	endogenous small interfering RNA
exRNA	extracellular RNA
gRNA	guide RNA
hc-siRNA	heterochromatic small interfering RNA
hcsiRNA	heterochromatic small interfering RNA
hnRNA	heterogeneous nuclear RNA
lincRNA	long intergenic non-coding RNA
lncRNA	long non-coding RNA
LSU rRNA	large subunit ribosomal RNA
miRNA	micro RNA
mRNA	messenger RNA
mrpRNA	mitochondrial RNA processing ribonuclease
msRNA	multicopy, single-stranded RNA
nat-siRNA	natural antisense short interfering RNA
NATs	natural antisense transcripts
natsiRNA	natural antisense short interfering RNA
ncRNA	non-coding RNA
nmRNA	non-messenger RNA
NoRC RNA	nucleolar remodeling complex associated RNA
OxyS RNA	oxidative stress response RNA
pcRNA	protein-coding RNA
piRNA	Piwi-interacting RNA
pre-mRNA	precursor messenger RNA
pRNA	promoter RNA
qiRNA	QDE-2 interfering RNA
rasiRNA	Repeat associated siRNA
RNAi	RNA interference

(Continued)

TABLE 3.1 (CONTINUED)
Types of RNAs

Designation	Type
RNase MRP	mitochondrial RNA processing ribonuclease
RNase P	ribonuclease P
rRNA	ribosomal RNA
scaRNA	small Cajal body-specific RNA
scnRNA	small-scan RNA
scRNA	small conditional RNA
scRNA	small cytoplasmic RNA
SgrS RNA	sugar transport-related sRNA
shRNA	short hairpin RNA
siRNA	small interfering RNA
SL RNA	spliced leader RNA
smnRNA	small non messenger RNA
SmY RNA	mRNA trans-splicing
snoRNA	small nucleolar RNA
snRNA	small nuclear RNA
snRNP	small nuclear ribonucleic proteins
SPA lncRNA	5′ small nucleolar RNA capped, and 3′ polyadenylated long noncoding RNA
sRNA	small RNA
sRNA	soluble RNA
SRP RNA	signal recognition particle RNA
ssRNA	single-stranded RNA
SsrS RNA	small RNA regulator of RNA polymerase
SSU rRNA	small subunit ribosomal RNA
stRNA	small temporal RNA
tasiRNA	trans-acting siRNA
tmRNA	transfer-messenger RNA
tracrRNA	trans-activating crRNA
tRNA	transfer RNA
uRNA	U spliceosomal RNA
vRNA	vault RNA
vtRNA	vault RNA
Xist RNA	X-inactive specific transcript
Y RNA	Y RNA

3.5 RNA THERAPIES

The Shine-Dalgarno sequence, found at the 5t end (5t UTR) of the mRNA chain, is transcribed directly from DNA in bacteria as it aids mRNA binding to ribosomes. Gene expression in eukaryotic species, on the other hand, is more complex, requiring the use of RNA Polymerase II (Pol II) enzyme for messenger RNA production.

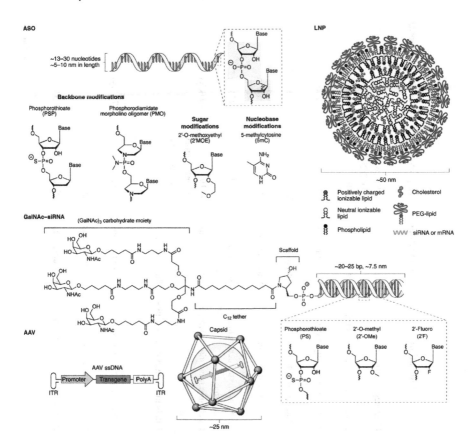

FIGURE 3.1 Four nucleic acid platform technologies. ASOs, backbone, sugar, or nucleobase modifications enhance affinity to target RNA, improve nuclease resistance, alter circulation characteristics, and modulate immunological properties. The LNP containing siRNA or mRNA includes key lipid components. At the 3′ end of the sense strand, a trivalent ligand containing terminal GalNAc moieties is covalently attached to siRNA. The (GalNAc)3 ligand's multivalency and excellent spatial organization enable hepatocyte-specific siRNA targeting via the asialoglycoprotein receptor. GalNAc-siRNA treatments also use chemical modifications such as 2′-OMe, 2′-fluoro, and phosphorothioate linkages. The AAV vector containing a 4.7-kb ssDNA is shown with inverted terminal repeats (ITR).

A pre-mRNA (primary transcript) is generated in this situation, which is then processed to yield mature mRNA. In the mature mRNA molecule, each amino acid is encoded by a codon, a group of three nucleotides. Specific sections of RNA determine the translation process and mRNA stability, which are critical for the biomolecule's greater durability in the cell. The first, the 5t UTR, is a sequence of nucleotides at the 5t end of the mRNA that does not encode for amino acids in both prokaryotic and eukaryotic mRNAs, as shown in Figure 3.1. The insertion of a guanine nucleotide with a methyl group (CH3) to the 5t end (Cap-5t) during pre-mRNA processing boosts mRNA stability and aids in mRNA transport to the cytoplasm

TABLE 3.2

Approved Nucleoside Products

Products	Gene target	Indication	Administration	Approval year	Cost ($/ treatment)
ASOs					
Vitravene, fomivirsen (Ionis Pharmaceuticals)	Cytomegalovirus gene (UL123)	Cytomegalovirus infection	Intravitreal	1998 (withdrawn 2002/2006)	10.4 k/yr
Exondys 51, eteplirsen (Sarepta Therapeutics)	Dystrophin (exon 51)	Duchenne muscular dystrophy	Intrathecal	2016	300 k/yr
Tegsedi, inotersen (Ionis Pharmaceuticals)	Transthyretin (TTR)	TTR-mediated amyloidosis	Subcutaneous	2018	450 k/yr
Spinraza, nusinersen (Ionis Pharmaceuticals)	Survival of motor neuron 2 (SMN2)	Spinal muscular atrophy	Intrathecal	2016	750 k/yr, 375 k/yr
Kynamro, mipomersen (Ionis Pharmaceuticals)	Apolipoprotein B-100	Hypercholesterolemia	Subcutaneous	2013	176 k/yr
Waylivra, Volanesoren (Ionis Pharmaceuticals / Akcea)	Apolipoprotein CIII	Familial chylomicronemia syndrome	Subcutaneous	2019	395 k/yr
Vyondys 53, golodirsen (Sarepta Therapeutics)	Dystrophin (exon 53)	Duchenne muscular dystrophy	Subcutaneous	2019 (confirmatory trial required)	300 k/yr
Amondys 45, casimersen (Sarepta Therapeutics)	Dystrophin (exon 45)	Duchenne muscular dystrophy	Subcutaneous	2021	
GalNAc–siRNA conjugates					
Givlaari, Givosiran (Alnylam Pharmaceuticals)	ALAS1	Acute hepatic porphyrias	Subcutaneous	2019	575 k/yr
Leqvio, inclisiran (Novartis/Alnylam Pharmaceuticals)	PCSK9	Hypercholesterolemia	Subcutaneous	2020	
Oxlumo, lumasiran (Alnylam Pharmaceuticals)	Glycolate oxidase	Primary hyperoxaluria type 1	Subcutaneous	2020	493 k/yr

(Continued)

TABLE 3.2 (CONTINUED)
Approved Nucleoside Products

Products	Gene target	Indication	Administration	Approval year	Cost ($/ treatment)
LNP-RNA					
Onpattro, patisiran (Alnylam Pharmaceuticals)	TTR siRNA	TTR-mediated amyloidosis	Intravenous	2018	450k/yr
Comirnaty, tozinameran (BioNTech/ Pfizer)	SARS-CoV-2 spike protein mRNA	COVID-19 (FDA, emergency use; Switzerland, full approval)	Intramuscular	2020	30–40/dose
mRNA-1273 (Moderna/NIAID/BARDA)	SARS-CoV-2 spike protein mRNA	COVID-19 (FDA, emergency use)	Intramuscular	2020	30–36/dose
AAV vectors					
Glybera, alipogene tiparvovec (uniQure)	Lipoprotein lipase (LPL) (AAV1)	LPL deficiency	Intramuscular	2012 (withdrawn 2017)	1 M
Luxturna, voretigene neparvovec-rzyl (Spark Therapeutics)	RPE65 (AAV2)	Leber congenital amaurosis	Subretinal	2017	850 k
Zolgensma, onasemnogene abeparvovec (AveXis/Novartis)	SMN1 (AAV9)	Spinal muscular atrophy	Intravenous	2019	2.1M
Adenovirus (Ad) vectors					
Vaxzevria, AZD1222, ChAdOx1 nCoV-19 (AstraZeneca)	SARS-CoV-2 spike protein DNA (ChAdOx1)	COVID-19 (FDA, and EMA emergency use)	Intramuscular	2021	4–8/dose
Ad26.COV2.S (Johnson & Johnson)	SARS-CoV-2 spike protein DNA (Ad26)	COVID-19 (FDA, and EMA emergency use)	Intramuscular	2021	8.5–10/dose
Convidecia, Ad5-nCoV (CanSinoBIO)	SARS-CoV-2 spike protein DNA (Ad5)	COVID-19 (Approved in China)	Intramuscular	2021	30/dose

Note: ASO, antisense oligonucleotide; ALAS1, 5'-aminolevulinate synthase 1; PCSK9, proprotein convertase subtilisin–kexin type; RPE65, retinal pigment epithelium-specific 65 kDa. Referenced to 2020 US$.

and further binding of the mRNA to the de adenylation ribosome. This alteration aids translation, nuclear export, intron elimination, and immunogenicity reduction, making it useful for some therapies, such as target protein replacement. Changes to the Cap-5t end, which prevent it from being removed, may also improve mRNA stability and resistance to enzymatic degradation. The protein-coding region, which contains the codons that determine the amino acid sequence, is the second portion of the mRNA. The protein-coding region begins with a methionine-encoding first codon and ends with a stop codon. Optimization of codons replaces unusual codons in protein-coding sequences with more common synonymous codons, leading to changes in expression and immunogenicity. In eukaryotic cells, both coding and non-coding RNA can be susceptible to epi-transcriptomic alterations, which involve the modification of particular nucleotides. These changes are significant because they can influence RNA translation, initiation, stability, localization, and function.

The third region is a non-coding nucleotide sequence that occurs at the 3t end of the mRNA, comparable to the 5t UTR (3t UTR). The creation of a polyadenylated "tail" (poly(A)) on the 3t UTR is the result of a process called polyadenylation, which is seen in Figure 3.1. The poly (A) tail encourages nuclease deadenylation inhibition, improving stability and translation efficiency. Furthermore, this sequence has been extensively investigated for the purification of mRNA. Both the 5t and 3t UTR sections boost mRNA's stability, extend its half-life in the cell, and potentially enhance protein synthesis. Furthermore, mRNA UTRs and microRNAs (miRNAs) are responsible for recruiting RNA-binding proteins and can significantly impact translation activity (Figure 3.2). There are several types and functions of RNAs. There are two types of RNA in cells: coding RNAs, including messenger RNA (mRNA); and non-coding RNAs, such as ncRNA, miRNA, and lncRNA (www.non-code.org). Only 2% of the RNA produced from the human genome encodes proteins. The mRNA is simply a complementary copy of DNA that serves as a template for the production of proteins since it carries information about the amino acid sequence that will make up the target protein. In addition, each mRNA molecule contains non-coding or untranslated regions that regulate mRNA processing and reading processes (Figure 3.3).

3.6 NONCODING RNA

Noncoding RNA therapies are divided into two categories. First, short oligonucleotides bind to complementary sequences in endogenous RNA transcripts and change their processing (to replace faulty proteins or existing antigens in vaccines, for example). Several significant obstacles have been overcome in developing RNA therapeutics, including the transport of negatively charged RNA across the hydrophobic cytoplasmic membrane; and exogenous RNA immunogenicity, which cause cell toxicity and impaired translation into therapeutic proteins. However, recent advances in RNA biology, bioinformatics, separation science, and nanotechnology have significantly reduced these barriers, allowing for the rapid production of RNA therapies such as the ability to act on targets that would otherwise be "undruggable" for a

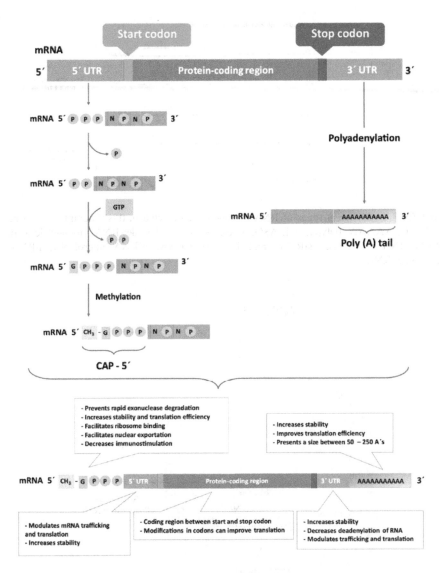

FIGURE 3.2 The basic sections for eukaryotic mRNA processing, such as the 5t UTR, protein-coding region, and 3t UTR, are represented schematically in this diagram. The schematization of the polyadenylation process, and introduction of Cap at the 5t end and its biological and structural functions. P—Phosphate group; N—Nucleotide; CH3—Methyl group; A—Adenine; G—Guanine; UTR—Untranslated region.

small molecule or a protein; their rapid and cost-effective development compared to small molecules or recombinant proteins; and the ability to change the sequence of an mRNA construct quickly for tailored treatments or to adapt to a changing pathogen—all advantages of RNA-based drugs that are propelling development (see Antisense Oligonucleotide (ASO) in Figure 3.1 and Figure 3.4).

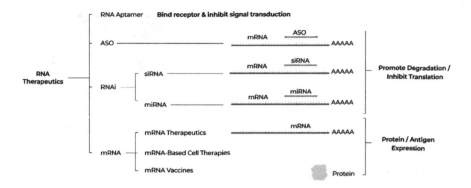

FIGURE 3.3 Different types of RNA therapies are depicted in this diagram. Adenosine molecule; AAAAA, poly(A) tail; ASO, antisense oligonucleotide; RNA, ribonucleic acid; RNAi, RNA interference; siRNA, small interfering RNA; miRNA, microRNA; mRNA, messenger RNA;

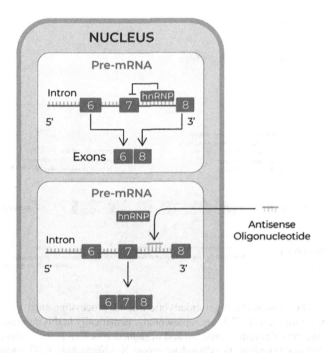

FIGURE 3.4 An antisense drug's route of action for treating spinal muscular atrophy is depicted in this diagram. The antisense drugs reach the nucleus, displace hnRNP proteins, and increase the synthesis of transcripts containing exon 7, thereby generating full-length SMN protein. SMN, motor neuron survival; hnRNP, heterogeneous nuclear ribonucleoprotein; pre-mRNA, precursor mRNA; mRNA, messenger RNA; RNA, ribonucleic acid.

Steric block ASOs are created to prevent polyadenylation, impede or promote translation, or change splicing by physically inhibiting or preventing translation or splicing.

A new class of antisense RNA known as splice-switching oligonucleotides (SSOs) alters gene expression through splicing. It can also correct aberrant splicing patterns in genetic disorders instead of siRNAs, which simply knock down protein expression. However, it is challenging to measure splice-switching activities in cells quantitatively.

The capacity of ASOs to interact with pre-mRNA allows them to target splicing processes and dramatically expands the number of RNA sequences that can be selected for ASO binding, reducing off-target effects. For example, only 7% of the 2842 known single nucleotide polymorphisms in the HTT gene, which codes for the huntingtin protein, could be targeted in mature mRNA (using siRNAs). Still, PCR could target these single nucleotide polymorphisms 100% of the time.

The US Food and Drug Agency (FDA) and European Medicines Agency (EMA) have approved 10 ASOs (see Table 3.3).

3.6.1 SMALL INTERFERING RNA

Small interfering RNAs (siRNAs) are noncoding RNA duplexes derived from precursor siRNAs. The latter range in size from 30 to more than 100 bp and are either transcribed or artificially added. Dicer breaks down the precursor siRNA duplex into 20–30 bp long siRNA with two base overhangs in the 3 region, which interacts with RISC to generate RNA interference (RNAi). The RISC's endonuclease argonaute 2 (AGO2) component cleaves the sense strand while leaving the antisense strand intact, allowing the active RISC to find its target mRNA. The phosphodiester backbone of the target mRNA is then cleaved by AGO2. Because the antisense strand is entirely complementary to the coding area of the target mRNA, siRNA blocks the production of the unc-22, unc-54, fem1, and hlh-1 genes in C. elegans, causing RNAi. In addition, they demonstrated that dsRNA is more successful than ssRNA for inducing RNAi and destroying an mRNA target artificially. Patisiran was the first siRNA-based medication to reach the market. It is used to treat polyneuropathy in adults caused by inherited TTR-mediated amyloidosis.

Patisiran is a dsRNA that promotes the degradation of TTR-encoding mRNA via RNAi. Another siRNA medication, Givosiran treats acute hepatic porphyria. It decreases the amounts of disease-causing neurotoxic intermediates, aminolevulinic acid and porphobilinogen, by targeting aminolevulinate synthase mRNA in the liver Figure 3.5.

Small interfering RNA (siRNA) are double-stranded RNA molecules that engage in the RNA-induced silencing complex (RISC) to silence genes. They are 19–23 base pairs long (with a two-nucleotide 3' overhang). The RISC complex binds siRNA, which is then unraveled via ATP hydrolysis and guided by the enzyme "Slicer" to target mRNA breakdown based on complementary base-pairing. As a therapeutic product, siRNA can be delivered through the eye or nose, enhancing bioavailability. However, because intravenous injections require significant amounts (around

TABLE 3.3
Approved ASOs FDA/EMA and Others

Drug	Disease/disorder	Mechanism	FDA approval	EMA approval
2'-O-(2-methoxyethyl) modified antisense oligonucleotide	Lafora disease	targeting glycogen synthase 1 pre-mRNA		2020
Casimersen	DMD	bind to exon 45 of the dystrophin pre-mRNA	Feb 2021	n/a
Eteplirsen	DMD	Splicing modulation	2016	Rejected 2018
Fomivirsen	CMV induced retinitis	Translation block	1998 (discontinued)	1999 (withdrawn)
Givosiran	Acute hepatic porphyria	RNAi	2019	2020
Golodirsen	DMD	Splicing modulation	2019	Awaited
Inclisiran	Hypercholesterolemia	blocking the production of PCSK9	Awaited	2020
Inotersen	FAP/hATTR	RNase H	2018	2018
Mipomersen	Hypercholesterolemia	RNase H	2013 (discontinued)	Rejected 2012
Nusinersen	SMA	Splicing modulation	2016	2017
Patisiran	FAP/hATTR	RNAi	2018	2018
Pegaptanib	Age-related macular degeneration	antagonist to VEG	2004 (discontinued)	2006 (withdrawn)
Ty777	Batten disease	MFSD8 gene block (one patient only)	2018	n/a
Valonesorsen	Hyper triglycidemia, familial chylomicronemia syndrome, familial partial lipodystrophy	RNase H	Rejected	2019
Viltolarsen	DMD	bind to exon 53 of dystrophin pre-mRNA	2020	Awaited
Volanesorsen	Familial chylomicronemia syndrome (FCS)	binds to apoC-III mRNA	Rejected	2019

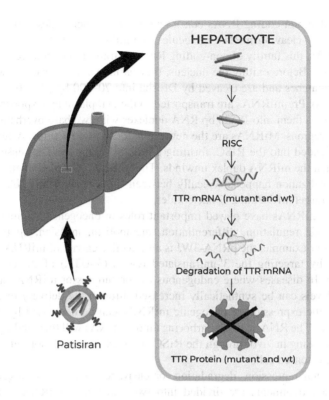

FIGURE 3.5 The mechanism of action of the small interfering RNA (siRNA) medication patisiran is depicted in this diagram. The medications are delivered intravenously after being encapsulated in lipid nanoparticles. The medications finally reach the hepatocyte after delivery and are released into the cytoplasm, where they are loaded onto the RISC. The antisense strand binds to target mRNA and inhibits protein synthesis (TTR). RISC, RNA-induced silencing complex; mRNA, messenger RNA; RNA, ribonucleic acid.

20–30% of total blood volume), targeted distribution to treat malignancies is difficult. Direct tissue/organ electroporation, conjugation to membrane-permeable peptides, and in vivo liposome packing exogenous siRNAs only persist a few days (at most a few weeks in non-dividing cells). However, when it gets to its target, it can use the RISC system to control gene expression by base-pairing to mRNA targets and promoting their destruction.

The FDA approved two siRNA therapeutic products: Givosiran targets ALAS1 to treat AHP; and Patisiran targets polyneuropathy to treat hereditary transthyretin-mediated amyloidosis.

3.6.2 Micro RNA

Similar to siRNA, micro-RNAs (miRNA) sequences can be fused onto each branch of the RNA scaffold and delivered to the diseased cells. MiRNAs are small single-stranded non-coding RNAs consisting of 19–25 nucleotides that can silence target genes by cleaving mRNA molecules or inhibiting their translation. As primary miRNAs, this family of non-coding RNAs is transcribed from genomic DNA (pri-miRNAs). Before exiting the nucleus, they assume a loop structure with intermittent mismatches and are cleaved by Drosha into 70–100 bp precursor miRNAs (pre-miRNAs). Pre-miRNAs are transported to the cytoplasm by Exportin 5, where Dicer processes them into 18–25 bp RNA duplexes with two base overhangs in each of the three regions. MiRNAs are the new name for these structures. After that, the miRNA is loaded into the RISC, forming a miRISC complex. The sense strand is released when the miRNA duplex unwinds. The miRISC is guided by the antisense strand. Hybridization happens typically between the 5 ends of miRNA and the 3 UTR of the target mRNA at 2–7 nucleotides.

Recently, miRNAs have played important roles in oncogenesis, tumor progression, cell cycle regulation, differentiation, metabolism, invasion, apoptosis, and metastasis. For example, the pRNA-3WJ is an effective carrier of miRNA to silence viral genes by targeting the 3′-untranslated region (3′-UTR) of the coxsackievirus genome. In diseases where endogenous tumor suppressor miRNAs are downregulated, levels can be synthetically increased through the delivery of miRNAs. Conversely, the expression of oncogenic miRNAs can be decreased by delivering anti-miRNAs. The RNA scaffold harboring (anti)miRNAs will then undergo normal DICER processing in vivo through the RISC complex, returning normal gene regulation in the diseased cells.

Translational repression, degradation, or cleavage suppress the target mRNA. miRNA-based treatments are divided into two categories: miRNA mimics and miRNA inhibitors. The latter are single-stranded RNA oligos meant to interfere with miRNAs; whereas the former are double-stranded RNA molecules that imitate miRNAs. Although no miRNA-based product has been approved, there are many potential candidates in clinical testing, such as Cobomarsen (MRG-106), remlarsen (MRG-201), MRG-229 (miR-29 mimic; pre-clinical), and MRG-110 are miR-92 inhibitors.

Abnormal miRNA expression is linked to a wide range of illnesses. Targeting dysregulated miRNAs with small-molecule medicines has emerged as a promising new treatment option for various human disorders, particularly cancer. For gene regulation, miRNAs have been identified as high-value targets for therapy. Because different gene expression profiles of the same condition could produce differential transcriptional responses, functional profiles are usually more reproducible.

3.6.3 Long Non-coding RNA

Long non-coding RNA (lncRNA) therapeutics involves applying specifically designed siRNAs against lncRNAs. For example, siRNAs designed against PANDA (a lncRNA that plays a significant role in DNA damage response) substantially reduced the expression of PANDA and consequently sensitized human fibroblasts to apoptosis induced by doxorubicin. Both miRNA and lncRNA present many future possibilities for basic research, biomarker discovery, and therapeutic applications.

3.6.4 Antisense RNA

Antisense RNA (asRNA) is a non-coding, single-stranded RNA complementary to a coding mRNA sequence. It prevents mRNA from translating into proteins. The enzyme Dicer cleaves double-stranded RNA precursors into 21–26 nucleotides-long RNA species, producing short asRNA transcripts within the nucleus. Antisense medications are based on the idea that asRNA hybridizes with mRNA and renders it inactive. These medications are short RNA sequences that bind to mRNA and prevent a gene from making the protein it codes for. Antisense medicines are being developed to treat lung cancer, diabetes, and disorders with a high inflammation component, such as arthritis and asthma.

Antisense RNA is transferred beyond the cell membrane into the cytoplasm and nucleus using nonviral vectors and virus vectors, such as retrovirus, adenovirus, and liposomes. Because of its high transfection effectiveness, viral vector-based delivery is the most advantageous of the many delivery techniques. However, it is difficult to distribute antisense RNA solely to the targeted regions, and there are numerous restrictions to its application due to antisense RNA's size and stability difficulties. In addition, improving delivery will require chemical modifications and designing new oligonucleotides.

3.6.5 Interfering RNA

Interfering RNA (RNAi) is a short, noncoding RNA that suppresses gene expression during or after translation. The RNAi system was identified when color genes were introduced into petunias, with the theory that it evolved as a means of innate immunity against double-stranded RNA viruses. However, there is no approved RNAi product on the market.

3.6.6 Aptamers

Aptamers are molecules made up of oligonucleotides or peptides that bind to a specific target molecule. Aptamers are usually made by picking them out of a huge pool of random sequences; however, natural aptamers can also be found in riboswitches. Aptamers can be employed as macromolecular medicines for fundamental research and clinical usage. Aptamers can be combined with ribozymes to self-cleave in the presence of their target molecule. Additional academic, industrial, and therapeutic applications exist for these chemical compounds. Aptamers are divided into DNA, RNA, and XNA aptamers. They are made up of (typically short) oligonucleotide strands. The peptide aptamers comprise one (or more) short variable peptide domains connected to a protein scaffold on both ends.

Aptamers are tiny molecules of single-stranded DNA or RNA that are 20–100 nucleotides long or 3–60 kDa in size. Due to their single-stranded nature, aptamers can generate various secondary structures, such as pseudoknots, stem-loops, and bulges, via intra-strand base-pairing interactions. The secondary structures included in an aptamer combine to form a unique tertiary structure, which determines which target the aptamer will selectively attach to. As a result, aptamers have a high affinity for their targets, with dissociation constants in the pM to nM range. As a result, they can connect to targets that tiny peptides, made by phage display or antibodies, cannot help; they can distinguish between conformational isomers and amino acid changes. Furthermore, because aptamers are based on nucleic acids, they may be directly manufactured, removing the need for cell-based expression and extraction required in antibody manufacturing. RNA aptamers, for example, may produce a wide range of configurations, leading to the conjecture that they are more discriminating in terms of target affinity than DNA aptamers.

Pegaptanib, a 28-nucleotides RNA aptamer targeting VEGF165, is the only approved therapy for age-related macular degeneration (AMD).

Slow off-rate modified aptamers (SOMAmers) are a new family of aptamers in which the deoxyribose thymine (dT) base in the heterocyclic ring in the oligonucleotide pool is replaced by the deoxyribose uridine (dU) base at the 5′ position. Several substitutions at the 5′ position can generate a wide range of aptamers with varying binding affinity and kinetic characteristics, improving the chances of discovering a good aptamer. D-oligonucleotides are naturally occurring nucleotides that form a right-handed helix. L-oligonucleotides form a left-handed helix, and mirror-image aptamers (spiegelmers) are L-oligonucleotides. To create spiegelmers, conventional D-oligonucleotides are first selected against a mirror-image target. Then the selected D-oligonucleotides are chemically produced as L-oligonucleotides in reverse configuration. Modifications can be made during the selection process (SELEX) or after (post-SELEX).

In comparison to modified aptamers, non-modified aptamers are less stable and immunogenic. Modifications prevent aptamers from being degraded by nucleases, improve binding affinity, and enable coupling with other molecules, medicines, or nanoparticles. Aptamers undergo many analytical assays after initial alteration to determine the effect of the modification on their binding affinity with the target. As a result, the final aptamer product differs from the original and may have single or numerous structural alterations (Figure 3.6).

RNA aptamers can act as antagonists, agonists, or "RNA decoy aptamers," depending on their function. When it comes to antagonists, the RNA aptamer is employed to either block a protein from binding to its cell membrane receptor or execute its function by binding to its target. RNA aptamers can also act as agonists to act as a co-stimulatory molecule, promoting immune cell activation and assisting in mobilizing the body's defense system. The synthetic RNA aptamer looks like a native RNA molecule for RNA decoy aptamers. As a result, proteins that bind to the natural RNA target instead bind to the RNA aptamer, potentially interfering with a disease's biomolecular pathway. RNA aptamers are being examined for alternative therapeutic applications and their use as direct therapeutic agents. The RNA aptamer, for example, can be conjugated to a therapeutic component and used as a targeted delivery mechanism for that medicine. ApDCs (aptamer-drug conjugates) are RNA aptamers of this type. RNA aptamers may also be effective in diagnostic imaging when conjugated to a radioisotope or a fluorescent dye molecule.

Vascular endothelial growth factor, osteoblasts, and C-X-C Chemokine Ligand 12 are examples of RNA aptamer molecular targets and prospective targets (CXCL2).

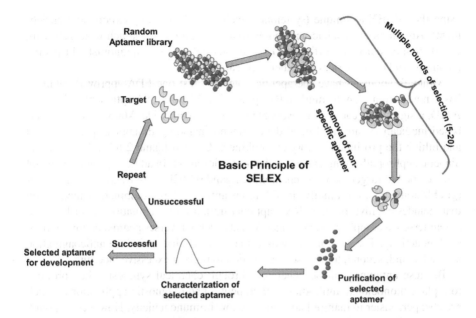

FIGURE 3.6   Basic principle of SELEX. (Source: https://www.frontiersin.org/files/Articles /656421/fcimb-11-656421-HTML/image_m/fcimb-11-656421-g001.jpg)

There are several hindrances to using aptamers: nucleases degrade RNA aptamers once they are injected into the body in minutes if they are not modified; in addition, RNA aptamers are eliminated from the bloodstream by the renal system due to their tiny size; and RNA aptamers also bind proteins in the circulation, resulting in non-target tissue distribution and toxicity. When isolating RNA aptamers, it is important to know that aptamers with repetitive Cytosine-Phosphate-Guanine (CpG) sequences will activate the immune system via the Toll-like receptor pathway.

To overcome some of the in vivo limitations of RNA aptamers, several alterations to the nucleotides can be made to improve the aptamer's potency. A polyethylene glycol (PEG) moiety, for example, can be added to increase the size of the aptamer, preventing it from being removed from the bloodstream by the renal glomerulus. During in vivo testing, however, PEG has been linked to allergic responses. Additionally, changes such as a 2′ fluoro or amino group and a 3′ inverted thymidine can be introduced to avoid nuclease breakdown. Furthermore, the aptamer can be made with the ribose sugar in the L-form rather than the D-form, which prevents nuclease recognition. Spiegelmers are aptamers like this. Finally, the cytosine nucleobases within the aptamer can be methylated to avoid Toll-like receptor pathway activation; nevertheless, despite these potential remedies to lower in vivo efficacy, chemically altering the aptamer may diminish its binding affinity towards its target.

Aptamers are single-stranded nucleic acids with a tertiary structure that allows them to bind to a range of substrates, including proteins, peptides, carbohydrates, and other compounds, rather than their sequence. Aptamers were discovered in 1990 using the SELEX technique (systematic evolution of ligand by exponential enrichment). Aptamers are nucleic acid pools that have evolved to attach to targets with excellent specificity and affinity. They can act as agonists, antagonists, bispecific aptamers, and even carriers for other medications.

Although aptamers have therapeutic potential, just one FDA-approved aptamer-based medication is on the market. Pegaptanib is a 27-base RNA aptamer used to treat AMD, a significant cause of irreversible blindness worldwide. Many more aptamer-based medications are in clinical development, including Emapticap pegol to bind and inhibit the pro-inflammatory chemokine C-C motif-ligand 2 (CCL2) in treating diabetic nephropathy, lung cancer, and pancreatic cancer. In addition, olaptesed pegol is developed to target the CXC chemokine ligand (CXCL12) in treating brain cancer (glioblastoma/glioma). Finally, REG1 is an anticoagulant combination medication that includes pegnivacogin, an RNA aptamer inhibitor of coagulation factor IXa, and anivamersen, a complementary sequence that quickly reverses pegnivacogin's anticoagulant activity. The goal of this two-part aptamer is, first, to induce anticoagulation as needed and, second, to reverse it as needed to prevent excessive bleeding.

Because aptamers can be generated through chemical synthesis, they promise to replace monoclonal antibodies in therapeutic and diagnostic applications, which are cheaper, easier to manipulate, and have low immunogenicity. However, although aptamers offer many benefits over antibodies, clinical translation is difficult due to inferior pharmacokinetic qualities (particularly sensitive to nucleases, easily eliminated by kidneys) and the complexity of selection processes (a time-consuming process with low success rates).

3.7   CODING RNA

3.7.1   MRNA AS THERAPEUTICS

mRNAs are essentially temporary blueprints for genes encoded in genomic DNA (Figure 3.7). These genes' mRNA transcripts convey genetic information to the

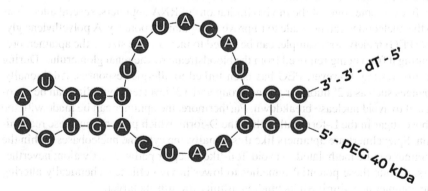

FIGURE 3.7   The sequence of pegaptanib with its secondary structure is depicted in this diagram. dT, deoxthymidine; PEG, polyethylene glycol; Messenger RNAs (mRNAs) serve as a link between genomic DNA that codes for proteins and the proteins that are encoded.

translational machinery, which produces the encoded proteins. Exogenous mRNA was first used to produce a protein in vivo by injecting luciferase, chloramphenicol acetyltransferase, or beta-galactosidase-encoding synthetic mRNA into mouse skeletal muscle resulting in proteins translated from at the injection site. The therapeutic impact of mRNA in a mouse model of central diabetes insipidus was proven when the degree of expression produced from RNA was comparable to that obtained from injection of a DNA vector expressing the same proteins. Vasopressin insufficiency is hereditary in Brattleboro rats. The researchers isolated cytoplasmic mRNA from wild-type rat hypothalamus or generated vasopressin-encoding mRNA. Injecting either mRNA into the hypothalamus of Brattleboro rats stimulated the production of vasopressin and corrected diabetic insipidus for a short time.

The challenges for mRNA come from its size ($10^5 \sim 10^6$ Da) and instability as nucleases quickly degrade it and activate the immune system. In addition, since mRNA has a large negative charge density, it is less permeable across cell membranes. Therefore, researchers have used microinjection, RNA patches (mRNA loaded in a dissolving micro-needle), gene gun, protamine condensation, RNA adjuvants, and encapsulating to stabilize and facilitate entry into the cytoplasm mRNA in nanoparticles containing lipids.

Synthetic or in vitro-translated mRNA looks like natural mRNA; It has a 3 poly(A) tail for stability and a 5 cap for translation. It comprises a single-stranded open reading frame flanked by untranslated sections. Exogenous mRNA is transcribed into protein in the cytoplasm and then degrades within minutes to hours, posing a low risk of genome integration as systemically administered mRNA expresses protein.

Compared to recombinant proteins or small molecules, the development and manufacture of RNA therapies are a comparatively easy and cost-effective alternative; mRNA sequences can also be easily changed, allowing for personalized RNA therapy. mRNA is used in a variety of therapeutic approaches: i) replacement therapy, in which mRNA is given to a patient to replace a missing gene or protein or to provide therapeutic proteins; ii) vaccination, in which mRNA encodes specific antigen(s) and is given to induce protective immunity; iii) mRNA is transfected into cells ex vivo to alter cell phenotypic or function, and then these cells are transferred into the patient as cell therapy.

3.7.2 MRNA AS REPLACEMENT THERAPY

Several products are under development as gene therapy and to treat metabolic illnesses, heart ailments, and immunomodulators for immuno-oncology applications (Figure 3.8):

- AZD8601 is a naked mRNA that encodes vascular endothelial growth factor (VEGF-A) and is designed to be injected into the heart during coronary artery bypass surgery. The goal is to improve local angiogenesis in ischemic heart disease patients, lower myocardial ischemia, and enhance left ventricular systolic performance.

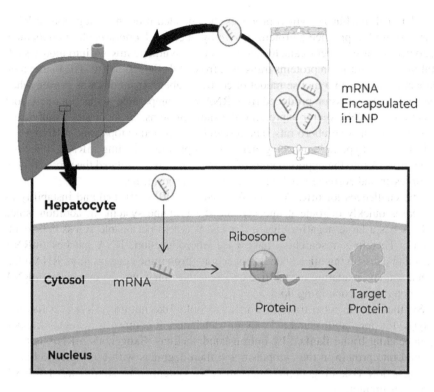

FIGURE 3.8 Intravenous delivery of mRNA encapsulated in lipid nanoparticles (LNP) to repair missing/defective protein in hepatic cells is depicted in this diagram. RNA, ribonucleic acid; mRNA, messenger RNA.

- mRNA-3704 encodes methyl malonyl-CoA mutase and is intended to treat methylmalonic aciduria caused by this enzyme deficiency.
- MRT5005 was developed to treat cystic fibrosis, a genetic condition caused by a mutation in the chloride channel cystic fibrosis transmembrane conductance regulator (CFTR). When the epithelium is damaged, thicker mucus accumulates in various organs, including the pancreas and the lungs. MRT5005 is a fully functional CFTR gene given to lung epithelial cells by nebulization.
- mRNA-2416, mRNA-2752, and MEDI1191 are mRNA-based immunomodulators.
- OX40 Ligand is a membrane-bound co-stimulatory protein that increases T-cell proliferation, activity, and survival to initiate an attack against cancer cells. When this ligand is administered intravenously (solid tumors/lymphoma/advanced ovarian carcinoma), tumor cells may express it on their surfaces, resulting in a greater T cell onslaught against tumor cells.
- mRNA2416 could have an abscopal effect in metastatic cancer, where localized injection into a tumor and cytolytic release of tumor antigens would

trigger a secondary immune response and affect metastases throughout the body.

- mRNA2752, another therapeutic possibility, delivers OX40L into tumors and mRNAs, encoding immunostimulatory cytokines IL-23 and IL-36 to boost T cell-mediated cytotoxicity.
- MEDI1191, which encodes IL-12, one of the most potent cytokines in mediating anticancer activity, is also indicated for solid tumors.
- BNT131 (SAR441000) is an mRNA-based intra-tumoral immunomodulator as a monotherapy in patients with advanced melanoma in conjunction with Sanofi. This immunomodulator is made up of IL-12sc, IL-15sushi, IFN, and GM-CSF mRNAs, the increased concentration of which in the local tumor microenvironment can enhance the activation of natural killer cells and the induction of cytotoxic T-cell responses, culminating in immune-mediated tumor cell destruction
- CV8102 is a TLR7/8/RIG1 agonist that promotes a systemic immune response against the injected primary tumor and distant cancer metastases; this drug is used to treat advanced melanoma, cutaneous squamous cell carcinoma, and head and neck squamous cell carcinoma.
- mRNA-based therapies, including treatment of r-1-antitrypsin deficiency; a hereditary condition marked by neutrophil elastase destruction of lung tissue due to a lack of its natural inhibitor 1-antitrypsin, as well as liver damage due to alhpa-1 antitrypsin deficiency.
- Another mRNA medication for urea cycle disorders, ARCT-810, encodes ornithine transcarbamylase (OTC) to treat ornithine transcarbamylase deficiency.
- Glycolipid derivatives (globotriaosylceramide, globotriaosylsphingosine) accumulate in multiple tissues in Fabry disease, causing various clinical symptoms. In GLA-deficient animals, a single dosage of GLA mRNA delivered intravenously decreased the buildup of globotriaosylsphingosine in plasma and tissues. Furthermore, this favorable effect of mRNA was seen for up to 6 weeks following treatment, which is noteworthy.

3.7.3 mRNA Vaccines

Antigens and/or adjuvants encoded by mRNAs can be employed as vaccines to elicit protective immunity against infectious diseases (prophylactic vaccinations) or to harness the immune system to combat cancer (therapeutic vaccines). mRNA can be used for passive immunization as well as for building active immunity. mRNA-1944 is an example of mRNA therapies expressing human monoclonal neutralizing antibodies (mAb) that provide passive protection against the chikungunya virus (Figure 3.9).

Self-amplifying RNA vaccines are another RNA-based immunization technique. The latter's backbone sequence is derived from an alphavirus, a positive-sense single-stranded RNA virus with a high reproduction ability. An antigen-encoding sequence and a viral RNA polymerase-dependent RNA-encoding sequence, and

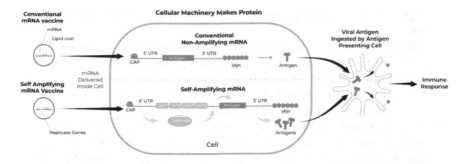

FIGURE 3.9 Diagrams depicting the usage of mRNA in ex vivo editing cells. Ex vivo, T cells obtained from the peripheral blood of ill patients are transformed with mRNA encoding the chimeric antigen receptor (CAR). The patient is subsequently given modified cells; mRNA, messenger RNA; RNA, ribonucleic acid.

other elements essential for replication are included in such mRNA vaccines. The self-replicating technique has the advantage of allowing substantially more antigens to be expressed with lower mRNA dosages. After transitory expression, both forms of RNA vaccines break down; however, self-replicating RNA produces extended antigen expression.

CV9202 (CureVac), a self-adjuvanting RNA vaccine targeting six antigens typically expressed in non-small cell lung cancer, is one of several RNA cancer vaccines under clinical trials. The mRNA-5671 gene is used to study patients with KRAS-mutant advanced or metastatic non-small cell lung cancer, colorectal cancer, or pancreatic adenocarcinoma. The mRNA-4157 is another cancer vaccine, but unlike mRNA-5671, it is a customized melanoma therapeutic vaccine. In this method, a patient's tumor is genetically sequenced and bioinformatically analyzed to find 20 patient-specific neoantigen epitopes encoded by an mRNA construct made for a single patient.

Another example of the individualized cancer vaccine is BNT122 (phase II) for locally progressed or solid metastatic cancers (including melanoma, non-small cell lung cancer, bladder cancer, and others). BNT111 is for advanced melanoma; BNT112 is for metastatic castration-resistant prostate cancer and high-risk localized prostate cancer; BNT113 is for HPV16-derived oncoproteins E6 and E7, which are found in HPV16-positive solid cancers like head and neck squamous cell carcinoma; BNT114 is for triple-negative breast cancer, and BNT115 is for ovarian cancer.

There are a few distinct forms of IVT mRNA-based vaccines for infectious diseases under development. Self-amplifying IVT mRNA with sequences of positive-stranded RNA viruses was originally designed to treat a flavivirus and is administered via intradermal injection. However, injecting a two-component vaccine containing an mRNA adjuvant and naked IVT mRNA encoding influenza hemagglutinin antigen alone or in conjunction with neuraminidase encoding, IVT mRNA is one of the other options.

Vaccines for HIV treatment, for example, use DCs transfected with IVT mRNA, which encodes HIV proteins. In March 2022, the NIAID launched a Phase 1 clinical trial evaluating three experimental HIV vaccines based on an mRNA platform, called HVTN 302.

3.7.4 MRNA-ENHANCED CELL THERAPIES

Although mRNA is utilized to achieve transient protein expression in the therapies mentioned above, it can also be tailored to function as a gene-editing tool to achieve regular protein expression. A treatment that combines mRNA and DNA is also possible. A transposon system is employed in one strategy to change cells for therapy genetically. A DNA plasmid encoding a gene of interest flanked by a mirrored set of inverted repeats (transposon) and mRNA encoding the transposase enzyme make up this system. In a single electroporation reaction, the plasmid DNA encoding the transposon is supplied alongside the mRNA transposase enzyme. The transposase, made from mRNA, attaches to the inverted repeats and breaks the DNA, releasing the transposon. The transposon then joins a strand of genomic DNA with a TA dinucleotide, causing a double-stranded break, which allows the transposon to integrate. P-BCMA-101 is a cell treatment for multiple myeloma; a transposon encoding the anti-BCMA CAR is integrated into resting T cells using the company's unique mRNA-based transposon technology.

CRISPR-Cas9 is a component of the adaptive immune system of bacteria. In bacteria, two RNA molecules and the protein Cas9 bind to a foreign target. Transactivating CRISPR RNA (tracrRNA), one of these molecules acts as a scaffold and attaches to Cas9, a DNA endonuclease. The other component, CRISPR RNA (crRNA), has sequence homology with the foreign DNA and provides cleavage specificity. This natural immune system has been tweaked to allow for genome editing. Both RNA molecules are coupled into a single guide RNA in one variant of the improved CRISPR-Cas9 technology (sgRNA). An adjacent protospacer motif (PAM), commonly known as the "NGG" sequence, is a short (2–6 bp) DNA sequence that follows the target DNA sequence. Cas9 creates a double-strand break by cleaving the target DNA sequence 3 bases upstream of the PAM. Nonhomologous end joining (NHEJ) and homology-directed repair are two ways of repairing the latter (HDR). However, NHEJ is a risky mechanism that disturbs the targeted locus by introducing small deletions or insertions (indels) (gene knockout). HDR is a more precise technique that uses a short donor DNA sequence to repair double-stranded breaks, making gene knock-in easier.

CRISPR-associated protein 9, or CRISPR-Cas9, is a genome editing technology that uses clustered, regularly interspaced short palindromic repeats. Genome editing techniques are used to add, remove, or change genetic material in specific regions throughout the genome. Gene therapy was proposed almost half a century ago, suggesting the use of nucleosides to cure diseases. Because DNA and mRNA both serve as models for protein synthesis, the cell can generate missing or faulty proteins rather than relying on external proteins. There are no protein size constraints or the difficulty of synthesizing proteins in vitro; hence this is a speedier and less expensive treatment.

Furthermore, proteins can undergo post-translational changes that are challenging to achieve in heterologous systems. In addition, in vivo protein delivery aids in chemical and physical protection of the protein once it reaches the target. When introducing exogenous mRNA into cells to alter protein expression, the cost of synthesis is also a consideration. The primary difference between DNA and RNA is that the latter does not integrate into the cell's genome but undergoes spontaneous breakdown and activity (Figure 3.10).

CRISPR-Cas9 gene-editing tools allow for precise genome editing and have a variety of applications. The two components necessary for CRISPR-Cas9-mediated gene editing are Cas9, a nuclease responsible for DNA cleavage, and sgRNA, a short single-stranded RNA guide (sgRNA), which directs DNA cleavage by the nuclease. A pDNA comprising the Cas9 protein and sgRNA genes is typically utilized to deliver these two components to cells. Cas9 nuclease is a nuclease that breaks down DNA; as a result, Cas9 mRNA is widely utilized in both cell culture and model organisms, such as Drosophila, zebrafish, Xenopus, and mouse.

mRNA can be utilized for gene editing by encoding nucleases. The precision of "cutting" and "pasting" genomic DNA in specific locations is a promising therapeutic area for applying mRNA technology. mRNA translates nucleases such as zinc-finger nucleases (ZFNs), transcription activator effector nucleases (TALENs), and CRISPR-Cas9. These genetic engineering technologies allow for the replacement

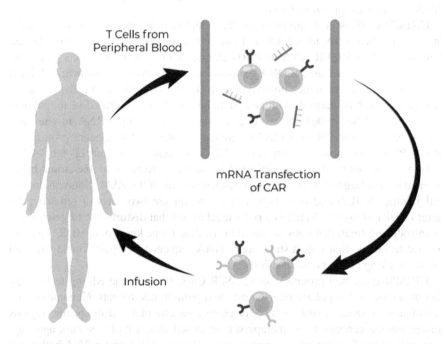

FIGURE 3.10 Conventional (BioNTech and Moderna COVID-19 vaccines) and self-amplifying mRNA vaccines have different mechanisms of action. Antigen-presenting cells convert the mRNA vaccine into protein, which subsequently triggers immune responses. N7-methylated guanosine is covalently linked to the first nucleotide of the mRNA via a reverse 5 to 5 triphosphate bond. Adenosine molecule; poly(A) tail (A)n; untranslated region (UTR); cap, non-structural protein

or adjustment of gene expression by introducing or deleting predefined modifications in the genome of target cells. By joining the nonhomologous end (NHEJ) or performing a homology-directed repair or insertion, a target gene can be corrected by deleting disease-causing mutations or adding protective mutations (HDR). ZFNs and TALENs make it easier for proteins to recognize a sequence via protein DNA interactions, but the extensive engineering required to generate particular DNA recognition and binding domains in proteins limits their use. The CRISPR-Cas9 system, which is the most frequently used, and gene-editing technology, is depicted in Figure 3.11.

Since the nucleic acid RNA is a transient biomolecule, it is preferred over pDNA CRISPR-Associated Protein 9 (CRISPR-Cas9) to reduce the presence of nucleases inside cells. In this method, the risk of non-specific cleavages is reduced, lowering the immunological response to the Cas9 protein. Furthermore, compared to the

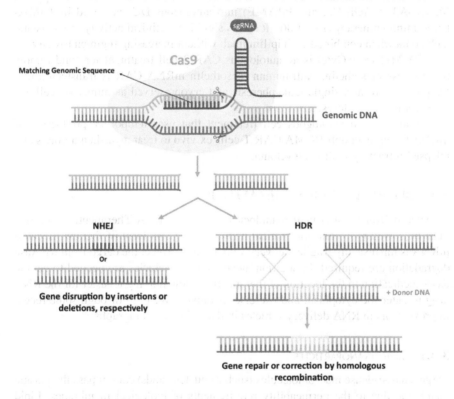

FIGURE 3.11 CRISPR-Cas9-mediated genome editing diagram. A single guide RNA sequence (sgRNA) directs a CRISPR-Cas9 endonuclease to a DNA sequence, resulting in double-strand cleavage. They are then repaired using nonhomologous final union (NHEJ) or homology-directed repair techniques (HDR). However, NHEJ repair produces mistakes, which frequently result in insertion or deletion mutations, resulting in genomic instability. Alternatively, if an external donor DNA model is present, it can be repaired using error-free HDR, which projects precise DNA alterations.

injection of the Cas9/sgRNA ribonucleoprotein complex, the intracellular presence of the Cas9 protein is more stable after mRNA production (Cas9-RNP). As a result, co-delivery of Cas9-encoding mRNA and sgRNA is a viable option. Cas9 can be delivered in mRNA, plasmid DNA, or even a protein. However, plasmid DNA Cas9 must cross cell and nuclear membrane barriers to operate. As a result, using Cas9 mRNA is a viable option. This technique becomes desirable because mRNA simply needs to cross the cell membrane to be functional.

mRNA also improves cell treatment. The cells can come from either the patient or a cell bank. Ex vivo therapeutic modification with mRNA encoding the desired proteins follows (CARs, reprogramming or trans-differentiation factors, telomerase, etc.). The patient's mRNA-enhanced cells are then reinfused to treat the condition. There are now several cell-based therapeutics in clinical trials that use mRNA. Ex vivo transfection of mRNAs expressing DC-activating molecules (CD40L, CD70, and caTLR4) and melanoma-specific tumor-associated antigens (tyrosinase, gp100, MAGE-A3, MAGE-C2, and PRAME) into autologous DCs are used in TriMix-based immunotherapy (ECI-006). It shows significant clinical activity in metastatic melanoma when combined with ipilimumab without increasing regimen toxicity.

MCY-M11 (MaxCyte) is an autologous CAR T-cell treatment for solid tumors that express mesothelin. Anti-human mesothelin mRNA CAR is transfected into lymphocytes from a single leukapheresis and cryopreserved as numerous cell aliquots for recurrent doses.

Descartes is an autologous cell treatment that uses temporary production of mRNA to engineer anti-BCMA CAR T-cells ex vivo to treat myasthenia gravis and relapsed/refractory multiple myeloma.

3.8   DELIVERY OF RNA THERAPEUTICS

Targeted delivery is a critical roadblock for effective RNA Therapeutics, one that must be solved to expand the clinical application of this form of therapy. Because mRNA is intrinsically fragile, delivery vehicles that protect the cargo from RNAase degradation are required. In addition, novel delivery vehicles are needed to get the RNA medication to the location of therapeutic action, making it easier for the RNA drug to enter the cytoplasm and exercise its impact. We'll go through some recent improvements in RNA delivery vehicles in the following paragraphs.

3.8.1   LIPID NANOPARTICLES

Large, charge-dense macromolecules (such as nucleic acids) cannot pass the plasma membrane due to the permeability requirements of biological membranes. Lipid polymorphic phase characteristics may momentarily impair the cell's permeability barrier, allowing nucleic acids to penetrate. Lipid nanoparticles (LNPs) provide a haven away from serum nuclease activity, immunological components, and a drug-biodistribution profile specified by the carrier. This review's topic is the authorized LNP technology developed for hepatic siRNA delivery following intravenous treatment. Identifying ionizable cationic lipids was critical for the clinical translation of LNP-based RNA therapies. These lipids ensure effective siRNA encapsulation (>85%), keep the surface charge of LNPs neutral at physiological pH, and aid endosomal escape. After systemic injection, Apolipoprotein E (ApoE) adsorbs to the LNP surface and enhances hepatocyte uptake via the low-density lipoprotein receptor, resulting in a cumulative dosage of >80% in the liver.

The development of LNP systems is the result of a 25-year progression from phospholipid and cholesterol-only formulations. These advancements were based on previous research into lipid carriers for small-molecule therapies. Enabling efficient trapping, retaining neutral surface charge, and evading the immune system were essential when translating such systems to nucleic acids.

LNPs are made up of four primary components: ionizable cationic lipids, phospholipids, cholesterol, and polyethylene glycol (PEG)-lipids. In hepatocyte gene silencing, LNP formulations entrap siRNA at a ratio of 0.095 (w/w, siRNA/lipid) and produce 50 nm particles with narrow size distributions; this size is crucial for permitting these particles to pass through the fenestrated hepatic vasculature.

The ionizable lipid structure and acid-dissociation constant adjustment increased LNP potency substantially, allowing clinical translation. Permanently cationic lipids, such as DOTMA, have shown toxicity in vivo, preventing fast translation. On the other hand, ionizable tertiary amine moieties in the lipid headgroup provided a net-positive charge at acidic pH and a neutral charge in circulation; the lesser toxicity and immunological stimulation suggested increased therapeutic value. DLinMC3DMA was discovered by rational design and iterative screening utilizing the murine factor VII (FVII) model; its development has been discussed elsewhere. The therapeutic index was improved 8000-fold by optimizing previous-generation lipids like DLinDAP.

The PEG-lipid, which was essential to prevent aggregation during particle formation, is another important factor determining LNPsiRNA transfection competency. On the other hand, PEG-lipids impeded absorption into target cells and were ineffective for transfection. Therefore, diffusible PEG-lipids with C14 alkyl chains were created to obtain the best balance of stability and transfection competency. These lipids quickly disassociate from the LNP in the presence of a lipid sink, resulting in transfection-competent systems. LNP containing diffusible PEG-lipids rapidly accumulates in the liver, with circulation half-lives of less than 15 minutes, according to preclinical research. ApoE adsorption was responsible for hepatocyte transfection's rapid accumulation and efficacy.

LNPsiRNA is generated via an ethanol-loading technique that involves mixing manufactured LNP (at pH 4) with nucleic acids in the presence of high ethanol concentrations (40% v/v). The researchers next devised a high-throughput fast mixing process that combined lipids dissolved in ethanol with nucleic acids in an aqueous buffer (pH 4), resulting in efficient nucleic acid loading into LNP systems. As a result, LNPsiRNA systems with high entrapment efficiency (>85%) and limited size distributions were created using rapid mixing procedures. According to recent research, such structures feature a hydrophobic oil core predominantly composed of neutral ionizable lipids, surrounded by siRNA complexed to lipids in a bilayer arrangement, with variation in the number of siRNA copies per particle.

Patisiran (Onpattro) is an RNAi therapy for treating hereditary transthyretin amyloidosis that uses LNP delivery technology (hATTR). Mutations in the transthyretin (TTR) gene cause the TTR protein to assemble and accumulate abnormally, resulting in this condition. As a result, the disease expresses itself in various systemic disorders that impact multiple organ systems. For example, hepatocytes in the liver produce transthyretin, which is then released into the bloodstream (similar to the FVII screening model).

Onpattro is 50/10/38.5/1.5 D-LinMC3DMA, phosphatidylcholine, cholesterol, and PEG-lipid (mol percent). When Onpattro was created, liver transplantation was the sole therapy option for people with hATTR, much as with the ASO Tegsedi. To decrease mutant TTR expression, Onpattro takes advantage of the high LNPsiRNA accumulation in hepatocytes (the source of TTR) and the potency of gene silencing in these cells. Onpattro accomplishes this by dramatically reducing the amount of nucleic acid necessary for effective gene silencing.

3.8.2 LIPOSOMES

Liposomes develop when materials with polar head groups and non-polar tails (phospholipids) are dispersed in the aqueous phase. They are spherical vesicles with at least one phospholipid bilayer and an aqueous core. They are versatile drug delivery particles that can be modified on the surface to deliver a range of therapeutic payloads. Doxil, a liposome-encapsulated version of doxorubicin for cancer treatment that lowers drug-related cardiac damage, is notable for these applications. This groundbreaking approach revealed the efficacy of using nanoparticles to alter drug biodistribution and improve safety.

Liposomes benefit from mimicking cell membrane composition and, when paired with cationic lipids, can encapsulate mRNA. Positively charged lipids can generate RNA and liposome complexes by electrostatically interacting with negatively charged mRNA. RNA is contained within liposomes in this fashion. Negatively charged RNA rapidly forms complexes with cationic lipids such as DOTMA (1,2-di-O-octadecenyl-3-trimethylammonium-propane) and DOTAP (1,2-dioleoyl-3-trimethylammonium-propane). The introduction of cholesterol-modified lipid increases transfection and makes the resultant complex more stable. Hattori et al. (2015) demonstrated the delivery of siRNA into mouse liver using cationic cholesterol-modified liposomes. Liposomes are used to transfer mRNA vaccines by encoding four tumor antigens, NY-ESO-1, MAGE-A3, tyrosinase, and TPTE, to dendritic cells (DCs) in patients with advanced malignant melanoma, effectively expressing the antigens in spleen cells. Liposome delivery systems, on the other hand, have flaws: i) they are less stable and may fuse or leak RNA, resulting in low delivery effectiveness; ii) they entrap less RNA; iii) they can be toxic if oxidized; and iv) their size is not uniform. The particle heterogeneity grows from batch to batch.

Advances in liposome surface modification have addressed some of the challenges mentioned above. LNPs with a hydrophilic inner core consisting of cationic and other lipids, cholesterol, and polyethylene glycol (PEG) preserve the ability to carry anionic RNA, protect it from degradation, and extend its circulation. Patisiran, the siRNA-based therapy against hereditary transthyretin-mediated amyloidosis, is an example of the LNP platform's efficacy. The dsRNA in patisiran is encased in four lipid excipients: cholesterol (DLin-MC3-DMA) [1,2-distearoyl-sn-glycero-3-p hosphocholine]; DSPC [1,2-distearoyl-sn-glycero-3-phosphocho (6Z,9Z,28Z,31Z) -heptatriacontane-6,9,28, 31-tetraen-19-yl-4-(dimethylamino) butanoate]; **DMG-PEG 2000: [1,2-dimyristoyl-rac-glycero-3-methoxypolyethylene glycol-2000]; MPEG 2000-DMD** [Methoxypoly(ethylene glycol) dimyristoyl glycerol].

-(3 -[1,2-di(myristyloxy)proponoxy] carbonyl-aminopropyl)—methoxy, polyoxyethylene]; and PEG-2000-C-DMG [-(3 -[1,2-di(myristyloxy). The PEG functionalization is critical for this platform because it permits the medication to circulate and be targeted in the liver.

PEG-liposome mRNA vaccines for the treatment of COVID-19 are another example. However, minor concerns have been raised since the proprietary lipid is slowly removed from target tissues. Research is ongoing to see if this lipid accumulation poses a safety risk (Figure 3.12).

3.8.2.1 Leukosomes

More complex surface modalities construct "biomimetic" nanoparticles that functionalize membrane proteins on the surface of nanoparticles and PEG-functionalized liposomes. By integrating leukocyte membrane proteins into the surface of liposomes, we were able to create "leukosomes." LFA-1 and CD-45 are endothelial adhesion molecules that allow these particles to adhere to active endothelium, localizing at inflammation areas. Furthermore, this biomimetic platform has exhibited intrinsic

Lipid Nanoparticle-Based Drug Delivery Strategies

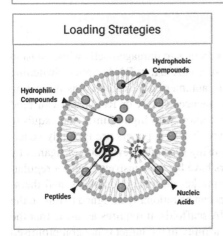
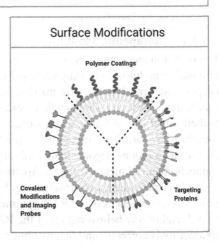

FIGURE 3.12   Therapeutic payloads such as hydrophobic and hydrophilic small molecules, genetic materials, and proteins can all be carried in lipid-based nanoparticles. The ability to functionalize the surface with various proteins that can target and localize nanoparticles over specific targets, imaging probes, or covalent modification is one of the platform's features.

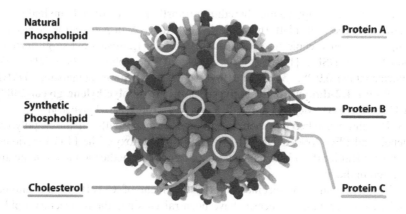

FIGURE 3.13   Biomimetic Nanoparticles—"Leukosome" Technology. These particles are made up of a liposome and proteins generated from leukocytes. They have anti-inflammatory characteristics and preferentially bind to active endothelium at locations of inflammation.

anti-inflammatory effects on the endothelium through its interaction with macrophages. Administration of biomimetic nanoparticles generated from macrophages lower pro-inflammatory genes (IL-6, IL-1b, and TNF-) and boost anti-inflammatory genes (IL-10 and TGF-) in a lipopolysaccharide (LPS)-induced mouse model of sepsis. Other illness models, such as inflammatory bowel disease (IBD), atherosclerosis, and cancer, have shown that these biomimetic leukosomes have inherent anti-inflammatory properties (Figure 3.13).

3.8.3   NANOTECHNOLOGY

3.8.3.1   Therapeutic Modules

The goal of nanotechnology is to deliver medicines to damaged cells while causing minimal or no harm to healthy cells and tissues (siRNA, miRNA, Splice-Switching Oligos, and CpG Motifs). Toward this goal, aptamers have emerged as promising candidates. These are short nucleic acid sequences (DNA or RNA) that can bind to their target (for instance, a cell surface receptor) with high affinity and exquisite specificity by forming a recognition structure. These aptamers are typically generated from a random oligonucleotide library using systematic evolution of ligands by exponential enrichment (SELEX). Aptamers have been extensively used for regulating cellular processes, cancer-targeting, biomarker discovery, diagnosis, and therapeutics. The sequences of the RNA aptamers can be rationally designed to link to the 5' or 3' end of any helical region of the RNA scaffolds. It requires assuring that the aptamer folds correctly and that its binding affinity to the target is not compromised after incorporation into the RNA scaffold.

   RNA interference (RNAi) is a critical post-transcriptional gene regulation mechanism. Short interfering RNAs (siRNAs) are typically 21–25 bp dsRNA that bind to RNA-induced silencing complex (RISC), a protein complex in the cytoplasm. The siRNA/RISC complex intercepts intracellular mRNA containing a complementary sequence to the bound siRNA. In the process, it cleaves and degrades the mRNA resulting in silencing the expression of that gene. Since the siRNA is double-stranded, the incorporation of siRNA into RNA nanoparticles is readily accomplished by simply fusing the siRNA sequences at any of the helical stems of the RNA scaffold, such as the pRNA-3WJ triangular structures. If necessary, the siRNA sequences can be easily separated from the scaffold sequence by inserting a UU or AA bulge. The 3' end 2-nt overhang of the siRNA should be retained for DICER recognition, binding, and processing. For increased serum stability, typically, 2'-F nucleotides are used to modify the sense strand. While incorporating chemical modifications, care should be taken so that DICER processing is not compromised.

CpG is an FDA-approved immunomodulator popularly tested for cancer immunotherapy. Unfortunately, many drug candidates do not reach the cancer cells, are rapidly cleared from the bloodstream, and exhibit significant side effects by accumulating nonspecifically in healthy organs and tissues. Nanotechnology offers several advantages over traditional drug delivery methods: improved drug formulations with increased plasma solubility, prolonged drug half-life, targeted delivery, and drug release specifically in the cancer cell, maximizing antitumor activity while significantly minimizing nonspecific toxicity of the drugs.

Several methods are widely used for post-synthetic conjugation of modules to RNA, and these methods can be used for the conjugation of chemotherapeutic drugs to RNA. Methods include Periodate chemistry, N-hydroxysuccinimide (NHS) chemistry, 5'-phosphate activation, Thiol chemistry, and "Click" chemistry, to name a few. For chemotherapeutics, it is very important to analyze the structure of the drug in detail to identify possible conjugation sites (such as a hydroxyl functional group). In addition, care should be taken to account for steric hindrances, which can interfere with site-specific labeling, the possibility of losing the drug functionality after conjugation, and linker properties to achieve optimal drug release at the target sites.

Since RNA nanoparticles employ a modular design, one of the component strands can be labeled with an imaging molecule, such as a fluorophore. Typically, varieties of fluorescent dyes can be added during solid-phase synthesis. Alternatively, enzymatic methods can incorporate modified nucleotides harboring fluorophores to RNA at the 5'- (using T7 RNA polymerase) or 3'-end (using T4 RNA ligase). Modified nucleotides can also harbor reactive groups used for conjugation to RNA after transcription. RNA is oxidized at the 3'-end to generate a dialdehyde, which is then reacted with a fluorophore-carbazide through a condensation reaction to label the RNA at the 3'-end fluorescently.

RNA nanotechnology uses RNA as a construction material to build homogeneous nanostructures by bottom-up self-assembly with defined size, structure, and stoichiometry. This is currently one of the most widely investigated topics. Nanomedicine is a powerful tool, as demonstrated by the new class of mRNA vaccines used to prevent COVID-19; this would not have been possible without nanotechnology applications. RNA is stable thermodynamically, displaying both canonical and noncanonical base-pairing properties, base-stacking capabilities, and tertiary interactions. There are several ways to make RNA fragments, including transcription, termination, self-processing, and splicing, that undergo self-assembly in vivo with special functionalities, such as siRNA, miRNA, RNA aptamers, riboswitches, and ribozymes.

Loops, helices, bulges, stems, junctions, and pseudoknots all exist in natural RNA molecules. These structural motifs can be employed as building blocks for assembling 3D RNA constructions with exact shape, structure, and stoichiometry control.

Intramolecular and intermolecular interactions allow RNA molecules to fold into specified shapes that self-assemble into multifunctional nanoparticles. The flexibility of RNA secondary structures and tertiary connections, the low free energy of RNA self-assembly, and the ease with which functional RNA sequences can be included make RNA a suitable nanomaterial for a wide range of applications. The field of RNA nanotechnology is still in its infancy but will play an increasingly important role in nanomedicine, nanobiotechnology, and industry.

Size restrictions (80 nt), limited yield, and high costs of large-scale production of chemically produced oligonucleotides are current limitations of RNA nanotechnology. These constraints may be resolved shortly thanks to developments in RNA chemistry. The ability of RNA to fold into complex structures is well recognized. Computational tools to anticipate 3D structures and the effects of intermolecular interactions are on the way, making it easier to build RNA nanoparticles for a wider range of applications.

RNA nanotechnology platform is unique compared to other nano-delivery systems (e.g., lipid, polymer, dendrimer, inorganic, viral, etc.) in several aspects:

- The central part of pRNA contains a 3WJ (three-way Junction) motif, which can be assembled from three short RNA fragments with unusually high affinity. The pRNA-3WJ is highly programmable and can be used to form highly branched architectures and multimeric structures with desired geometry. The pRNA-3WJ constructs are thermodynamically stable, resistant to denaturation by 8 M urea, and do not dissociate at ultra-low concentrations in vivo; their RNase resistance is achieved by 2'-Fluoro (2'-F) chemical modification while retaining the original folding, authentic biological activities of the scaffold, and incorporated functional modules. pRNA-3WJ nanoparticles display favorable pharmacokinetics and biodistribution profiles in vivo are non-toxic and do not induce interferon-I or cytokine production. The pRNA-3WJ nanoparticles strongly bind to cancer cells after systemic injection with little accumulation in the healthy liver, lungs, spleen, and kidneys. Branched RNA using junction motif: RNA is a polyanionic polymer and thus can avoid nonspecific cell entry across negatively charged cell membranes and, in the process, reduce the toxic effects of organ accumulation due to entrapment by liver Kupffer cells and lung macrophages;
- RNA nanoparticles have defined size, structure, and stoichiometry; therefore, unpredictable side effects arise from heterogeneous particles. Some RNA nanoparticles have favorable shapes that facilitate tumor penetration and enhanced permeability and retention (EPR) effects;

- Typically RNA nanoparticles are 10–100 nm in size, which is sufficient to harbor chemotherapeutic agents, siRNAs, miRNAs, and RNA aptamers. They are large enough to avoid excretion by kidneys while small enough to enter target cells via receptor-mediated endocytosis;
- RNA nanoparticles are highly soluble, not prone to aggregation, and do not require linkage to PEG or serum albumins that are typically used for a wide range of common nanoparticles;
- The multivalent nature of RNA nanoparticles allows for a modular design, and the truly unique aspect is that it enables the design of distinct functions in the RNA fragment sequences that can self-assemble into intact hyperstable particles;
- RNA nanoparticles do not contain protein and do not induce host-antibody responses, which will allow for repeated treatment of cancer, and chronic diseases. This is particularly applicable to patients who develop neutralizing antibodies over time in response to protein-based reagents.

3.8.3.2   Construction of Multifunctional RNA Nanoparticles

The construction of RNA nanoparticles is a multi-step process for use in nanotechnology and nanomedicine:

- Conception
  - Global structure and desired functionalities: imaging (fluorophores, radiolabels), targeting (RNA aptamers, chemical ligands), and therapeutic (siRNA, miRNA, ribozyme, riboswitches, etc.) modules.
- Computation folding prediction
  - Programmable and addressable building blocks: junction motifs, sticky ends (palindrome sequences), loop–loop interactions, polygons, and branched architectures. Palindrome sequences (foot–foot interactions): a palindrome sequence reads the same from the $5' \rightarrow 3'$ direction on one strand and $5' \rightarrow 3'$ direction on the complementary strand. Introducing palindrome sequences at the helical ends of pRNA can promote the self-assembly of bridged RNA structures (foot-to-foot intermolecular interactions) with high efficiency.
- Synthesis
  - Building blocks: IVT using tRNA polymerase or chemical synthesis using phosphoramidite chemistry. RNA is highly susceptible to degradation in the serum. To enhance chemical stability, modifications can be made on the bases (e.g., 5-BrU and 5-IU), the phosphate linkage (e.g., phosphorothioate and boranophosphate), or at the ribose $2'$ hydroxyl group (e.g., $2'$-Fluoro, $2'$-O-Methyl, or $2'$-NH2). $2'$-Fluoro ($2'$-F) modification is more commonly used for in vivo applications and results in RNA nanoparticles that exhibit authentic structure and biological functions in most cases. It not only enhances chemical stability but also increases the melting temperature.

- Assembly
  - Template or non-templated approach: assemble multifunctional RNA nanoparticles in any bottom-up approach from individual RNA fragments.
- Purification
  - Individual fragments and assembled RNA nanoparticles: gel electrophoresis (native and denaturing PAGE and Agarose gels). Ultracentrifugation, HPLC.
- Characterization
  - Physical, chemical, and biological assays: nanoparticle assembly, structure, shape, size, composition, purity, thermodynamic, chemical stability, in vitro, and in vivo functional assays.

3.8.4 Polymer Nanomaterials

Synthetic compounds made up of a few basic components to form complex structures are known as polymer nanomaterials. Synthetic polymers, such as poly (lactic-co-glycolic acid) (PLGA), polylactic acid (PLA), chitosan, gelatin, polycaprolactone, and polyalkyl-cyanoacrylates are commonly used in these materials. These materials have a long shelf life, the capacity to encapsulate both hydrophilic and hydrophobic chemicals and proteins, and the ability to distribute therapeutic molecules in a controlled manner. Small chemical alterations of the basic polymeric units allow for precise control of the release profile, giving polymeric nanomaterials flexibility. Polymers can be produced to form injectable nanoparticles that can be injected intravenously or supplied as drug depots in the intramuscular, subdermal, or intraperitoneal areas and disintegrate over months or weeks.

Encapsulation of nucleic acids is also simple. Cationic hydrophilic polymers with hydrophobic modifications can self-assemble to encapsulate RNA in the aqueous phase. To transmit HIV-1 gag encoding mRNA to dendritic cells (DC2.4 cells) and BALB/c mice, a cationic polyethyleneimine-stearic acid (PSA) copolymer is utilized. According to transfection efficiency, the best mass ratio of PSA to mRNA is 4:1. The pH sensitivity of nucleic acid carriers that activate endosomal delivery is stable across a narrow pH range (7–9). Green fluorescence protein (GFP) siRNA was delivered in A549 cells using poly(allylamine) phosphate supramolecular nanocarriers to successfully mute GFP protein expression.

In addition, polymers have an inherent tendency to cause inflammation in the immediate microenvironment, either due to a lack of breakdown—as in the case of PLA—or through by-products. Breakdown of PLGA into its basic monomers, lactic acid and glycolic acid, causes a drop in pH at the degradation site, which promotes inflammation. This isn't a problem that cannot be solved. The usage of lipid-polymer hybrids is a common and viable solution. For example, a nanoparticle with a lipid surface and a polymer core combines the best of both worlds by allowing precise control over the polymer core and lipid surface release patterns, which more closely resemble the cell membrane, as well as the ability to modify it to improve targeting to diseased tissues. Preclinical data with xenograft tumors show that using this technology to deliver RNA therapies is promising. In a psoriatic plaque murine model, the combination of lipid and polymer allows for combination therapy, delivering anti-TNF siRNA (siTNF) together with capsaicin—the therapeutic interference RNA delivered via the epidermal barrier by polymer nanoparticle.

3.8.5 SILICA NANOPARTICLES

Mesoporous silica nanoparticles (MSNPs) comprise an amorphous silica (silicon dioxide) matrix with mesoporous ordered porosity. This nanoparticle's unique qualities include huge surface areas with enormous pore contents, simplicity of customization, and established silanol chemistry. To transport negatively charged RNA, the surface of the nanoparticles is changed by positively charged moieties. Pore diameters in MSNPs are adjusted across a wide range and are quite consistent. The particles have a high nucleic acid loading capacity and effective delivery. To transfer the RNA to the target region, RNA can be placed into pores for transport, and the surface can be changed with cancer-specific ligands and antibodies. Particle aggregation is a challenge that must be overcome before the product may be used. Aggregation might result in thrombosis or tissue damage. However, PEGylation of the nanoparticles' surfaces significantly reduces aggregation and tissue damage. These nanoparticles break down into non-toxic compounds and are excreted safely. MSNPs with a large pore and a bi-continuous cubic mesostructure is used for siRNA delivery in human colon cancer cells (HCT116). Researchers created hybrid particles with a positive charge structure with large pores to load anionic siRNA drug (knockdown B cell lymphoma 2, Bcl-2) and a negatively charged structure with small pores to load the anticancer drug, doxorubicin, to improve the efficiency of silica particles in drug delivery and tumor protein suppression. They delivered siRNA and doxorubicin to HeLa cells using their hybrid particles. The platform's adaptability in manufacturing dual pore hybrid silica nanoparticles for treating cancer with genetic and chemotherapeutic medications was demonstrated in their research.

3.8.6 CARBON AND GOLD NANOMATERIALS

Gold nanoparticles, quantum dots, nanographene oxide, and carbon nanotubes are synthetic nanostructures that can hold RNA, protect it from degradation, and deliver it to the disease site of interest. Quantum dot siRNA complexes were employed to suppress a target gene (HPV18 E6 gene) in HeLa cells using gold nanoparticles for topical delivery of therapeutic nucleic acids (siRNA, knockdown EGFR) in animal and human skin. Nanographene oxide modified with gadolinium (Gd-NGO) is used to deliver a small molecule anti-cancer drug, epirubicin, in combination with Let-7g miRNA (tumor suppressors that decrease expression of the Ras oncogene family to image and treat glioblastoma in mice), to discover that functionalized carbon nanotubes could deliver siRNA against lamin A/C to suppress the expression of this protein in He.

3.8.7 N-Acetylgalactosamine (GalNAc)

GalNAc is a three-dimensional ligand that interacts with ASGPR receptors in hepatocytes. GalNAc conjugated siRNAs appear to be particularly effective at knocking down gene expression in the liver, according to clinical research. Revisuran, a GalNAc conjugated siRNA medication, was used in the first clinical trial to treat transthyretin-mediated amyloidosis (ATTR). However, the investigation of Revisuran siRNA-treated patients in phase III clinical trials was halted due to an imbalance in deaths. Givosiran is the first GalNAc conjugated siRNA medication to receive FDA approval; It works by inhibiting aminolevulinate synthase mRNA expression in the liver, preventing acute attacks of hepatic porphyria. This reduces neurotoxic aminolevulinic acid and porphobilinogen levels, which can cause convulsions, paralysis, respiratory failure, brain damage, and death. A few more GalNAc conjugated siRNA products are available (Fitusuran, Lumasiran, Vutrisiran, and Inclisiran).

GalNAc conjugation is an effective technique to increase siRNA target organ accumulation and make cellular uptake easier. To maintain stability in the circulation after parenteral treatment without a protective transport vector, siRNA must be chemically modified. These treatments are made up of siRNA conjugated to a triantennary GalNAc moiety that targets the asialoglycoprotein receptor (ASGPR) to silence disease-causing genes in hepatocytes. Because this receptor is mainly expressed on hepatocytes, it allows access to a specific cell type in the liver. ASGPR binds carbohydrates with terminal galactose or GalNAc residues selectively. After ligand interaction, the receptor-ligand complex is internalized by clathrin-dependent receptor-mediated endocytosis. Because it is abundant (about 500,000 ASGPR per cell) and largely expressed (>95%) on the hepatocyte sinusoidal membrane, ASGPR is a suitable receptor for hepatic siRNA delivery. Additionally, quick internalization and recycling (within minutes) allow for continuous siRNA uptake, resulting in higher target cell concentration. All species have a comparable carbohydrate recognition pattern, which is important in preclinical and translational study design. After ligand binding, the receptor-ligand complex is internalized by clathrin-dependent receptor-mediated endocytosis. ASGPR is a suitable receptor for hepatic siRNA delivery because of its abundance (about 500,000 ASGPR per cell) and mostly expressed (>95% of total expression) on the hepatocyte sinusoidal membrane.

GalNAcsiRNA is efficient in ASGPR targeting ligands, optimal siRNA design, and a convenient delivery method. ASGPR is a hetero-oligomeric receptor complex with carbohydrate recognition domains consisting of several subunits. The avidity of a substance increases exponentially as the number of carbs that bind to many receptor subunits simultaneously increases (the cluster glycoside effect). For selective and efficient ASGPR binding, the spatial organization of carbohydrates and sugar moieties is critical. Compared to galactose, ASGPR has a greater affinity for GalNAc (up to 100-fold). To increase affinity, triantennary GalNAc ligands with dissociation constants in the nanomolar range were created instead of the millimolar range for monovalent ligands. The compatibility of the triantennary GalNAc ligand with siRNA production further simplified large-scale manufacturing methods.

Backbone chemistry advances developed initially for ASO therapies have now been utilized for siRNA treatments. To improve metabolic stability, minimize recognition by Toll-like receptors 3 and 7, and increase binding to target mRNA, siRNAs have been modified with 2'-OMe, 2'-fluoro, and phosphorothioate linkages. Alnylam's patented Enhanced Stabilization Chemistry (ESC) was developed through iterative siRNA design optimization. The improved stability of ESCGalNAcsiRNA conjugates resulted in ten times better efficacy than traditional template chemistry in liver exposure and gene silencing duration. Hepatocytes' acidic intracellular compartments must be stable for sustained action (long-term depot). Hybridization-dependent off-target effects can be reduced by carefully selecting siRNA sequences, especially seed regions. Future conjugates may include additional siRNA alterations, such as glycol nucleic acid substitution in the seed region (ESC+) or altriol nucleic acid residues, to improve RNAi effectiveness and reduce side effects. Additional functionality could be provided through chirality-dependent characteristics. The next generation of siRNA therapies will balance additional chemical changes with compatibility with RNAi machinery.

Finally, the delivery method has altered patient compliance and the clinical translation of GalNAcsiRNA conjugates. GalNAcsiRNA conjugates can be administered subcutaneously due to their low molecular weight. However, due to the high-capacity recycling of ASGPR, this slows siRNA delivery to the liver, although effective and consistent knockdown is still obtained. Several GalNAcsiRNA conjugates are being tested in late-stage clinical trials to treat cardiometabolic and genetic diseases.

Givosiran (marketed as Givlaari) is an FDA-approved RNAi therapy based on GalNAcsiRNA technology to treat acute hepatic porphyria caused by mutations in heme biosynthesis pathway genes55. Physical stimuli that stimulate the expression of aminolevulinic acid synthase (ALAS1) result in the accumulation of hazardous intermediates such as aminolevulinic acid (ALA) and porphobilinogen, which harm nervous tissue, and contribute to the onset of severe abdominal pain, neuropathy (central, and peripheral), and neuropsychiatric symptoms.

3.8.7.1 Testing

Cryogenic electron microscopy (cryo-EM) can reveal the 3D conformation of assembled RNA complexes at ~10 Å resolution. The RNA samples are deposited on an EM grid, blotted with filter papers, and then flash-frozen using liquid nitrogen. Raw images are then acquired, followed by single-particle reconstructions using software packages. The computed projections from the 3D reconstructions should match well with the class averages of observed nanoparticles with similar views. Alternatively, transmission electron microscopy (TEM) can be used.

Dynamic light scattering (DLS) is a simple method for determining RNA nanoparticle hydrodynamic radius under native conditions. If the nanoparticles are homogeneous, the experimental values should agree with the predicted radii of circumscribed spheres around the RNA complexes.

Flow cytometry with appropriate negative controls can verify the functionality of the RNA aptamers or chemical ligands targeting cell surface receptors. Briefly, the cells are maintained in a culture medium, followed by trypsinization and incubation with RNA nanoparticles harboring imaging fluorophores and targeting modules. The cells are then assayed by flow cytometry.

Alternatively, the assay can be performed using confocal microscopy. The cells are grown on glass cover slides in a culture medium, followed by incubation with RNA nanoparticles harboring imaging fluorophores and targeting modules.

Target gene regulation effects of siRNAs and miRNAs can be evaluated by RT-PCR assay on the mRNA level and western blot to assay at protein levels. In addition, cell proliferation and apoptosis can be assayed by MTT, and flow cytometry, respectively, with appropriate controls.

Subcutaneous cancer xenografts are good model systems since they mimic the tumor–extracellular matrix interactions, inflammation, and angiogenesis. On the other hand, orthotopic cancer models more closely mimic the tumor's microenvironment and, more importantly, enhance the possibility of distant metastatic spread compared to subcutaneous transplants. These xenografts are established by injecting tumor cells directly into the flank or target organs.

3.8.7.1.1   Development testing

The intended indication of a new vaccine is simulated in species close to human responses. Testing includes:

- High doses are administered.
- A high level of exposure is obtained.
- Toxicology is the result of a pharmacological effect that is too strong.
- Some instances of possible damages are as follows:
- Specific functions are lost or decreased.
- Biomarkers are used to identify people (e.g., hematology, clinical chemistry, urinalysis, and immune system markers).
- Lesions are morphologically identified (visualized, for example, by histopathology).

However, it is not always possible to study all risks. Treatment duration, the endurance of toxic symptoms, the slope of the dose-effect curve, and the affection of critical organs, for example, all enhance the risk of toxicity. Therefore, toxicological testing aims to characterize the profile thoroughly and assess and evaluate the vaccine's expected and unforeseen dangers.

3.9   CONCLUSION

RNA therapeutics is a wide field, including therapies and prevention of infection and autoimmune disorders. The role of RNA and its dozens of types are now well recognized, and a few applications have been introduced. The consistency with which RNA operates at all levels of its operation, from translation to its limited life cycle, makes it an ideal modality for preventing and treating diseases. Unlike chemical drugs, its toxicity is limited to a localized distribution site. Unlike DNA therapies, it does not enter the nucleus, reducing the risk of any damage to the genes in the nucleus. It is anticipated that RNA therapeutics will be the most forthcoming branch of new drug discovery, and for this reason, a contemporary understanding of RNA developments is essential for developers.

4 Nucleoside Vaccines

4.1 BACKGROUND

Vaccines save millions of lives every year and add substantially to human longevity. Their impact on the economic viability of the healthcare system is also very large since vaccines lower the treatment costs of diseases and reduce the impact and risk of outbreaks. For example, the most recent episode of the SARS-CoV-2 virus has already cost trillions of dollars. Additionally, vaccines can impact antimicrobial resistance by preventing infection and, subsequently, reducing the need for antibiotic treatment. The use of vaccines goes beyond the prevention of infectious diseases. For example, technological advances coupled with progress in target selection and understanding of the immunosuppressive mechanisms have led to the development of therapeutic cancer vaccines.

Traditional vaccines take years, often decades, to develop and bring to patients. The nucleoside vaccines, the mRNA and DNA vaccines that force the body cells to produce a targeted antigen rather than introducing an exogenous antigen into the body, have transformed the field of vaccinology. Besides the fast development, nucleic acid vaccines have a much better safety profile, particularly the mRNA vaccines. With the first regulatory approvals of mRNA vaccines, it is anticipated that the focus of vaccines will make an irreversible shift towards nucleoside vaccines. A unique application of nucleic acid vaccines involves preventing or treating autoimmune disorders that will speed up developing preventive measures against 100+ autoimmune disorders, including diabetes type 1, Alzheimer's, and Parkinson's diseases, for which no treatment or prevention exists. Additional applications of nucleoside vaccines will include cancer vaccines and treatments and many cell therapy applications. The main hurdle in the delivery of nucleoside vaccines has also been resolved through lipid nanoparticles instead of using viral vectors, leading to simpler, non-biological, low-cost manufacturing of these vaccines. To date, no DNA vaccine has been approved due to the risk of possible alterations to the genetic code in the nucleus, and, for this reason, I do not see any approvals soon by regulatory agencies. This chapter describes the technology for these vaccines and how the regulatory guidance is evolving to develop these therapeutic possibilities.

4.2 HISTORY

The first documented method of vaccination, the process of exposing people to little amounts of disease to build up immunity, is the written record of Chinese practitioners breaking up smallpox scabs and having other people inhale them. Even though there were methods to keep doses minimal, the risk of a person contracting the disease from these small inoculations remained, and people were desperate for an alternative. The first time a distinct disease was used to prevent infection was when

DOI: 10.1201/9781003248156-5

cowpox was used to develop immunity against smallpox, a live attenuated vaccine. After eliminating smallpox with a live attenuated vaccine, we now utilize these vaccinations for MMR (measles, mumps, rubella), Chickenpox, and Rotavirus vaccines.

Vaccines comprise the most dramatic healthcare breakthrough and a significant public health tool. They prevent infection, morbidity, and mortality individually and reduce and eliminate disease prevalence locally, ultimately leading to the eradication of disease globally. For example, when the smallpox vaccine came into practice in 1798 and the rabies vaccine in 1885, vaccine technology progressed from inactivated and attenuated pathogens to subunits that only contain those pathogen components that can trigger an immunologic response (Figure 4.1). Key milestones include the development of virus-like particle vaccines, recombinant viral-vectored vaccines, and toxoids, polysaccharides, or protein-based vaccines, which can be conjugated with different protein carriers to improve immune response.

Toxoid vaccines stimulate an immunological response by using a bacteria's toxin. Researchers discovered that exposing guinea pigs to diphtheria toxins helped prevent diphtheria infection in the early 1900s, which led to the development of these vaccinations. The pathogen can be recognized and removed by educating the immune system to recognize a toxin produced by a pathogen. Diphtheria is still prevented by

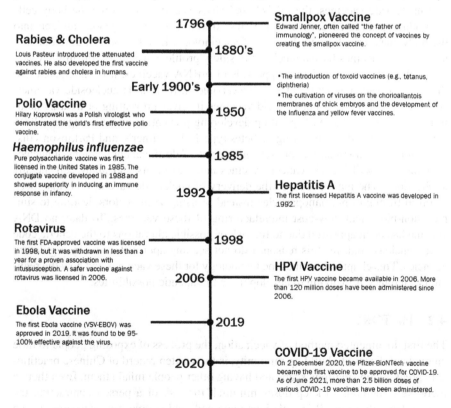

1796

Smallpox Vaccine
Edward Jenner, often called "the father of immunology", pioneered the concept of vaccines by creating the smallpox vaccine.

Rabies & Cholera
Louis Pasteur introduced the attenuated vaccines. He also developed the first vaccine against rabies and cholera in humans.

1880's

Early 1900's

• The introduction of toxoid vaccines (e.g., tetanus, diphtheria)
• The cultivation of viruses on the chorioallantois membranes of chick embryos and the development of the Influenza and yellow fever vaccines.

Polio Vaccine
Hilary Koprowski was a Polish virologist who demonstrated the world's first effective polio vaccine.

1950

Haemophilus influenzae
Pure polysaccharide vaccine was first licensed in the United States in 1985. The conjugate vaccine developed in 1988 and showed superiority in inducing an immune response in infancy.

1985

1992

Hepatitis A
The first licensed Hepatitis A vaccine was developed in 1992.

Rotavirus
The first FDA-approved vaccine was licensed in 1998, but it was withdrawn in less than a year for a proven association with intussusception. A safer vaccine against rotavirus was licensed in 2006.

1998

2006

HPV Vaccine
The first HPV vaccine became available in 2006. More than 120 million doses have been administered since 2006.

Ebola Vaccine
The first Ebola vaccine (VSV-EBOV) was approved in 2019. It was found to be 95-100% effective against the virus.

2019

2020

COVID-19 Vaccine
On 2 December 2020, the Pfizer-BioNTech vaccine became the first vaccine to be approved for COVID-19. As of June 2021, more than 2.5 billion doses of various COVID-19 vaccines have been administered.

FIGURE 4.1   Vaccination targets and milestones.

toxoid vaccinations. Meanwhile, a subunit vaccine is a component of a pathogen, a protein, sugar, or a bit of the pathogen's shell, known as a capsid, that is used to train the immune system. While these vaccines produce powerful reactions to the part of the pathogen delivered, they do not produce significant reactions if the virus mutates, which is exceedingly improbable. Because of their robustness and stability, vaccines that have been attenuated or inactivated in the past, such as Bacillus Calmette–Guérin vaccine (BCG) and Inactivated Polio vaccine (IPV), are frequently utilized. However, because they use whole viruses and, in many cases, lack recognizable traits, they create safety concerns.

Vaccines developed on the basis of traditional technology have failed, such as those developed for malaria, tuberculosis, AIDS, or flu. Furthermore, SARS and Ebola epidemic outbreaks and, more recently, the COVID-19 pandemic show that many of the current platforms are not well suited for a fast, efficient, and cost-effective response.

Another approach is to produce a spike protein of a virus through recombinant engineering, preferred over introducing an attenuated virus. However, an even more effective pathway involves making mRNA that will translate the same protein within the body—the mRNA technology that should soon replace other technologies when combined with efficient chemical vectors creating one of the lowest cost solutions to vaccines (Table 4.1).

TABLE 4.1
A Brief History of mRNA Vaccines

Date	Event
1961	mRNA discovered
1965	Liposome formulation discovered
1969	First protein translated in a lab from mRNA
1974	Liposome for mRNA vaccine delivery formulated
1978	Liposomal mRNA delivered to cells
1984	mRNA synthesized in lab
1987	mRNA + fat droplets allowed entry and protein production in human cells (Malone)
1989	Cationic liposomes deliver mRNA in human cells and frog embryo
1990	Liposomal mRNA delivered to mice
1992	mRNA vaccine tested as treatment in rats
1994	First mRNA vaccine tested for influenza in mice
1995	mRNA vaccine tested for cancer in mice
2001	The first four-lipid formulation for DNA delivery
2005	Discovered that modified RNA avoids immune detection
2005	Commercial-scale production of nano LPS
2010	First mRNA vaccine in LNP tested in mice
2013	A first clinical trial of mRNA rabies vaccine
2015	First mRNA vaccine in LNP tested for influenza
2018	First LNP iRNA product, Patisiran approved
2021	First mRNA COVID-19 vaccine approved

Patisiran is a double-stranded small interfering RNA that targets a sequence within the transthyretin (TTR) messenger RNA that is conserved across wild-type and all TTR variants to decrease hepatic production of mutant and wild-type TTR.

4.3 IMMUNOGENICITY

Every living species is endowed with a system of protecting itself against agents foreign to it and those that can cause harm. This is part of our internal pharmacy that has helped life on Earth survive millions of years of evolution. The immune system comprises an innate and adaptive system containing humoral and cellular activity.

The humoral system or antibody-mediated beta cellular immunity involves macromolecules in extracellular fluids—antibodies, complement proteins, and antimicrobial peptides ("humor" refers to body fluids). Humoral immunity involves antibodies, activation of cytokines, isotype switching, germinal center formation, cell generation, and affinity maturation. Additionally, it includes the effector function of antibodies, including toxic and pathogen neutralization, opsonin promotion of phagocytosis, and complement activation.

Antibodies are Y-shaped proteins with two large, heavy chains and two small light chains formed in plasma cells to provide the immune system; antibodies identify and neutralize pathogens. Antibodies are glycoproteins with a molecular weight of around 150 kDa, with sugar chains added to some amino acid residues. Immunoglobulins are another name for antibodies. There are several antibody isotypes, IgA (dimeric), IgD, IgE, IgG, and IgM (tetrameric or pentameric). The Ig prefix is to abbreviate immunoglobulin.

4.3.1 ANTIGENS

The word "antigen" means an *antibody* generator molecule, which provokes an adaptive immune response. Antigens bind to the immune response components, such as lymphocytes and their receptors, antibodies, and T-cell receptors. Antigens are structural molecules or fragments of molecules that bind uniquely to antibodies and are identified by adaptive immune system antigen receptors (B-cell receptor or T-cell receptor). Antigens do not elicit the immune response without the help of an immunologic adjuvant. Antigens are proteins or polysaccharides and, less often, lipids that come from the cell walls, coats, capsules, flagella, toxins, or fimbriae of pathogens. Nucleic acids and lipids become antigenic only when combined with proteins and polysaccharides. Besides the sources being pathogens, antigens can be egg white, pollen, proteins from transplanted tissues, or elements on the surface of transfused blood cells. An excellent example of antigens are vaccines administered to induce an immune response. Antibodies are designed or produced to interact with antigens based on the antibody's complementary determining region (Figure 4.2).

T-Cell Receptor (TCR) recognition must be processed into small fragments inside the cell and presented to a T-cell receptor by a major histocompatibility complex

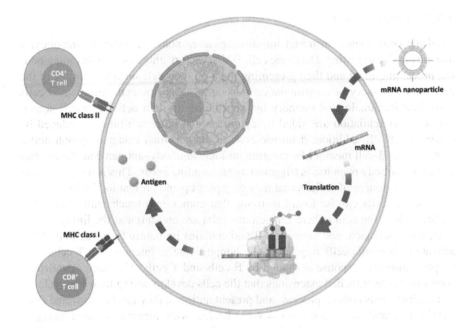

FIGURE 4.2 Antigen processing and presentation by dendritic cells, following subcutaneous injection of an mRNA vaccine for adaptive immune system activation. A synthetic mRNA is internalized by antigen-presenting dendritic cells, where the mRNA is translated. Then, the antigen is exposed to class I or II major histocompatibility complex (MHC) molecules and is later recognized by CD8+ or CD4+ T cells, activating chemical and humoral responses.

(MHC). For example, a hapten is a small molecule attached to a large carrier molecule, such as protein, to become antigenic.

The immune system is generally not reactive against the antigens produced in the body—called self or endogenous—but primarily against the non-self or exogenous sources. However, there are many exceptions to the differentiation between exogenous or endogenous proteins. An excellent example of this is the body's autoimmune response in treating type I diabetes, resulting from an autoimmune reaction that develops against pancreatic β-cells.

Cells present their antigenic structures through a histocompatibility molecule to the immune system, activating several immune cells. Other attributes of antigens and immunogens are their high molecular weight, molecular complexity, and the degradability of antigens to fragments that can bond "MHC" ("major histocompatibility complex") proteins (or MHC antigens) on the surface of the APC ("antigen-presenting cell"), and this whole complex then binds to T-cells. Carbohydrate antigens are not processed or presented, as they can bind to B-cells directly and activate them to produce antibodies. The route of immunization determines the nature of responses; for instance, antigens that encounter mucous membranes generally induce one type of antibodies, whereas intramuscular and intravenous immunization often induces a different type.

4.3.2 DENDRITIC CELLS

Dendritic cells trigger an initial immunological response in naive T lymphocytes that are passive or resting. Dendritic cells (DCs) capture antigens from invading bodies, processing them and then presenting them on their cell surface, along with the necessary accessory or co-stimulation molecules. Dendritic cells also help B cells keep their immunological memory by contributing to their activity. B-cell activation and differentiation are aided by cytokines and other substances produced by dendritic cells. In addition, dendritic cells in the germinal center of lymph nodes contribute to B-cell memory by creating multiple antibody–antigen complexes after an initial antibody response is triggered by an invading entity. This is done to give B cells a stable source of antigen that they may pick up and present to T cells.

Dendritic cells can be found in tissue that comes into touch with the outside world, such as the skin (where Langerhans cells are present) and the linings of the nose, lungs, stomach, and intestines. Blood contains immature forms as well. After activation, dendritic cells migrate to the lymph tissue to interact with T cells. The adaptive immune response is shaped by B cells and T cells. The name "dendrites" comes from the branched extensions that the cells develop during their life cycle.

Dendritic cells collect, process, and present antigens; they can be cultivated from CD14+ patients' autologous monocytes, loaded with tumor-associated antigens (TAAs), matured, and given back to them. The maturation process is critical for the generation of robust anticancer immune responses. Many approaches achieve an optimal DC maturation status, including an mRNA-based platform to activate the autologous DCs by electroporation with three mRNA molecules. CD40L and a constitutively active version of Toll-like receptor 4 (caTLR4) and the co-stimulatory protein CD70 are encoded by this mRNA combination, which can be supplemented with TAA mRNA molecules. The intra-tumoral injection of mRNA is a variant of this in situ mRNA administration that allows the body to act directly on tumor-infiltrating T cells (via DC–T-cell interaction) and the suppressive tumor microenvironment (by using tumor resident DCs as "factories" for the secretion of mRNA-encoded immunomodulatory factors). Importantly, by directly activating tumor-resistent DCs that are already laden with antigens produced from dying tumor cells, intra-tumoral mRNA injection provides a TAA-independent immunization strategy (Figure 4.2).

The first therapeutic applications of mRNA vaccines were in dendritic cells for adaptive immunotherapy against cancer and protein replacement therapies. Although DC therapies still account for the bulk of mRNA vaccine clinical trials, nonviral vector immunization and gene editing are increasingly being researched in the search for new medicines against a variety of diseases.

4.3.3 RNA VIRUS

Because of their straightforward gene expression and replication strategies, positive-strand RNA viruses were the first RNA viruses to be susceptible to direct genetic modification. The genomic RNA (vRNA) is an mRNA that controls the creation of all viral proteins required for virus replication to begin. The initial round of viral genomic RNA translation results in forming a replicase complex, which polymerizes a minus strand complementary to the genome (cRNA) to serve as a template for the synthesis of new mRNA molecules. As a result, the components of the replicase complex for all positive-strand RNA viruses must be translated directly from genomic RNA. Depending on the kind of virus, viral polypeptides not essential for RNA replication, such as structural proteins, can be translated either from genomic RNA or from one or more subgenomic mRNAs transcribed from the negative sense cRNA template. Members of the group who used the former expression technique have one lengthy open reading frame in their genomes (ORF). This RNA is translated into a polyprotein, which is then processed by viral and host cellular proteases both cotranslationally and posttranslationally. This first category includes members of the Picornaviridae and Flaviviridae families. The families Togaviridae, Coronaviridae, Arteriviridae, and Caliciviridae make up the second group. These viruses are distinguished by the subgenomic RNAs employed to express a portion of their genes (Figure 4.1). These viruses' replicase genes are positioned in the 5′ region of the genome, upstream of the structural genes, in contrast to the first group. Subgenomic RNAs are 3′ coterminal with genomic RNA in all of these viruses.

4.4 MESSENGER RNA

Messenger RNA (mRNA) is a single-stranded RNA molecule providing the information of a DNA sequence in the form of a series of ribonucleotide bases (adenine, uracil, guanine, and cytosine) are converted into one or more proteins in the cell by the ribosome. mRNA is synthesized in the cell by the enzyme RNA polymerase using a DNA molecule as a template, in a transcription process; in this context, mRNA is sometimes referred to as the transcript. The coding region of the mRNA molecule is called the coding sequence (CDS); in this region, each triplet of nucleotides is called a codon and corresponds to a specific amino acid. When the ribosome processes mRNA, these amino acids are recruited and linked to each other through peptide bonds, forming a protein; this process is called translation. A DNA sequence that may be transcribed into mRNA and then translated into a protein is called a gene.

In eukaryotic organisms, in addition to the CDS, the mRNA strand includes a modified guanosine nucleotide at the 5′ end of the RNA, called a 5′ cap; a poly(A) denosine sequence at the 3′ end, called a poly(A) tail; and untranslated regions (UTRs) on both sides of the CDS, as shown in Figure 4.3.

In nature, the addition of the 5′ cap ("capping") is facilitated by a set of enzymes during transcription; it is crucial for recognition of the mRNA by the ribosome (and therefore for translation) and helps to protect the mRNA from ribonucleases

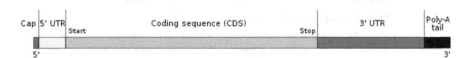

FIGURE 4.3   Structure of a typical eukaryotic mRNA.

(i.e., increases its stability). The inclusion of the poly(A) tail happens at the end of transcription, in a process catalyzed by another set of enzymes. The poly(A) tail is essential for mRNA stability, protecting the transcript from ribonucleases, and aids translation. The 5' UTR and the 3' UTR contain regulatory sequences that affect translation efficiency and mRNA stability; for instance, specific nucleotide sequences in the 5' UTR can interact with the first transfer RNA (initiator tRNA) to increase the translation rate. Table 4.2 shows the comparison of mRNA with siRNA structure.

The mRNA provides the gene of a pathogenic protein (antigen) to human cells; these cells can synthesize the antigenic protein themselves and thus generate an immune response that protects the individual from the actual pathogen.

4.4.1 TYPES

There are two types of RNA vaccines—conventional and self-amplifying—capable of preventing multiple infectious diseases, including influenza, RSV, Rabies, Ebola, and HIV-1. Self-amplifying RNAs have enhanced antigen expression at lower doses compared to conventional mRNA (Figure 4.4).

Incorporating chemically modified nucleotides, sequence optimization, and different purification strategies improve the efficiency of mRNA translation efficiency and reduce intrinsic immunogenic properties. On the other hand, antigen expression is proportional to the number of conventional mRNA transcripts delivered effectively during immunization. Substantial doses or multiple administrations may be required to achieve enough expression for protection or immunomodulation. This issue is addressed by saRNA vaccines, which are genetically designed replicons produced from self-replicating single-stranded RNA viruses. They are given as viral replicon particles (VRPs), including the saRNA, or as fully synthetic saRNA synthesized after in vitro transcription. During manufacturing, envelope proteins are given in trans as faulty assistance constructions to form replication-defective VRPs. Following a first infection, the resulting VRPs lack the ability to create infectious viral particles, and only the RNA can be amplified further. Positive-sense and negative-sense RNA viruses both produce VRPs. On the other hand, the latter is more complicated and requires reverse genetics to save the VRPs.

TABLE 4.2
Comparison of the Structures of mRNA and siRNA

Property	mRNA	siRNA
Molecular weight (g/mol)	$\geq 10^6$	10^4
Molecular conformation	Single-stranded	Double-stranded
5' end	5' cap	Phosphorylated 5' end
3' end	Poly(A) tail	Hydroxylated 3' end

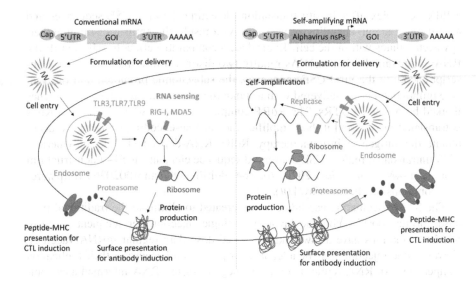

FIGURE 4.4   Two types of RNA vaccines.

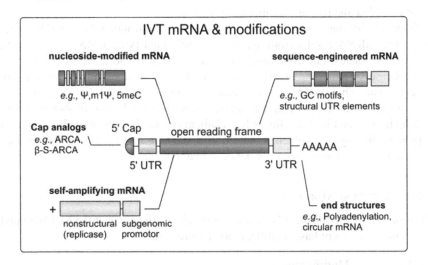

FIGURE 4.5   In vitro transcribed (IVT) mRNA structural elements. To modify mRNA's stability, translation capability, and immune-stimulatory profile, these elements can be tuned and manipulated.

All RNA transcripts have a 5′ cap (m7G) and a poly(A) tail (Figure 4.5). Traditional mRNAs encode the vaccine immunogen and flanking 5′ and 3′ UTRs. The nonreplicating transcript is used to create an antigen or immunotherapy. B 5′ and 3′ CSE sequences, the nsP1-4 genes, a subgenomic promoter, and the vaccine immunogen are encoded by self-amplifying RNA. The nsP1-4 proteins create a RdRP complex after in situ translation, detecting flanking CSE sequences and amplifying vaccine-encoding transcripts. As a result, the antigen or immunotherapy accumulates within the cell. To produce a comparable effect to self-amplifying RNAs, trans-amplifying mRNAs require two distinct transcripts. A distinct transcript encoding the viral CSE sequences, the subgenomic promoter, and the vaccine immunogen is co-delivered with a standard mRNA encoding the nsP1-4 genes flanked by 5′ and 3′ UTRs. The RdRP complex is formed when ordinary mRNA is translated in situ, and it then amplifies the vaccine-encoding transcript to accumulate the antigen or immunotherapy. RdRP RNA-dependent RNA polymerase, UTR untranslated region, CSE conserved sequence elements, nsP1–4 nonstructural proteins 1–4*Nanomaterials* **2020**, *10*, 364; doi:10.3390/nano10020364 (http://creativecommons.org/licenses/by/4.0/).

The SAM vaccination candidates were created to eliminate the traditional two-dose "prime-boost" technique favoring a single injection per recipient. Instead, SAM vaccinations have a lower administered dose than regular mRNA vaccines. However, one injection may be adequate for protection because of their replication competency. An RNA replicase produces negative-sense RNA intermediates complementary to the coding mRNA template when SAMs are translated into the host cell. These are subsequently translated into many coding mRNA molecules, resulting in extended and increased antigen expression.

Trans-amplifying mRNA (taRNA) is a new structural modality of mRNA vaccines. The taRNA results from splitting the self-amplifying mRNA in a system with two templates, one containing the gene of interest and a second containing the replicase system. The amplification is performed in trans by the replicase in the cytoplasm. This system presents some advantages over saRNA since it is safer, more versatile, and cost-effective to manufacture. The production of shorter RNAs with high yield and high quality is less challenging. taRNA has already been used to protect mice against influenza, with results showing induction of antibodies and protection but has not yet been developed for human use.

4.4.2 Chemical Modifications

The term "RNA modification" refers to chemical modifications of the backbone and sugar modifications of base modifications (Figure 4.5).

4.4.2.1 Sugar Modifications

The sugar moiety alters the nucleosides and nucleotides in a modified RNA molecule. For example, the 2′ hydroxyl group (OH) can be replaced or modified with several "oxy" or "deoxy" substituents. Alkoxy or aryloxy (e.g., R = H, alkyl, cycloalkyl, aryl, aralkyl, aralkyl, aralkyl, aralkyl, aralkyl, heteroaryl, or sugar); polyethyleneglycols (PEG),-O(CH2CH2O)nCH2CH2OR; "locked" nucleic acids (LNA), where the one or more carbons in the sugar group can have the stereochemical configuration that is the polar opposite of the corresponding carbon in ribose. Nucleotides having arabinose as the sugar, for example, can be included in a modified RNA molecule.

4.4.2.2 Backbone Modifications

Modified nucleosides and nucleotides have a modified phosphate backbone integrated into a modified RNA molecule. One or more of the oxygen atoms in the phosphate groups of the backbone are replaced with a new substituent. Furthermore, as stated above, the modified nucleosides and nucleotides can involve the complete replacement of an unmodified phosphate moiety with a modified phosphate. Phosphorothioate, phosphoroselenates, borano phosphates, borano phosphate esters, hydrogen phosphonates, phosphoroamidates, alkyl or aryl phosphonates, and phosphotriesters are examples of modified phosphate groups. Both non-linking oxygens are replaced by sulfur in phosphorodithioates. Linking oxygen can alternatively be replaced by nitrogen (bridged phosphoroamidates), sulfur (bridged phosphorothioates), or carbon (bridged phosphorothioates) (bridged methylene-phosphonates).

4.4.2.3 Base Modifications:

The UTRs are mRNA portions that border the coding region and influence the mRNA's stability and translation. Because its shortening and eventual removal cause mRNA degradation, the poly(A) tail also affects stability. The 5' cap structure is required for protein synthesis and the recruitment of translation initiation components. Codon optimization, which entails choosing "frequent codons" in the coding region, improves the stability and translation of mRNA with a high GC (guanine–cytosine) content. The secondary structure of mRNA can be stabilized by changing the fundamental sequence utilizing codon optimizations and computational approaches. There are various advantages of using highly structured mRNA vaccines to build secondary structures in mRNA (save in the 5' UTR region).

The modified nucleosides and nucleotides, incorporated into a modified RNA molecule, can further be modified in the nucleobase moiety. Examples of nucleobases found in RNA include adenine, guanine, cytosine, and uracil. For example, the nucleosides and nucleotides are chemically modified on the major groove face, including an amino group, a thiol group, an alkyl group, or a halo group.

The common nucleotide analogues/modifications include:
1-carboxymethyl-pseudouridine; 1-methyl-1-deaza-pseudoisocytidine; 1-methyl-1-deaza-pseudouridine; 1-methyl-6-thio-guanosine; 1-methyl-inosine; 1-methyl-pseudoisocytidine; 1-methyl-pseudouridine; 1-methyladenosine; 1-methylguanosine; 1-propynyl-pseudouridine; 1-tauri-nomethyl-pseudouridine; 1-taurinomethyl-4-thio-uridine; 2-amino-6-chloro-purine; 2-amino-6-chloropurineriboside-5'-triphosphate; 2-aminopurine-riboside-5'-triphosphate; 2-aminoadenosine-5'-triphosphate; 2-methoxy-4-thio-uridine; 2-methoxy-5-me thylcytidine; 2-methoxy-adenine; 2-methoxy-cytidine; 2-methoxyuridine; 2-methylthio-adenine; 2-methylthio-N6-(cis-hydroxyisopentenyl) adenosine; 2-methylthio-N6-threonyl carbamoyladenosine; 2-thio-1-methyl-1-deaza-pseudouridine; 2-thio-1-methyl-pseudouridine; 2-thio-5-aza-uridine; 2-thio-5-methyl-cytidine; 2-thio-cytidine; 2-thio-dihydrop-seudouridine; 2-thio-dihydrouridine; 2-thio-pseudouridine; 2-thio-zebularine; 2-thiocyti-dine-5'-triphosphate; 2-thiouridine; 2-thiouridine-5'-triphosphate; 2'-amino-2'-deoxycytidine-triphosphate; 2'-fluorothymidine-5'-triphosphate;

2'-O-methyl inosine-5'-triphos-phate 4-thiouridine-5'-triphosphate; 3-methyl-cytidine; 3-methyluridine; 4-methoxy-2-thio-pseuddine; 4-methoxy-I-methyl-pseudoisocytidine; 4-methoxy-pseudoisocytidine; 4-methoxy-pseudouridine; 4-thio-1-methyl-1-deaza-pseudoisocytidine; 4-thio-1-methyl-pseudoisocytidine; 4-thio-1-methyl-pseudouridine; 4-thio-pseudoisocytidine; 4-thio-pseudouridine; 4-thio-uridine; 5-aminoallyl-uridine; 5-aminoallylcytidine-5'-triphosphate; 5-amino-allyluridine-5'-triphosphate; 5-aza-2-thio-zebularine; 5-aza-cytidine; 5-aza-uridine; 5-aza-zebularine; 5-bromo-2'-deoxycytidine-5'-triphosphate; 5-bromo-cytidine-5'-triphosphate; 5-bromouridine-5'-triphosphate; 5-carboxymethyl-uridine; 5-for-mylcytidine; 5-hydroxy-uridine; 5-hydroxymethylcytidine; 5-hydroxyuridine; 5-iodo-2'-deoxycytidine-5'-triphosphate; 5-iodo-uridine; 5-iodouridine-5'-tri-phos-phate; 5-methyl-cytdine; 5-methyl-uridine; 5-methyl-zebularine; 5-methylcyti-dine-5'-triphosphate; 5-methyluridine-5'-triphosphate; 5-propynyl-2'-deoxycytidi ne-5'-triphosphate; 5-propynyl-uridine; 5-taurinomethyl-2-thio-uridine; 5-tau-rinomethyluridine; 5'-O-(1-thiophosphate)-cytidine; 5'-O-(1-thiophosphate)-guanosine; 5'-O-(1-thiophosphate)-uridine or 5'-O-(1-thiophosphate)-pseudouridine; 6-aza-cytidine; 6-aza-uridine; 6-azauridine-5'-triphosphate; 6-chloro-purine; 6-chloropurineriboside-5'-triphosphate; 6-diaminopurine; 6-dihydrouridine; 6-methoxy-guanosine; 6-methyl-guanosine; 6-thio-7-deaza-8-aza-guanosine; 6-thio-7-deaza-guanosine; 6-thio-7-methyl-guanosine; 6-thio-guanosine; 7-deaza-2-aminopurine; 7-deaza-8-aza-2-aminopurine; 7-deaza-8-aza-adenine; 7-deaza-8-aza-guanosine; 7-deaza-adenine; 7-deaza-adenosine.; 7-deaza-guanosine; 7-deazaadenosine-5'-triphosphate; 7-deazaguano-sine-5'-triphosphate; 7-deaza-guanosine-5'-triphosphate; 7-methyl-8-oxo-guanosine; 7-methyl-guanosine; 7-methyladenine; 7-methylinosine; 8-azaadenosine-5'-triphosphate; 8-azido-ade-nosine; 8-azidoadenosine-5'-triphosphate; 8-oxo-guanosine; benzimidazole-ribo-side-5'-tri-phosphate; deoxy-thymidine; dihydropseudouridine; dihydrouridine; inosine; N1-methyl-adenosine; N1-methyl-pseudouridine; N1-methyladenosine-5'-triphosphate; N1-methylguanosine-5'-triphosphate; N2-dimethyl-6-thio-guanosine; N2-dimethylguanosine; N2-methyl-6-thio-guanosine; N2-methylguanosine; N4-acetylcytidine; N4-methylcytidine; N6-(cis-hydroxyisopente-nyl)adenosine; N6-dimethyladenosine; N6-glycinylcarbamoyladenosine; N6-isopentenyladenosine; N6-methyl-2-amino-purine; N6-methyl-adenosine; N6-methyladenosine; N6-methyladenosine-5'-tri-phosphate; N6-threonylcar-15 bamoyladenosine; O6-methylguanosine-5'-triphosphate; pseudo-iso-cytidine; pseudouridine-5'-tri-phosphate; puromycin-5'-triphosphate; pyridin-4-one ribonucleoside; pyrrolo-cyti-dine; pyrrolo-pseudoisocytidine; wybutosine; wyosine; xantho-sine-5'-triphosphate; zebularine; □-thio-adenosine; 5-thio-cytidine; 5-thio-guanosine; 5-thio-uridine.

Chemical modifications can be added to the mRNA molecule to improve efficacy and translation efficiency when employed as a vaccine (e.g., nucleoside modification and codon optimization). Toll-like receptors (TLR) 3, 7, and 8 can activate innate immune cells when foreign mRNA is present. TLR ligation triggers the creation of cytokines, which in turn trigger adaptive T- and B-cell responses. TLR7 signaling boosts the production of proinflammatory cytokines, improves antigen presentation, and extends the life of memory B cells.

In eukaryotic cells, naturally occurring mRNA is created by RNA polymerase, which transcribes DNA in the nucleus into mRNA molecules, which are then transferred to the cytoplasm and used as templates to translate into specific proteins passing through the ribosomes. After injection, mRNA has an estimated half-life of 8–10 hours before degrading and being broken down by native RNase in the body. To be functional, mRNA does not need to enter the nucleus.

4.4.3 MHC

An mRNA vaccine provides acquired immunity through an mRNA containing vectors, such as lipid nanoparticles, wherein the mRNA sequence codes for antigens and identical proteins resembling the pathogens. Upon delivering the vaccine into the body, this sequence is translated by the host cells to produce the encoded antigens, which then stimulate the body's adaptive immune system to produce antibodies against the pathogen (Figure 4.6).

The purpose of major histocompatibility complex (MHC) molecules is to bind pathogen-derived peptide fragments and display them on the cell surface for identification by T lymphocytes (Figure 4.7). Virus-infected cells are killed, macrophages are triggered to kill bacteria dwelling in their intracellular vesicles, and B cells are activated to create antibodies that remove or neutralize extracellular pathogens, all of which damage the pathogen. As a result, any pathogen that has changed so that it avoids being presented by an MHC protein faces tremendous selective pressure. Pathogens find it challenging to elude immune responses in this fashion due to two distinct features of the MHC. To begin with, the MHC is polygenic, containing many MHC class I and MHC class II genes. Every person has a collection of MHC molecules with varied peptide-binding specificities. Second, the MHC is highly polymorphic, implying that each population gene has several versions. As a result, MHC genes are the most polymorphic genes ever discovered. This section will describe the organization of the genes in the MHC and discuss how the variation in MHC molecules arises. Also discussed is the effect of polygeny and polymorphism on the range of peptides that can contribute to the immune system's ability to respond to the multitude of diverse and rapidly evolving pathogens.

The difference between the two classes of the MHC is shown in Figure 4.8.

4.4.4 STABILITY

mRNA has a negative charge due to its phosphate group. At the physiological pH, a naked mRNA molecule's structure is specifically engineered to increase the target antigen's translation in vivo. A unique property of mRNA is that even a single alteration (strand break or base oxidation) in the lengthy mRNA strand (usually between 1000 and 5000 nucleotides long) can interrupt translation. This distinguishes mRNA vaccines from other vaccinations in which minor antigen changes do not always affect their efficacy. As a result, monitoring the integrity of the entire molecule is crucial for mRNA vaccines.

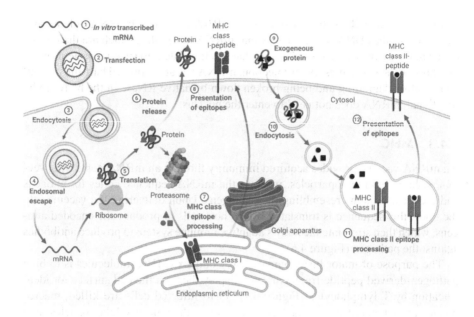

FIGURE 4.6 Mechanism of action of mRNA vaccines. 1. MRNA is in vitro transcribed (IVT) from a DNA template in a cell-free system. 2. IVT mRNA is then transfected into dendritic cells (DCs) by (3) endocytosis. 4. Endosomal escape allows entrapped mRNA to be released into the cytoplasm. 5. The mRNA is translated into antigenic proteins using the translational machinery of the host cell (ribosomes). Posttranslational modifications are made to the translated antigenic protein. It has the ability to act in the cell where it is produced. 6. The protein can also be secreted by the host cell. 7. The proteasome is the cytoplasm degrades the antigen protein. Antigenic peptide epitopes are synthesized and transported to the endoplasmic reticulum, loaded onto MHC class I molecules (MHC I: cell-mediated). 8. After T-cell receptor recognition and proper co-stimulation, the loaded MHC I-peptide epitope complexes are displayed on the surface of cells, finally leading to the production of antigen-specific CD8+ T-cell responses. DCs can take in exogenous proteins. 10. They're destroyed in endosomes before being delivered through the MHC II (antibody-mediated) route. Furthermore, the protein should be directed through the MHC II pathway to get cognate T-cell assistance in antigen-presenting cells. 11. The antigenic peptide epitopes that have been created are next loaded onto MHC II molecules. 12. The antigen-specific CD4+ T-cell responses are induced once the loaded MHC II-peptide epitope complexes are displayed on the cell surface. Cross-presentation is a mechanism that allows exogenous antigens to be processed and loaded onto MHC class I molecules. (Source: Pharmaceutics 2020, 12(2), 102; https://doi.org/10.3390/pharmaceutics12020102)

mRNA is quickly degraded by ribonucleases (RNase), which are abundant in the extracellular environment of the injection site. Intracellular RNA sensors, such as endosomal Toll-like receptors (TLR) and cytoplasmic nucleic acid sensors, detect mRNA internalization inside the cell. Binding mRNA to these host defense receptors activates innate immune pathways, resulting in the activation of hundreds of genes. This technique enhances vaccination potency by inducing an antiviral state

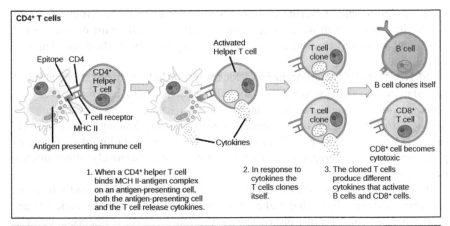

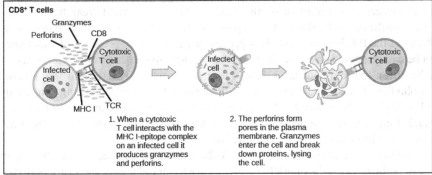

FIGURE 4.7 Role of major histocompatibility complex (MHC) in neutralizing antigens.

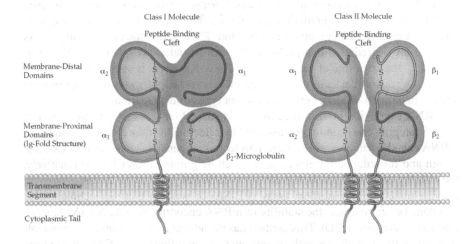

FIGURE 4.8 Difference between MHC Class I and MHC Class II molecules. (Source: https://microbenotes.com/differences-between-mhc-class-i-and-class-ii/)

in cells, significantly lowering mRNA intracellular stability and translation. To enable the expression of the encoded protein, mRNA strands must be transported into the ribosomes after internalization. mRNA engineering can help speed up this process.

mRNA degradation can occur in various ways, including chemical and physical degradation. The changes in bonds in the mRNA molecule are referred to as chemical degradation. Physical instability includes denaturation (the loss of secondary and tertiary structure), which has different—and presumably less significant—effects on mRNA activity than protein biologics. However, denaturation also comprises processes such as aggregation and precipitation, which negatively affect mRNA translation.

In vitro, mRNA degradation is primarily caused by hydrolysis and oxidation. The phosphodiester links that make up the backbone of the mRNA molecule are primarily responsible for hydrolysis. The 2'OH group on ribose is important because the transesterification mechanism that leads to an mRNA strand break begins with a nucleophilic attack by the 2'OH group on the phosphate ester link, which results in a break at the P-O5' ester bond. This process necessitates the presence of water and can be catalyzed by nucleases, the mRNA molecule, and other external components such as Brønsted acids and bases. Base-stacking, in particular, may reduce the rate of phosphodiester bond breaking. As a result, an mRNA molecule's "average unpaired probability" can be reduced. Algorithms that pick nucleotide sequences for single-stranded mRNA with the most double-stranded areas are available. Following this method, in vitro stability is significantly increased.

In contrast, oxidation affects the nucleobases and, to a lesser extent, the sugar groups of the ribose units of mRNA. Base cleavage, strand break, and changes in the secondary structure of mRNA can all be caused by oxidation. On the other hand, hydrolysis is the primary cause of mRNA degradation.

The reverse transcription-quantitative polymerase chain reaction can also be used to investigate mRNA degradation (RT-qPCR). This method determines the total amount of mRNA that can be transcribed into PCR-ready intact cDNA targets. As a result, any degradation that prohibits this can be indirectly quantified. However, because of the error rate of the enzymes utilized, RT-qPCR is sometimes less trustworthy. Other drawbacks of this strategy include its lack of widespread application and the inability to discern between different types of degradation.

mRNA expression in vitro (in cells) is also used to assess mRNA integrity. The mRNA integrity can be indirectly assessed by detecting the fluorescence signal using mRNA encodes a fluorescent protein. This technique can help bioactive mRNA-LNP design and formulation development research by guiding principles. Alternatively, the stability of mRNA producing non-fluorescent antigens can be assessed using an enzyme-linked immunosorbent assay (ELISA) or western blotting techniques, as was done before to assess the stability of mRNA encoding the SARS-CoV-2 receptor-binding domain (RBD). This method has the advantage of combining the overall integrity of the formulation with everything that can influence mRNA transcription. However, the method's disadvantages include its lack of precision, inability to show the type of mRNA damage, and time-consuming nature.

4.4.5 PRODUCTION

mRNA vaccines have the benefit of being relatively quick to produce because mRNA-LNPs are a real platform technology. The mRNA can be generated within weeks of identifying the protective protein antigen(s) and sequencing the relevant gene(s). Because the mRNAs that code for different antigens is chemically and physically identical, the formulation design and manufacturing methods for novel mRNA vaccines are comparable. mRNA vaccines may be more effective for COVID-19 prevention than replication-deficient viral vectors. Unlike viral vector-based vaccines, they do not confer protection against the carrier. In this way, mRNA vaccines are analogous to desoxyribonucleic acid (DNA)-based vaccines. On the other hand, DNA immunizations have a small chance of becoming part of the human genome. Furthermore, in comparison to mRNA vaccines, DNA vaccines have shown little immunogenicity in early clinical experiments, possibly because DNA-based vaccinations require access to the nucleus to carry out their function, limiting efficient delivery. Because of their flexible design, constant production procedures, and short cytoplasmic presence, mRNA vaccines are extremely effective, especially in a pandemic situation with rapidly mutating viruses.

Currently, mRNA is produced by an enzyme reaction from a DNA template, in which the DNA serves as the mRNA's sequence, and the mRNA is converted to a DNA sequence and placed into plasmid DNA, which is easily duplicated in E. coli; the other option of chemical syntheses, such as PCR, is less practical, at least for the time being.

For years, mRNA purification has been difficult. Still, improved IVT reagent quality has allowed for better purification procedures that allow for qualities good enough to be employed in clinical trials and mass manufacture.

4.4.6 DELIVERY

Liposomes were used in the 1970s to transfer mRNA into cells for the first time. At that time, mRNA use was not possible for gene therapy purposes due to its instability and immunogenicity. Now we have much improved technologies that allow stable delivery through many routes of administration (Figure 4.9).

To achieve the goal of an efficient mRNA-based therapy, or gene silencing when treating with small interfering RNAs (siRNAs), miRNAs, oligonucleotides, or aptamers, mRNA must enter the cells at a necessary quantity to achieve expression (Figure 4.10).

In its free state, mRNA has limited cellular absorption due to its hydrophilicity, high molecular weight, and negative charge. While many optimizations are possible to improve the molecule's stability, increase translation efficiency, and reduce immunogenicity, overcoming many extracellular and intracellular obstacles is the target of RNA technology.

The main drawback of using mRNA is its vulnerability to enzymatic breakdown, exacerbated by the presence of ubiquitous RNases in the blood and tissues. This is most relevant to non-encapsulated mRNA. And then comes the obstacle of the cell

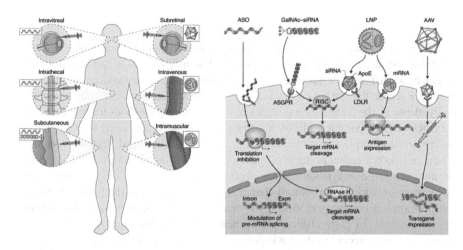

FIGURE 4.9 ASO administered subcutaneously, intravitreally, or intrathecally alters pre-mRNA splicing or causes RNAse H1 or interfering RNA (RNAi)-dependent transcript degradation. The asialoglycoprotein receptor (ASGPR) expressed on the sinusoidal surface is used to transfer GalNAcsiRNA conjugates to hepatocytes. When delivered intravenously, LNPs contain siRNA silence hepatocyte genes after internalization via the low-density lipoprotein receptor (LDLR). Target mRNA is cleaved when siRNA is loaded into the RNA-induced silencing complex (RISC). Following the production of virus antigen, LNP-mRNA vaccines delivered intramuscularly induce robust immune responses. AAV vectors for treating retinal illnesses are delivered locally into the eye by subretinal injection for therapeutic transgene delivery. Intravenous administration is used for other AAV vector therapeutic molecules in development. The capsid protein sequences determine the AAV tropism and uptake process.

membrane. Naked mRNA lacks the qualities required for passage through the phospholipid bilayer. It has a negative charge and a large size, making it difficult to carry into the cell without using a delivery system. Furthermore, naked mRNA delivered intravenously degrades quickly in vivo and may trigger an immunological response. The naked mRNA has a half-life of only around five minutes after intravenous delivery. As a result, encapsulation of mRNA by proper delivery mechanisms is required to overcome those obstacles. Adding specific ligands that recognize receptors on cell membranes improves mRNA distribution into target cells and tissues, improving efficiency and targeted transfection.

mRNA delivery is achieved by physical methods that temporarily breach the cell membrane, viral-based procedures that rely on the ability of a virus or viral components to transfect cells, and nonviral nanosystems (Figure 4.11).

Electroporation (EP) is the process of creating aqueous channels within the lipid bilayer membranes of mammalian cells using short electrical pulses. As a result, large molecules, such as DNA and other macromolecules, can now move through the cell membrane, which would otherwise be impossible. As a result, EP boosts drug and DNA absorption and the amount of medicines and DNA delivered to the target tissue of interest. EP has traditionally been used to treat muscle tissue, and several clinical trials are now being undertaken to utilize this method.

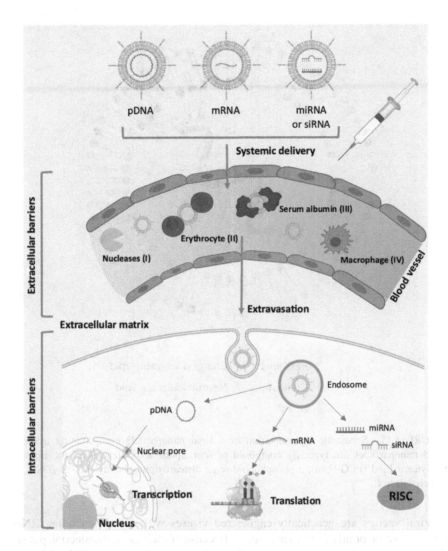

FIGURE 4.10 Extracellular and intracellular barriers to nucleic acid delivery are depicted in this diagram. (I) Endonuclease destruction; (II) Erythrocyte interaction and binding; (III) Serum protein complexation binding and aggregation; (IV) Immune activation to supplied nucleic acids

Physical approaches are straightforward and include applying physical force to the membrane barrier to distribute genetic material. The therapeutic application of naked mRNA ex vivo has been studied using physical methods such as electroporation and gene gun. However, cell mortality and limited access to target cells/tissues are the main drawbacks. In mouse models, for example, RNA complexed with gold particles has exhibited good expression in tissues when used with a gene gun; however, no efficiency data for larger animals or humans is available.

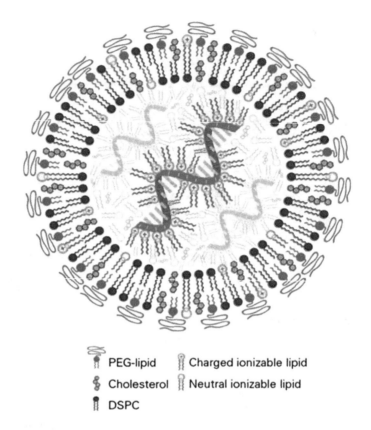

PEG-lipid   Charged ionizable lipid

Cholesterol   Neutral ionizable lipid

DSPC

FIGURE 4.11 Schematic representation of a lipid nanoparticle encapsulating mRNA. Lipid nanoparticles are typically composed of four lipids: an ionizable/cationic lipid; a PEGylated lipid (PEG-lipid); a phospholipid (e.g., distearoylphosphatidylcholine (DSPC)); and cholesterol.

Viral vectors are genetically engineered viruses with antigen-encoding RNA replacing some or all of the virus's genes. Because of their great transfection potential, viruses like picornaviruses and lentivirus have been chosen for mRNA delivery. However, using recombinant viruses comes with the risk of insertion into the genome, the difficulty of managing gene expression, the size of the sequence of interest is limited, and the presence of significant immunological side effects. Furthermore, viral vectors have considerable production costs and a limited packaging capacity.

The nonviral delivery techniques have great potential due to their biocompatibility, various features, their simple formulation with mRNA, and appropriate and controlled release kinetics. Nonviral systems are composed chiefly of synthetic or natural biocompatible components that form complexes with mRNA and vary in composition, physicochemical properties, shape, and size. The nonviral technologies include polymeric, lipid, and hybrid systems. Polyplexes are formed when biodegradable and predominantly cationic polymers are utilized to create nanoparticle formulations with nucleic acids. However, Polyethylenimine (PEI) usage has been limited due to its toxicity. Other polymers include polyethyleneimine stearic acid (PSA) copolymer. Chitosan, a biocompatible cationic glycopolymer that can deliver mRNA encoding luciferase, is another potential polymer.

Although cationic polymers have been extensively researched for mRNA complexation, they are not as clinically advanced as lipid systems for mRNA-based treatments. In mRNA delivery, various synthetic and naturally produced lipids are employed. Liposomes have an inherent advantage in that they can imitate the makeup of the cell membrane. However, because most lipoplex formulations cannot withstand the presence of serum and mRNA is more unstable, they are not widely used.

4.4.6.1 Lipid Nanoparticles

Lipid nanoparticles (LNPs) are currently among the most developed technologies for mRNA delivery, and clinical trials are underway. LNPs usually contain an ionizable lipid, a neutral/auxiliary lipid, cholesterol, and a PEG lipid. Ionizable lipids are lipids that become cationic at acid pH, allowing them to bind with mRNA via electrostatic interactions, forming a complex called lipoplex while remaining neutral at physiological pH, greatly lowering their toxicity. Patisiran (ONPATTRO), a clinically approved siRNA formulation against transthyretin mRNA, comprises Dlin-MC3-DMA-containing LNPs (MC3 ionizable lipid). In addition to ionizable lipids, N-[1-(2,3-dioleyloxy)propyl]], the first synthetic cationic lipid, is used to complex in vitro transcribed (IVT) mRNA. Another example is N, N,N-trimethylammonium chloride. In addition, 1,2-dioleoyl-3-trimethylammonium-propane (DOTAP) has also been developed.

Cationic lipids diminish efficacy due to nonspecific interactions in vivo and probable inflammatory reactions and toxicity. LNPs were once thought to be viable siRNA delivery techniques. Because LNPs are presently utilized to manufacture COVID-19 vaccines from both Moderna and Pfizer/BioNTech, they are now considered the practical standard of mRNA formulation.

The hybrid system, which combines multiple components such as polymers and lipids, offers higher functionality and flexibility than isolated systems to make use of various delivery mechanisms. Lipopolyplexes are an example of a hybrid system that combines the benefits of cationic polymers with lipids for nucleic acid complexation. Polyethylene glycol (PEG)ylated derivatives of histidylated polylysine and L-histidine-(N, N-di-n-hexadecyl amine)ethyl amide liposomes are the first example of this hybrid system. Other delivery techniques, including polypeptides and mineral-coated microparticles, have been investigated in addition to these most commonly utilized ones. The RNActive technology, developed by CureVac, uses protamine as an mRNA delivery mechanism. Nasal injection of mRNA vaccines can also be done with a cationic liposome/protamine complex (LPC).

mRNA must cross the cell membrane to reach the cytosol. This is challenging due to the negative charge of the molecule, its relatively large size (300–5000 kDa), and degradability, which can hamper its passive movement through the cell membrane. To overcome this, mRNA can be delivered using different strategies, including i) direct injection of naked mRNA; ii) conjugation with lipid-based carriers, polymers, or peptides; iii) via transfection of dendritic cells (DC).

The induction of an immune response by injection of naked mRNA in conventional and self-amplifying forms can be limited due to extracellular exonucleases in the target tissues, inefficient cell uptake, or unsuccessful endosomal release. Liposomes or lipid nanoparticles (LNPs) are among the most promising mRNA delivery tools. Although less explored, polymer-based delivery systems can also be used. Polyethylenimine (PEI) systems were successfully implemented as a strategy to deliver mRNA to cells, and intranasally. Additionally, PEI-based systems improved the response to sa-mRNA vaccines in skin explants and mice. Peptide-based delivery is a less explored system, as only protamine has been evaluated in clinical trials. New delivery approaches include cationic cell-penetrating peptides (CPPs) and anionic peptides. CPPs systems have improved T-cell immunity response in vivo, modulating the innate immune response and enhancing protein expression in both DC and human cancer cells in vitro. mRNA polyplexes conjugated with an anion peptide exhibited increased cellular uptake without inducing cytotoxicity in DC cells.

Additional immunological concerns include distribution formulations, inoculation sites, and adjuvants. RNA treatments and vaccines are delivered through nonviral formulations such as cationic lipids, LNPs, polymers, and protamine sulfate and physical means such as electroporation. In addition, because saRNAs contain the nsP1-4 replicon sequence, they are significantly longer than ordinary RNAs, which is critical for formulation.

Newer approaches to improve the delivery of saRNAs include using novel bioreducible polymer formulations with high molecular weight poly(CBA-co-4amino-1-butanol) (pABOL), ornithine dendrimers, mannosylated polyethyleneimine, or multiple linear peptides that help facilitate intracellular trafficking and endosomal release. Manosylation of polyethyleneimine improves delivery of saRNA reporter constructs to human skin explants. When saRNAs is delivered intramuscularly (IM) as neutral lipopolyplexes (LPPs), antigen-specific T lymphocytes rise while antigen-expressing cells decrease. These LPPs are made by encapsulating core RNA/polyethyleneimine polyplexes in PEGanionic liposome formulations with mannosylated lipids before encapsulation. Mannose helps vaccines reach antigen-presenting cells more effectively. SaRNAs, on the other hand, do not require encapsulation to protect them from RNAse degradation. The exterior of positively charged LNPs formed with dimethyl dioctadecyl ammonium (DAA) cationic lipids is entirely protected against RNaseA treatment when saRNAs are complexed outside.

The Pfizer-BioNTech COVID-19 Vaccine includes the following ingredients: mRNA, lipids ((4-hydroxybutyl)azanediyl)bis(hexane-6,1-diyl)bis(2-hexyldecanoate), 2 [(polyethylene glycol)-2000]-N,N-ditetradecylacetamide, 1,2-Distearoyl-sn-glycero-3- phosphocholine, and cholesterol), potassium chloride, monobasic potassium phosphate, sodium chloride, dibasic sodium phosphate dihydrate, and sucrose.

The Moderna COVID-19 Vaccine contains the following ingredients: messenger ribonucleic acid (mRNA), lipids (SM-102, polyethylene glycol [PEG] 2000 dimyristoyl glycerol [DMG], cholesterol, and 1,2-distearoyl-sn-glycero-3-phospho choline [DSPC]), tromethamine, tromethamine hydrochloride, acetic acid, sodium acetate, and sucrose).

Both enzymatic and chemical degradation mechanisms can degrade RNA. Formulation buffers are screened for contaminating RNases and may include buffer components like antioxidants and chelators to reduce the impact of reactive oxygen species and divalent metal ions on mRNA stability. Before being taken up by cells, mRNA is rapidly degraded by extracellular ribonucleases. Complexing compounds that protect RNA from degradation improve the efficacy of mRNA vaccinations. Complexation improves cellular absorption and delivery to the translation machinery in the cytoplasm. As a result, mRNA is frequently complexed with lipids or polymers. Packaging mRNA products in nanoparticles or co-formulation with RNase inhibitors may help boost their stability. At least six months of stability has been seen for lipid-encapsulated mRNA, but longer-term storage of such mRNA–lipid complexes in an unfrozen form has yet to be documented. Pfizer's first FDA-approved mRNA vaccine required storage at −90°C, while a similar vaccination from Moderna requires storage at −25°C to −15°C.

Both enzymatic and chemical degradation mechanisms can degrade RNA. Formulation buffers are screened for contaminating RNases and may include buffer components like antioxidants and chelators to reduce the impact of reactive oxygen species and divalent metal ions on mRNA stability. mRNA degrades rapidly by ubiquitous extracellular ribonucleases before being taken up by cells. Thus, the efficacy of mRNA vaccines benefits from complexing agents that protect RNA from degradation. Complexation enhances uptake by cells and improves delivery to the cytoplasm's translation machinery. mRNA is often complexed with either lipids or polymers. The stability of mRNA products might also be improved by packaging within nanoparticles or co-formulation with RNase inhibitors. At least six months of stability has been observed for lipid-encapsulated mRNA, but longer-term storage of such mRNA–lipid complexes in an unfrozen form has not yet been reported.

Not all complexing agents that promote DNA transfection are suitable for mRNA's complexation (Figure 4.12). In cell-free translation systems and inside cells, various big polycations, all established DNA transfection reagents, severely block mRNA translation. Only the tiniest polycations are useful. When mRNA is tied to big polycations, it is not released into the cytosol, but endogenous RNA releases DNA from large polycations into the cytosol.

mRNA encapsulated in liposomes is most common where cationic lipids are used for the intradermal and intravenous injection of antigen-encoding mRNA. However, mRNA's complexation with protamine, a small arginine-rich nuclear protein that stabilizes DNA during spermatogenesis, also stabilizes mRNA against degradation by serum components.

The RNA transfer to cells occurs within (in vivo) or outside (ex vivo) the organism, determining the vaccine delivery mechanism. Dendritic cells are immune cells that display antigens on their surfaces, leading to T cells' interactions to initiate an immune response. Dendritic cells are collected from patients and programmed with

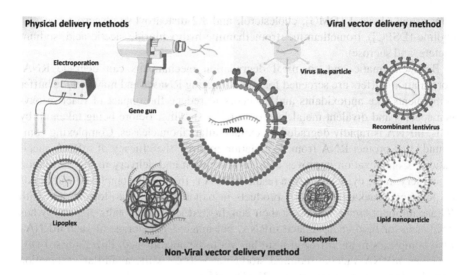

FIGURE 4.12 Schematic representation of different delivery strategies for mRNA therapies. There are represented 3 methods for the delivery of mRNA: physical methods, such as electroporation and gene gun; viral delivery systems that uses recombinant virus; and nonviral delivery systems, such as lipid nanoparticles, polyplex, lipoplex, and lipopolyplex.

the desired mRNA. Then, they are re-administered back to patients to create an immune response.

Ex vivo methods have various advantages over in vivo methods, most notably the expense of harvesting and adapting dendritic cells from patients and the ability to mimic a real infection. However, evolutionary processes that hinder the entrance of unfamiliar nucleic material and favor RNase destruction must be bypassed to start the translation. Furthermore, because RNA is too heavy to diffuse inside the cell, it is vulnerable to being found and removed by the host cell.

RNA viruses have been developed to achieve similar immune responses to nonviral delivery methods. Retroviruses, lentiviruses, alphaviruses, and rhabdoviruses are common RNA viruses employed as vectors, and each has its structure and function.

Adjuvants have long been used in vaccines to increase adaptive immunity and influence T-cell responses. Adjuvants currently used in licensed vaccines include aluminum salts, emulsions, lipid analogs, and virosomes, to name a few. The value of such adjuvants in RNA vaccinology is unknown, and it depends on the types of modifications made during design and production. Clinical experiments with traditional mRNA vaccines have thus far revealed only a limited level of humoral protection. Because saRNAs include native alphavirus motifs and can mimic viral translation in situ, they have the potential to boost immunity by stimulating PRRs. Adjuvants based on lipids are well-known adjuvants developed to promote RNA vaccine immuno-potentiation. By boosting receptor-mediated endocytosis of saRNA vaccines by dendritic cells, the inclusion of mannosylated conjugates and chitosan-based nanogel alginate helps influence the immune response.

4.5   DEVELOPMENT STRATEGIES

4.5.1   VACCINE DESIGN

The structure of mRNA vaccines is similar to eukaryotic mRNA, a single-stranded molecule with a cap at the 5' end, a poly(A) tail at the 3' end, and an open reading frame (ORF) flanked by untranslated regions (UTRs). The 5' cap is an essential component as it enables the translation initiation by binding to a eukaryotic translation initiation factor (eIF4E). The 5' cap can be built in a variety of ways. The most basic structure is Cap 0, which consists of a methyl-7 guanine nucleotide connected to the 5' position by a 5' triphosphate. The Cap 1 structure is formed when the first nucleotide of mRNA is methylated at the ribose 2' site. A synthetic cap analog or the patented Cap dinucleotide CleanCap can be used to add both caps during in vitro mRNA transcription. A post-transcriptional enzymatic reaction based on the vaccinia capping system is used in another capping method.

The construction of mRNA vaccines requires the insertion of the encoded antigen in a DNA template from where the mRNA is transcribed in vitro. Unlike DNA, mRNA simply has to reach the cytoplasm before being transcribed into the antigen by the cell machinery in vivo. This way, any desired sequence can be designed, produced in vitro, and delivered to any cell type. Inside the cells, RNA is recognized by endosomal or cytosolic receptors, which can activate the type I interferon (IFN-I) pathway and promote the production of chemokines and proinflammatory cytokines. In addition, these signal molecules lead to antigen-presenting cell (APC) activation and, subsequently, to a strong adaptive response.

Each part of the RNA can be tweaked to make as much protein as feasible while being as stable as possible within the cell. Here are some broad remarks on the various components of the RNA. The 5' untranslated region (UTR) provides translation signals to the cell, and it can even contain instructions that increase or limit translation. The 3' UTR serves a similar purpose, focused on stability signals. The protein that can be made is determined by what is encoded in the coding sequence, and using specific codes in the RNA can impede or speed up protein synthesis. The poly(A) tail at the end acts as a buffer to keep the RNA from being damaged.

When designing an mRNA for a vaccine, there are many options available. Extra unwanted signals in the 5' UTRs of natural RNAs vaccine are common; however, it's simple to delete the signals in undesirable sequences. Hundreds of mRNA variants may be evaluated before a single mRNA is selected. However, things left out of mRNAs can be significant if these do not add to the translation of an effective antigen. There is no need to encode the entire virus in the mRNA, only the target subunit for translation. mRNAs are currently developed to help treat rare diseases and develop cell-type-specific signals.

Modifying the pharmacokinetics of RNA can be done by changing the 5' cap structure, adjusting the length of the poly(A) tail, including modified nucleotides, codon, or sequence optimization, and changing the 5' and 3' UTRs. For longer saRNA transcripts, balancing the intrinsic and extrinsic immunogenic characteristics of the synthetic RNA, the vaccination antigen, and delivery formulation is equally crucial. The translation is improved, and RNA-associated immunogenicity is reduced by incorporating pseudouridine-modified nucleotides during transcription. Because saRNAs employ host-cell components to replicate mRNA, adding modified nucleotides is less useful because they are lost during amplification.

The optimization of 5′ and 3′ UTRs, which is based on the evolution of naturally occurring alphaviruses, is one feasible way to optimize the translation of saRNA vaccines. The single-stranded RNA genome creates a variety of secondary structures that allow alphaviruses to elude immune responses by bypassing the needs of regular host-cell translation processes. It is also beneficial to review the sequence encoding the nsP1-4 replicon genes.

Modifying the synthetic 5′ cap structure is one way to shield in vitro produced RNAs against nuclease digestion while also increasing translation. By capping transcripts in the forward orientation, the anti-reverse cap analog and phosphorothioate derivatives promote in situ translation of RNAs. Cap 1 structures that mimic normal eukaryotic mRNAs are generated when post-transcription capping enzymes originating from the vaccinia virus are coupled with 2′-O-methyltransferases.

The main strategies employed by vaccine design include:

- Capping modification. Improves translation initiation by engaging translation initiation factors, protects synthetic mRNA from exonuclease degradation, and prevents overactivation of innate immunity. The addition of a 3′ poly(A) tail also improves mRNA stability and translational activities, as it protects mRNA from nuclease degradation by the poly(A)-binding protein (PABP). This tail can be added to the transcript by inserting a poly(A) sequence in the DNA template or an enzymatic reaction. Tail size optimization is an essential factor for the stabilization and expression. Longer poly(A) tails can improve mRNA stability and translation. However, this effect is not linear, and the best tail size is dependent on cell type. The untranslated regions (UTRs) are responsible for transcription regulation and mRNA stability. These sequences significantly impact translation efficiency because they are involved in translation machinery recognition, recruitment, and mRNA trafficking. Strategies to influence the innate immune response, such as artificial nucleosides (NTPs), and to improve translation efficiency, such as codon optimization, are common in mRNA production.
- Nucleoside modification. Replacing ordinary nucleosides with naturally occurring modified nucleosides (e.g., replacing uridine with pseudo-uridine) reduces the immune response to exogenous mRNA and increases its stability. For example, both COVID-19 vaccines from Pfizer and Moderna employ modified N1-methylpseudouridine instead of uridine. The vaccine from the German company CureVac, on the other hand, relies on ordinary uridine, and it had failed in its efficacy testing.
- Capping. The 5′ cap is added to the mRNA strand either during in vitro transcription (IVT), by including a cap analog in the IVT reaction mixture, or after IVT, by using specialized enzymes (e.g., 2′-O-methyltransferase). Proprietary cap analogs with high capping efficiencies have been developed

for this purpose. Co-transcriptional capping tends to give lower yields than post-transcriptional capping but may be more cost-effective.

- Polyadenylation. The addition of the poly(A) tail at the 3′ end of the mRNA strand can be done enzymatically (mimicking the natural process to some extent), or a sequence of deoxythymidine nucleotides can be appended to the DNA template so that the poly(A) tail is naturally produced during transcription. The drawback of the latter approach lies in the production of the DNA template; this template is usually in the form of plasmid DNA (pDNA) replicated in bacteria, and a long stretch of identical nucleotides in pDNA makes it structurally unstable. Sequence optimization—the sequences of the UTRs and the coding region can be optimized to improve translation efficiency and mRNA stability. UTRs of natural mRNAs such as alpha- or beta-globin are commonly used as the basis for the UTRs of mRNA vaccines. In the CDS, the degeneracy of the genetic code (i.e., the fact that multiple codons code for the same amino acid) makes it possible to replace rare codons with frequent codons in human cells; this procedure is called codon optimization, and it generally improves mRNA stability and translation efficiency.

- Purification. Removal of double-stranded RNA (dsRNA) is formed during mRNA manufacturing that is immunogenic, and it should be removed. Purification steps such as hydrophobic interaction chromatography can distinguish and separate dsRNA from single-stranded RNA (ssRNA).

- Efficient mRNA vectors. A critical step for the maturation of mRNA vaccines was the development of efficient ways to transport mRNA into cells. mRNA itself is polyanionic and thus negatively charged, as is the surface of the mammalian cell membrane; consequently, they repel each other electrostatically. Together with mRNA's considerable size, this repulsion makes mRNA's natural uptake by cells deficient (less than 1 in 10,000 molecules). Moreover, naked mRNA is highly susceptible to degradation by ribonucleases and can provoke severe immune reactions. mRNA vectors include peptides, polymers, and dendritic cells; however, lipid nanoparticles (LNPs) have been the most successful in the two COVID-19 vaccines. LNPs are self-assembled spherical structures typically composed of four different lipids (a cationic/ionizable lipid; a PEGylated lipid; a phospholipid; and cholesterol) capable of encapsulating mRNA molecules. LNPs are engulfed by cells through endocytosis, forming vesicles inside the cell called endosomes. When the lipids of the LNP merge with the endosome membrane, they release the mRNA to the cytosol, where it can be translated.

4.5.2 Process Development

Once a pathogen is identified or an outbreak is declared, the pathogen and antigen(s) genome are determined, if not already available, by the combined sequencing, bioinformatics, and computational approach. Candidate vaccine antigen sequences are deposited electronically and globally for in silico design of mRNA vaccines, followed by constructing a plasmid DNA template by molecular cloning or synthesis. Pilot vaccine batches are generated in a cell-free system by in vitro transcription and capping the mRNA, purification, and formulation with the delivery system. In-process analytic and potency tests are performed to assess the quality of pilot mRNA vaccine batches. If needed, pilot mRNA vaccine batches can be further tested in the immunogenicity and disease animal model. The final mRNA vaccine is scaled up and manufactured through a generic process with minimal modifications, rapidly tested, and dispatched for use (Figure 4.13).

GMP mRNA production begins with creating a DNA template, which is then followed by enzymatic in vitro transcription. To start the production process, template plasmid DNA generated in E. coli is linearized using a restriction enzyme, and run-off transcripts with a poly(A) tract at the 3′ end are synthesized. A DNA-dependent RNA polymerase from a bacteriophage then synthesizes mRNA from nucleoside triphosphates (NTP) (T7, SP6, or T3). After that, DNase is used to breakdown the template DNA. Finally, the mRNA is capped, either chemically or enzymatically, to allow for efficient translation in vivo.

Alternatives to plasmid DNA, such as PCR-based DNA replication and circular DNA, are being developed. Polymerase-chain-reaction (PCR)-generated linear DNA is a cleaner, more effective alternative to plasmid DNAs created by bacterial fermentation [https://adnas.com/linearx-pcr-produced-linear-dna/] (Table 4.3).

Another alternate to bacterial-based growth of cDNA clones is in vitro amplification using rolling circle amplification (RCA), an isothermal, high yield method of DNA amplification that uses a highly processive polymerase to amplify DNA over 70kb. Importantly, the enzyme replicates DNA with high fidelity due to its 3′-5′exonuclease or proofreading activity [https://www.biorxiv.org/content/10.1101/2020.06.22.165241v1] (Figure 4.14).

While the in vitro methods described above are attractive, the economics of the construction of mRNA vaccines remains dependent on plasmid DNA.

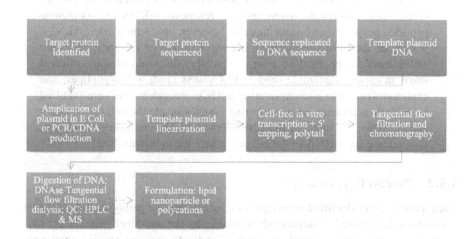

FIGURE 4.13 GMP Production of mRNA Vaccine.

TABLE 4.3

Comparison of Plasmid DNA and LineaRx PCR-Based Production of mRNA

Attribute	PCR DNA Production	Plasmid DNA Production
Risk of antibiotic resistance transfer	None	Yes
Endotoxin	None	Yes
Cellular purification	None	Required
Yield	Fixed	Variable
Cycle time	Hours	Days to weeks
Chemical modification of DNA by primer modification	Yes	No
Long homogenous Poly(A) tails (part of mRNA template)	Yes	No

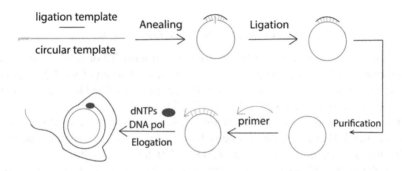

FIGURE 4.14   Rolling circle amplification of DNA.

After mRNA is generated, it is purified to remove reaction components such as enzymes, unbound nucleotides, leftover DNA, and truncated RNA fragments, among other things. While lithium chloride precipitation is commonly employed for laboratory-scale preparation, derivatized microbeads in batch or column formats, which are easier to handle on a large scale, are used for clinical purification. Because dsRNA is a significant inducer of interferon-dependent translation inhibition, eliminating it and other contaminants from various mRNA platforms is crucial for the final product's efficacy.

Various nucleotides, oligodeoxynucleotides, brief, abortive transcripts from abortive cycling during initiation, and protein make up the required mRNA transcript in a complicated combination. A mixture of precipitation and extraction processes eliminates these pollutants from the sample.

However, the sample contains other contaminating RNA species that are difficult to distinguish from the proper transcript using conventional methods: premature termination during elongation results in shorter transcripts than expected. Transcripts that are longer than indicated are produced when template DNA is linearized with an enzyme that leaves a 3'-overhang or vestiges of non-linearized template DNA. Bacteriophage polymerases' RNA-dependent RNA polymerase activity also generates unwanted transcripts. As a result, before mRNA may be used as a therapeutic ingredient, it must be further treated to remove such contaminated transcripts.

Shorter and longer transcripts were eliminated in a single chromatographic step (e.g., HPLC) that separated mRNA by size, yielding a pure single mRNA product. In addition, incorporating chromatographic purification into a GMP mRNA synthesis process enhanced the activity of mRNA molecules in terms of protein expression in vivo by a factor of several.

Protein expression from in vitro transcribed, enzymatically capped mRNA is increased by enzymatic 2'-O-methylation of the first transcribed nucleotide, resulting in protein expression from mRNA capped with ARCA co-transcriptionally.

In multi-gram scale operations, mRNA synthesis typically generates more than two g/l of full-length mRNA under optimal circumstances. The scale-up is also straightforward because the in vitro and upstream processes are not batch size-dependent.

4.5.3 CONSTRUCTION OF PLASMIDS FOR RNA TRANSCRIPTION

A promoter specific for a viral RNA polymerase (usually T7 or SP6) drives downstream transcription of the mRNA of interest in plasmid vectors for mRNA vaccine production. In most cases, elements that stabilize the transcribed RNA are included in the vector. Untranslated regions before (5' UTR) and/or after (3' UTR) the cDNA sequence encoding the gene of interest are examples. A synthetic poly(A) tail is also present in the 3' UTR, which is necessary for effective protein translation. Increased mRNA half-life and more effective protein translation are frequently associated with longer poly(A) tails. pTNT is a commercially available vector that incorporates these properties (Promega). This vector has a synthetic poly(A)30 tail, tandem SP6 and T7 promoters, and a 5' UTR from rabbit-globin.

These vectors are used to make genomic RNA, which contains the nonstructural proteins 1–4 of an alphavirus (Sindbis or Semliki Forest Virus) that make up the viral replicase. A sub-genomic promoter, also known as a 24-nucleotide (nt) conserved sequence element (CSE), is located downstream of the replicase and controls the production of the gene of interest. This is followed by a synthetic poly(A) tail and a viral 3' UTR with a conserved 19-nt CSE, which constitutes the central promoter for producing negative-strand RNA. The interaction of the viral 3' and 5' UTRs is required for replication to begin and for both minus and plus-strand synthesis to be regulated.

Thermo Scientific sells the pSFV and pSinRep5 (Figure 4.15) vectors, which can be used to make self-replicating RNAs using SFV and Sindbis virus replicases, respectively.

Figure 4.15 Commercially available vectors for in vitro transcription of self-replicating (pSinRep5) or conventional (pTNT) mRNA vaccines [Weiss R., Scheiblhofer S., Thalhamer J. (2017) Generation and Evaluation of Prophylactic mRNA Vaccines Against Allergy. In: Kramps T., Elbers K. (eds) RNA Vaccines. Methods in Molecular Biology, vol 1499. Humana Press, New York, NY. https://doi.org/10.1007/978-1-4939-6481-9_7].

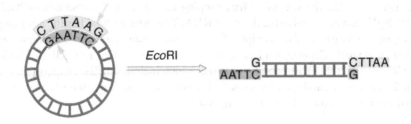

FIGURE 4.15   Plasmid DNA.

Standard recombinant DNA procedures can be used to construct the pTNT-P5 and pSin-P5 vectors. First, to prevent religation, the vectors pTNT and pSinRep5 are linearized with XbaI and treated with calf intestinal alkaline phosphatase (CIAP). Then, using the NheI/ XbaI enzymes, the cDNA encoding Phl p 5 is extracted from pCMV-Phl p 5 and ligated into the linearized vectors. pTNT-P5 and pSin-P5 are the names of the generated vectors.

4.5.4   PLASMID PURIFICATION AND LINEARIZATION

Plasmid templates can be made using any commercially available plasmid preparation kit that produces high-quality endotoxin-free plasmid DNA. However, before mRNA can be transcribed, the plasmid DNA must be linearized following the poly(A) tail (Figure 4.15).

To avoid circular transcription, which results in RNA of the wrong size, plasmid DNA must be completely linearized. Therefore, it is desirable to make a larger batch of linearized plasmid DNA that can be stored at 20 degrees Celsius.

4.5.5   IN VITRO TRANSCRIPTION OF RNA

T7 or SP6 RNA polymerase is used to in vitro transcribe RNA from linearized plasmid DNA. Using tailored buffers and high concentrations of rNTPs and inorganic pyrophosphatase, milligram amounts of RNA can be synthesized, avoiding the inhibitory effects of pyrophosphate generated during ribonucleoside triphosphate incorporation.

T7 or SP6 polymerase can be used to transcribe conventional mRNA encoding Phl p 5 from linearized pTNT-P5 template DNA. Approximately 2–5 mg of RNA is produced from a 1 mL reaction. Similarly, using SP6 polymerase, self-replicating RNA can be transcribed from linearized pSin-P5. A one-milliliter reaction yields about one milligram of self-replicating RNA.

4.5.6   RNA CAPPING

A 7-methylguanosine cap structure is required for mRNA stability and translation efficiency. Therefore, during the transcribing process, cap analog might be used.

Alternatively, using the vaccinia virus capping enzyme, cap 0 structures (m7G(5′) ppp(5′)NpN) can be added to the 5′ end of RNA. The latter method has the advantage of capping up to 100% of transcripts. The enzymatic capping technique employing the ScriptCap m7G Capping Kit is described in this chapter (CELLSCRIPT). The kit includes the vaccinia virus capping enzyme, which includes mRNA triphosphatase, guanylyltransferase, and guanine-7-methyltransferase, as well as all three enzymatic activities that are required for cap formation.

4.5.7 RNA QUALITY CONTROL

Quality control of capped mRNA is done using denaturing agarose gel electrophoresis, in vitro transfection, and western blot analysis

Denaturing agarose gel electrophoresis is used to evaluate the integrity and length of the transcribed RNA. Ideally, transcripts should appear as a single band of the expected size. Longer transcripts indicate a plasmid template with insufficient linearization or the presence of hidden antisense promoters. Conversely, secondary RNA structures such as poly(T) regions or repetitions might result in smaller transcripts.

Translation efficacy of the RNA can be tested by in vitro transfection of BHK-21 cells. The effective translation is dependent on the integrity and secondary structure of the RNA and the presence of a cap 0 structure. Also, codon usage may affect translation efficacy.

4.5.8 IMMUNIZATION AND ALLERGIC SENSITIZATION OF MICE

BALB/c mice are commonly used for allergy models because they are prone to developing TH2biased immunological responses. These animals have high titers of allergen-specific IgE and higher IL-4, IL-5, and IL-13 after sensitization with recombinant allergen plus adjuvants like aluminum hydroxide (Alu-Gel-S). Furthermore, the ratio of allergen-specific IgG1:IgG2a subclass antibodies is raised in sensitized mice, indicating a TH2-dominated response. Therefore, by immunizing mice with allergen-encoding mRNA vaccines before sensitization, the generation of IgE and IgG1 antibodies and the production of allergy-related cytokines can be avoided.

Two to three vaccinations at weekly intervals, followed by 2–3 sensitization rounds, is a standard experimental design for protective mRNA immunization against allergies. An interval of at least 2 weeks between vaccination and sensitization should be maintained to minimize antigen-independent inhibition of TH2 sensitization. Vaccine memory lasts at least 9 months, so longer intervals are possible. Groups of animals receiving mRNA expressing an irrelevant antigen/allergen and just sensitizations must be included for control purposes.

4.5.9 MEASUREMENT OF ANTIBODY SUBCLASSES

The easiest indicator to measure to see if preventive immunization succeeded is the ratio of IgG1:IgG2a in sera. A rise in IgG2a titers following allergic sensitization is a strong indicator of a TH1 bias created by the RNA vaccine and effective protection, even if the humoral responses after immunization are hardly detectable.

4.5.10 Basophil Release Assay

Basophils expressing FcRI, the high-affinity receptor for IgE, are passively loaded with IgE to determine the amount of free allergen-specific IgE in the sera of sensitized mice. The presence of the allergen causes IgE cross-linking and, as a result, mediator release. One of these mediators, -hexosaminidase, cleaves the substrate 4-MUG, resulting in fluorescence spectroscopy-detectable cleavage products.

The RBL release test provides a functional readout for IgE-mediated degranulation, unlike the ELISA detection of IgE. In addition, a basophil activation test, which has been described in detail elsewhere, can also be used to measure the quantity of cell-bound IgE in the blood of sensitized animals.

4.5.11 Culture of RBL Cells

The RBL-2H3 cells are adherent, fibroblast-like cells forming monolayers. They are cultured in a mixture of MEM and RPMI with supplements in an incubator at 37°C, 95% RH, and 5% CO_2.

Whereas most early work in mRNA vaccines focused on cancer applications, recently greater emphasis has been placed on preventing infectious pathogens, including influenza virus, Ebola virus, Zika virus, Streptococcus spp T. gondii, and Coronavirus.

mRNA synthesis avoids the frequent dangers associated with other vaccination platforms, such as live viruses, viral vectors, inactivated viruses, and subunit protein vaccines. It does not require hazardous chemicals or cell cultures that adventitious viruses could contaminate. Furthermore, the short synthesis period for mRNA prevents microbial contamination. The theoretical hazards of infection or vector integration into host cell DNA are not a worry for mRNA in the vaccinated population. For the reasons stated above, mRNA vaccines are thought to be a generally safe vaccination formulation.

Local and systemic inflammation, biodistribution and durability of produced immunogen, induction of autoreactive antibodies, and potentially harmful effects of any non-native nucleotides and delivery system components are all investigated in preclinical and clinical investigations. Some mRNA-based vaccine platforms have been linked to inflammatory and possible autoimmune type I interferon responses. Another potential hazard stemming from the presence of extracellular RNA during mRNA immunization could be the presence of extracellular RNA. Naked RNA from the extracellular environment has been demonstrated to alter the permeability of densely packed endothelial cells, contributing to edema. Blood coagulation and pathological thrombus development are also aided by extracellular RNA. As alternative mRNA methods and delivery systems are used first in people and tested in bigger patient groups, safety will need to be monitored.

mRNA promotes humoral and cellular immune responses and induces the innate immune system. Compared with DNA-based vaccines, mRNA is more effective since expression does not require nuclear entry and is safer since the probability of random genome integration is virtually zero. Additionally, expression of the coded antigens is transient since mRNA is quickly degraded by cellular processes, with no traces found after 2–3 days. The mRNA vaccine platform's flexibility is also useful in manufacturing since a change in the encoded antigen does not affect the mRNA backbone's physical–chemical characteristics, hence allowing production to be standardized. Additionally, since production is based on an in vitro cell-free transcription reaction, safety concerns regarding the presence of cell-derived impurities and viral contaminants commonly found in other platforms are minimized.

mRNA vaccines present numerous advantages vis-à-vis DNA vaccines and conventional vaccines, such as those based on inactivated/attenuated pathogens, pathogen fragments, or proteins:

- The manufacturing process of mRNA is cell-free and independent of the mRNA sequence, making it easy and fast to develop and mass-produce a new vaccine. Therefore, mRNA vaccines may be considered a platform technology, which makes them particularly advantageous for tackling pandemics. In contrast, to produce an inactivated or recombinant protein vaccine, it is necessary to develop specific microbial/cell culture processes with particular microbial strains or cell lines that usually require a series of long culture steps to generate the product as custom product recovery and purification steps. Moreover, cell-free manufacturing has a lower risk of microbial contamination.
- Since the antigenic protein is synthesized from the mRNA in the host cell by the host's cell machinery, the protein generated has precisely the same structural characteristics (including posttranslational modifications) that the actual pathogen's protein would have in the host. However, when the antigenic protein is produced industrially, for example, using bacteria or yeast cells, this is not always the case.
- In contrast to DNA vaccinations, mRNA does not require entry into the cell nucleus to be decoded, reducing the risk of DNA integration into the genome, which may exist for DNA vaccines.

mRNA does present, however, certain challenges for its use in vaccines:

- Cells' uptake of naked mRNA (i.e., mRNA that is not associated with some sort of delivery carrier such as lipid nanoparticles) is very low under normal circumstances.
- Naked mRNA is highly unstable in vivo, being rapidly degraded by ribonucleases.
- The organism perceives exogenous naked mRNA as antigenic itself and may elicit a strong immune reaction. Although this may be useful for vaccination to a certain extent, it may reduce the translation efficiency of mRNA and consequently hinder the development of an effective immune response against the antigenic protein.

4.6 NUCLEOSIDE VACCINES PERSPECTIVE

It is now conceivable to develop a universal flu vaccine that will protect against every viral strain without being altered every year. Since RNA vaccines can incorporate instructions for several antigens, either strung together in a single strand or packaged together in a single nanoparticle, essentially, a single vaccine in place of multiple sexually transmitted diseases including HPV, HIV, and chlamydia can be combined.

Another form of the mRNA vaccination can encode fully human IgG antibodies that are identical to or resembling the antibodies found in a patient with a prior history of potent immunity. This application can replace antibody therapy and allow the modulation of autoimmune responses. This new research area offers numerous opportunities to treat diseases currently considered not treatable, like Parkinson's disease, Alzheimer's, diabetes, and many rare cancers.

New applications of mRNA vaccines would include:

- Multiple mRNAs, strung or single, in a single nanoparticle for recalcitrant diseases like tuberculosis, HIV, and malaria.
- Continuous modulation, season flu vaccine.
- Monoclonal antibody replaced with innate antibody production.
- Antigens to produce antibodies against rogue antibodies: autoimmune disorders to prevent diabetes 1, Parkinson's disease, Alzheimer's, etc.
- Diabetes protection vaccine against the six strains of the Coxsackie B (CVB) virus and myocarditis and meningitis.
- For a vaccine to prevent diabetes type 1, the autoantigen is insulin, glutamic acid decarboxylase or heat shock protein, myelin oligodendrocyte glycoprotein, myelin antigens, zona pellucida 3, myoglobulin, type II collagen, thyroglobulin, cell membrane surface antigen, type II colloid antigen, acetylcholine receptor, thyrocyte cell surface antigen, salivary gland duct antigen, thyroglobulin, superantigen, or interphotoreceptor retinoid-binding protein. In addition, the vaccine can inhibit T-cell proliferation from inducing the occurrence of immune suppression and prevent and treat autoimmune diseases effectively.

4.6.1 SARS-CoV-2 VACCINE

SARS-CoV-2 is an RNA-enveloped single-stranded virus. Its genome, 29,881 bp in length (GenBank no. MN908947), encoding 9860 amino acids, was characterized using an RNA-based metagenomic next-generation sequencing technique. Gene fragments express structured and non-structural proteins. The ORF area encodes nonstructural proteins such as 3-chymotrypsin-like protease, papain-like protease, and RNA-dependent RNA polymerase, whereas the S, E, M, and N genes encode structural proteins (Figure 4.16).

The surface of SARS-CoV-2 is covered in glycosylated S proteins that bind to the host cell receptor angiotensin-converting enzyme 2 (ACE2) and mediate viral cell entrance. TM protease serine 2 (TMPRSS2), a type 2 TM serine protease found

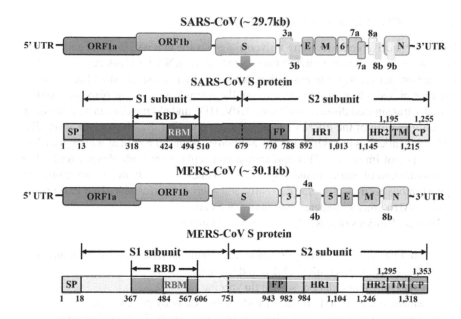

FIGURE 4.16   SARS-CoV protein structure. (Source: https://commons.wikimedia.org/w/index.php?curid=88420710Schematic of the SARS-CoV-2 S protein)

on the host cell membrane, stimulates virus entrance into the cell by activating the S protein when the S protein attaches to the receptor. The viral RNA is released, polyproteins are translated from the RNA genome, and replication and transcription of the viral RNA genome occur via protein cleavage and assembly of the replicase–transcriptase complex once the virus has entered the cell. Viral RNA is reproduced in the host cell, and structural proteins are created, assembled, and packaged before the release of viral particles (Figure 4.16).

These proteins are essential for the viral life cycle and could be used as therapeutic targets. Experiments have shown that ACE2-based peptides, 3CLpro inhibitors (3CLpro-1), and a new vinyl sulfone protease inhibitor are effective against SARS-CoV-2. The SARS-CoV-2 S protein is involved in receptor identification, viral attachment, and entry into host cells and is highly conserved among all human coronaviruses (HCoVs). One of the most important targets for COVID-19 vaccination and therapeutic research is its ability to produce antibodies withuot affecting the DNA.

The mRNA COVID-19 vaccines encode the viral spike (S) glycoprotein of SARS-CoV-2 that includes two proline substitutions (K986P and V987P mutations) to stabilize the prefusion conformation of the glycoprotein. The LNP method permits uptake by host cells and delivery of mRNA into the cytosol, where the mRNA sequence is translated into the S protein in the ribosomes after intramuscular (IM) administration. The S protein is delivered as a membrane-bound antigen in its prefusion conformation at the cellular surface after post-translation processing by the host cells, providing the antigen target for B lymphocytes. Part of the temporally generated Spike proteins also enters antigen presentation pathways, allowing T cells to recognize antigen via MHC presentation of T-cell epitopes. The mechanism of action is that LNP-formulated RNA vaccines are administered intramuscularly (IM), causing transitory local inflammation that attracts neutrophils and antigen presentation cells (APCs) to the delivery site. Recruited APCs can take up LNP, express proteins, and travel to the draining lymph nodes where T cells are primed. Because of this intrinsic, innate immune activity, no additional adjuvants are required to formulate mRNA vaccines. However, nucleoside-modified mRNA is used in licensed mRNA vaccines, which decreases (rather than enhances) mRNA immunogenicity, stressing the significance of balancing mRNA vaccines' innate immune activity. The ability of mRNA vaccines to create in vivo antigens after delivery, together with the self-adjuvant properties of mRNA-LNP vaccines, resulted in the generation of efficient neutralizing antibody responses and cellular immunity, reducing the risk of COVID-19 infection in vaccination recipients.

Table 4.4 lists the features of the BioNTech/Pfizer BNT-162b2 vaccine. Figure 4.17 lists the exact sequence of the mRNA nucleosides. (https://berthub.eu/articles/11889 .doc). (The WHO document is no longer available on the WHO website.)

The Moderna mRNA sequence is given in Figure 4.15; it is not complete but as best it could be deciphered by reverse engineering (Figure 4.18).

TABLE 4.4
Features of Pfizer BioNTech Vaccine

Element	Description	Position
cap	A modified 5'-cap1 structure ($m^7G^+m^{3'}$-5'-ppp-5'-Am)	1–2
5'-UTR	5'-untranslated region derived from human alpha-globin RNA with an optimized Kozak sequence	3–54
sig	S glycoprotein signal peptide (extended leader sequence), which guides translocation of the nascent polypeptide chain into the endoplasmic reticulum.	55–102
S protein_mut	Codon-optimized sequence encoding full-length SARS-CoV-2 spike (S) glycoprotein containing mutations K986P and V987P to ensure the S glycoprotein remains in an antigenically optimal pre-fusion conformation; stop codons: 3874-3879 (underlined)	103–3879
3'-UTR	The 3' untranslated region comprises two sequence elements derived from the amino-terminal enhancer of split (AES) mRNA and the mitochondrial encoded 12S ribosomal RNA to confer RNA stability and high total protein expression.	3880–4174
poly(A)	A 110-nucleotide poly(A) tail consisting of a stretch of 30 adenosine residues, followed by a 10-nucleotide linker sequence and another 70 adenosine residues.	4175–4284

```
GAGAAVAAAC VAGVAVVCVV CVGGVCCCCA CAGACVCAGA GAGAACCCGC   50
CACCAVGVVC GVGVVCCVGG VGCVGCVGCC VCVGGVGVCC AGCCAGVGVG  100
VGAACCVGAC CACCAGAACA CAGCVGCCVC CAGCCVACAC CAACAGCVVV  150
ACCAGAGGCG VGVACVACCC CGACAAGGVG VVCAGAVCCA GCGVGCVGCA  200
CVCVACCCAG GACCVGVVCC VGCCVVVCVV CAGCAACGVG ACCVGGVVCC  250
ACGCCAVCCA CGVGVCCGGC ACCAAVGGCA CCAAGAGAVV CGACAACCCC  300
GVGCVGCCCV VCAACGACGG GGVGVACVVV GCCAGCACCG AGAAGVCCAA  350
CAVCAVCAGA GGCVGGAVCV VCGGCACCAC ACVGGACAGC AAGACCCAGA  400
GCCVGCVGAV CGVGAACAAC GCCACCAACG VGGVCAVCAA AGVGVGCGAG  450
VVCCAGVVCV GCAACGACCC CVVCCVGGGC GVCVACVACC ACAAGAACAA  500
CAAGAGCVGG AVGGAAAGCG AGVVCCGGGV GVACAGCAGC GCCAACAACV  550
GCACCVVCGA GVACGVGVCC CAGCCVVVCC VGAVGGACCV GGAAGGCAAG  600
CAGGGCAACV VCAAGAACCV GCGCGAGVVC GVGVVVAAGA ACAVCGACGG  650
CVACVVCAAG AVCVACAGCA AGCACACCCC VAVCAACCVC GVGCGGGAVC  700
VGCCVCAGGG CVVCVCVGCV CVGGAACCCC VGGVGGAVCV GCCCAVCGGC  750
AVCAACACVC CCCGGVVVCA GACACVGCVG GCCCVGCACA GAAGCVACCV  800
GACACCVGGC GAVAGCAGCA GCGGAVGGAC AGCVGGVGCC GCCGCVVACV  850
AVGVGGGCVA CCVGCCAGCC AGAACCVVCC VGCVGGAAGVA CAACGAGAAC  900
GGCACCAVCA VCCGGCGCGV GGAVVGVGVC CVGGAVVCCVC VGAGCGGAGAC  950
AAAGVGCACC CVGAAGVCCV VCACCGVGGA AAAGGGCAVC VACCAGACCA 1000
GCAACVVCCG GGVGCAGCCC ACCGAAVCCA VCGVGCGGVV CCCCAAVAVC 1050
ACCAAVCVGV GCCCCVVCGG CGAGGVGVVC AAVGCCACCA GAVVCGCCVC 1100
VGVGVACGCC VGGAACCGGA AGCGGAVCAG CAAVVGCGVG GCCGACVACV 1150
CCGVGCVGVA CAACVCCGCC AGCVVCAGCA CCVVCAAGVG CVACGGCGVG 1200
VCCCCVACCA AGCVGAACGA CCVGVGCVVC ACAAACGVGV ACGCCGACAG 1250
CVVCGVGAVC CGGGGAGAVG AAGVGCGGCA GAVVGCCCCV GGACAGACAG 1300
GCAAGAVCGC CGACVACAAC VACAAGCVGC CCGACGACVV CACCGGCVGV 1350
GVGAVVGCCV GGAACAGCAA CAACCVGGAC VCCAAAGVCG GCGGCAACVA 1400
CAAVVACCVG VACCGGCVGV VCCGGAAGVC CAAVCVGAAG CCCVVCGAGC 1450
GGGACAVCVC CACCGAGAVC VAVCAGGCCG GCAGCACCCC VVGVAACGGC 1500
GVGGAAGGCV VCAACVGCVA CVVCCCACVG CAGVCCVACG GCVVVCAGCC 1550
CACAAAVGGC GVGGGCVAVC AGCCCVACAG AGVGGVGGVG CVGAGCVVCG 1600
AACVGCVGCA VGCCCCVGCC ACAGVGVGCG GCCCVAAGAA AAGCACCAAV 1650
CVCGVGAAGA ACAAAVGCGV GAACVVCAAC VVCAACGGCC VGACCGGCAC 1700
CGGCGVGCVG ACAGAGAGCA ACAAGAAGVV CCVGCCAVVC CAGCAGVVVG 1750
GCCGGGAVAV CGCCGAVACC ACAGACGCCG VVAGAGAVCC CCAGACACVG 1800
GAAAVCCVGG ACAVCACCCC VVGCAGCVVC GGCGGAGVGV CVGVGAVCAC 1850
CCCVGGCACC AACACCAGCA AVCAGGVGGC AGVGCVGVAC CAGGACGVGA 1900
ACVGVACCGA AGVGCCCGVG GCCAVVCACG CCGAVCAGCV GACACCVACA 1950
VGGCGGGVGV ACVCCACCGG CAGCAAVGVG VVVCAGACCA GAGCCGGCVG 2000
VCVGAVCGGA GCCGAGCACG VGAACAAVAG CVACGAGVGC GACAVCCCCA 2050
VCGGCGCVGG AAVCVGCGCC AGCVACCAGA CACAGACAAA CAGCCCVCGG 2100
AGAGCCAGAA GCGVGGCCAG CCAGAGCAVC AVVVGCCVACA CAAVGVCVCV 2150
GGGCGCCGAG AACAGCGVGG CCVACVCCAA CAACVCVAVC GCVAVCCCCA 2200
CCAACVVCAC CAVCAGCGVG ACCACAGAGA VCCVGCCVGV GVCCAVGACC 2250
AAGACCAGCG VGGACVGCAC CAVGVACAVC VGCGGCGAVV CCACCGAGVG 2300
CVCCAACCVG CVGCVGCAGV ACGGCAGCVV CVGCACCCAG CVGAAVAGAG 2350
CCCVGACAGG GAVCGCCGVG GAACAGGACA AGAACACCCA AGAGGVGVVC 2400
GCCCAAGVGA AGCAGAVCVA CAAGACCCCV CCVAVVCAAG ACVVCGGCGG 2450
CVVCAAVVVC AGCCAGAVVC VGCCCGAVCC VAGCAAGCCC AGCAAGCGGA 2500
GCVVCAVCGA GGACCVGCVG VVCAACAAAG VGACACVGGC CGACGCCGGC 2550
VVCAVCAAGC AGVAVGGCGA VVGVCVGGGC GACAVVGCCG CCAGGGAVCV 2600
GAVVVGCGCC CAGAAGVVVA ACGGACVGAC AGVGCVGCCV CCVCVGCVGA 2650
CCGAVGAGAV GAVCGCCCAG VACACAVCVG CVCVGCVGGC CGGCACAAVC 2700
ACAAGCGGCV GGACAVVVGG AGCAGGCGCC GCVCVGCAGA VCCCCVVVGC 2750
VAVGCAGAVG GCCVACCGGV VCAACGGCAV CGGAGVGACC CAGAAVGVGC 2800
VGVACGAGAA CCAGAAGCVG AVCGCCAACC AGVVCAACAG CGCCAVCGGC 2850
AAGAVCCAGG ACAGCCVGAG CAGCACAGCA AGCGCCCVGG GAAAGCVGCA 2900
GGACGVGGVC AACCAGAAVG CCCAGGCACV GAACACCCVG GVCAAGCAGC 2950
VGVCCVCCAA CVVCGGCGCC AVCAGCVCVG VGCVGAACGA VAVCCVGAGC 3000
AGACVGGACC CVCCVGAGGC CGAGGVGCAG AVCGACAGAC VGAVCACAGG 3050
CAGACVGCAG AGCCVCCAGA CAVACGVGAC CCAGCAGCVG AVCAGAGCCG 3100
CCGAGAVVAG AGCCVCVGCC AAVCVGGCCG CCACCAAGAV GVCVGAGVGV 3150
GVGCVGGGCC AGAGCAAGAG AGVGGACVVV VGCGGCAAGG GCVACCACCV 3200
GAVGAGCVVC CCVCAGVCVG CCCCVCACGG CGVGGVGVVV CVGCACGVGA 3250
CAVAVGVGCC CGCVCAAGAG AAGAAVVVVA CCACCGCVCC AGCCAVCVGC 3300
CACGACGGCA AAGCCCACVV VCCVAGAGAA GGCGVGVVCG VGVCCAACGG 3350
CACCCAVVGG VVCGVGACAC AGCGGAACVV CVACGAGCCC CAGAVCAVCA 3400
CCACCGACAA CACCVVCGVG VCVGGCAACV GCGACGVCGV GAVCGGCAVV 3450
GVGAACAAVA CCGVGVACGA CCCVCVGCAG CCCGAGCVGG ACAGCVVCAA 3500
AGAGGAACVG GACAAGVACV VVAAGAACCA CACAAGCCCC GACGVGGACC 3550
VGGGCGAVAV CAGCGGAAVC AAVGCCAGCG VCGVGAACAV CCAGAAAGAG 3600
AVCGACCGGC VGAACGAGGV GGCCAAGAAV CVGAACGAGA GCCVGAVCGA 3650
CCVGCAAGAA CVGGGGAAGV ACGAGCAGVA CAVCAAGVGG CCCVGGVACA 3700
VCVGGCVGGG CVVVAVCGCC GGACVGAVVG CCAVCGVGAV GGVCACAAVC 3750
AVGCVGVGVV GCAVGACCAG CVGCVGVAGC VGCCVGAAGG GCVGVVGVAG 3800
CVGVGGCAGC VGCVGCAAGV VCGACGAGGA CGAVVCVGAG CCCGVGCVGA 3850
AGGGCGVGAA ACVGCACVAC ACAVGAVGAC VCGAGCVGGV ACVGCAVCAC 3900
CGCAAVGCVA GCVGCCCCVV VCCCGVCVVC CCCVVCCVVV CVCCACCACC 3950
ACCVCGGGGV CCAGGVAVGC VCCCACCVCC ACCVGCCCCA CVCACCACCV 4000
CVGCVAGVVC CAGACACCVC CCAAGCACGC AGCAAVGCAG CVCAAAACGC 4050
VVAGCCVAGC CACACCCCCA CGGGAAACAG CAGVGAVVAA CCVVVAGCAA 4100
VAAACGAAAG VVVAACVAAG CVAVACVAAC CCCAGGGVVG GVCAAVVVCG 4150
VGCCAGCCAC ACCCVGGAGC VAGCAAAAAA AAAAAAAAAA AAAAAAAAAA 4200
AAAAGCAVAV GACVAAAAAA AAAAAAAAAA AAAAAAAAAA AAAAAAAAAA 4250
AAAAAAAAAA AAAAAAAAAA AAAAAAAAAA AAAA            4284
```

▼ = 1-methyl-3'-pseudouridylyl

FIGURE 4.17   Exact sequence of Pfizer-BioNTech mRNA vaccine.

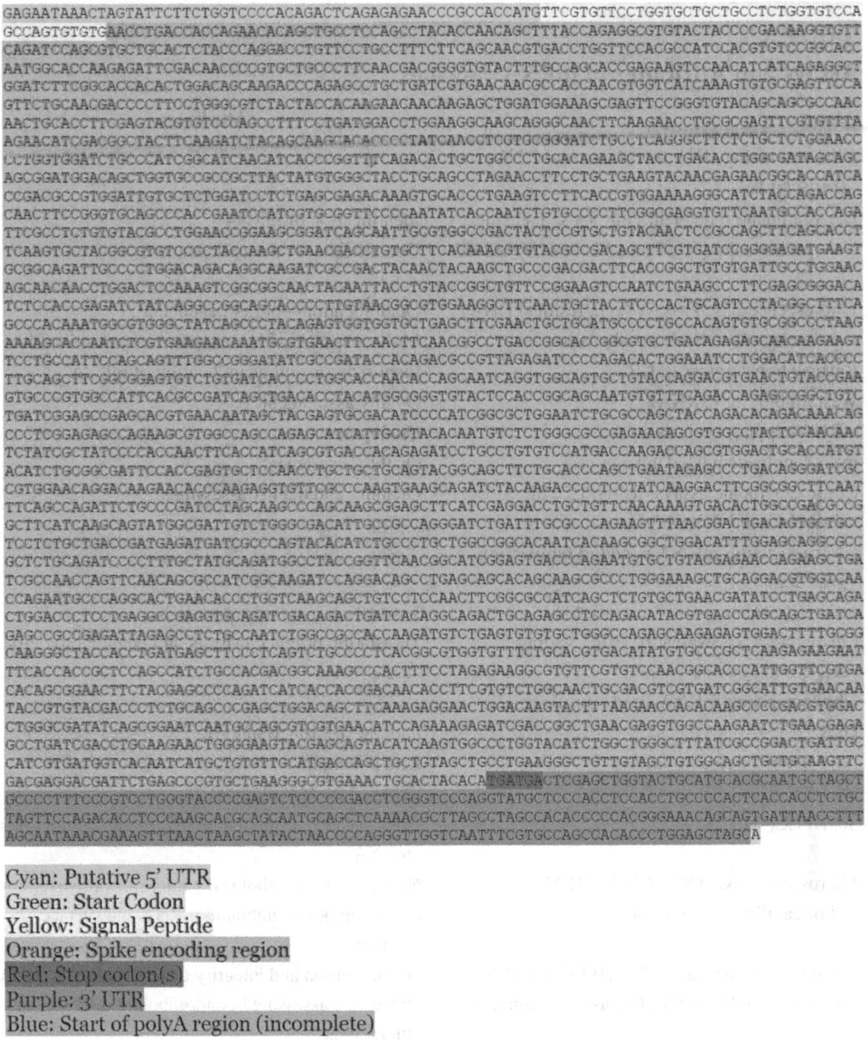

```
GAGAATAAACTAGTATTCTTCTGGTCCCCACAGACTCAGAGAGAACCCGCCACCATGTTCGTGTTCCTGGTGCTGCTGCCTCTGGTGTCCA
GCCAGTGTGTGAACCTGACCACCAGAACACAGCTGCCTCCAGCCTACACCAACAGCTTTACCAGAGGCGTGTACTACCCCGACAAGGTGTT
CAGATCCAGCGTGCTGCACTCTACCCAGGACCTGTTCCTGCCTTTCTTCAGCAACGTGACCTGGTTCCACGCCATCCACGTGTCCGGCACC
AATGGCACCAAGAGATTCGACAACCCCGTGCTGCCCTTCAACGACGGGGTGTACTTTGCCAGCACCGAGAAGTCCAACATCATCAGAGGCT
GGATCTTCGGCACCACACTGGACAGCAAGACCCAGAGCCCTGCTGATCGTGAACAACGCCACCAACGTGGTCATCAAAGTGTGCGAGTTCCA
GTTCTGCAACGACCCCTTCCTGGGCGTCTACTACCACAAGAACAACAAGAGCTGGATGGAAAGCGAGTTCCGGGTGTACAGCAGCGCCAAC
AACTGCACCTTCGAGTACGTGTCCCAGCCTTTCCTGATGGACCTGGAAGGCAAGCAGGGCAACTTCAAGAACCTGCGCGAGTTCGTGTTTA
AGAACATCGACGGCTACTTCAAGATCTACAGCAAGCACACACCCCTATCAACGTCGTGCGGGATCTGCCTCAGGGCTTCTCTGCTCTGGAACC
CCTGGTGGATCTGCCCATCGGCATCAACATCACCCGGTTTCAGACACTGCTGGCCCTGCACAGAAGCTACCTGACACCTGGCGATAGCAGC
AGCGGATGGACAGCTGGTGCCGCCGCTTACTATGTGGGCTACCTGCAGCCTAGAACCTTCCTGCTGAAGTACAACGAGAACGGCACCATCA
CCGACGCCGTGGATTGTGCTCTGGATCCTCTGAGCGAGACAAAGTGCACCCTGAAGTCCTTCACCGTGGAAAAGGGCATCTACCAGACCAG
CAACTTCCGGGTGCAGCCCACCGAATCCATCGTGCGGTTCCCCAATATCACCAATCTGTGCCCCTTCGGCGAGGTGTTCAATGCCACCAGA
TTCGCCTCTGTGTACGCCTGGAACCGGAAGCGGATCAGCAATTGCGTGGCCGACTACTCCGTGCTGTACAACTCCGCCAGCTTCAGCACCT
TCAAGTGCTACGGCGTGTCCCCTACCAAGCTGAACGACCTGTGCTTCACAAACGTGTACGTGCTGTACCCTTCGTGATCCGGGGAGATGAAGT
GCGGCAGATTGCCCCTGGACAGACAGGCAAGATCGCCGACTACAACTACAAGCTGCCCGACGACTTCACCGGCTGTGTGATTGCCTGGAAC
AGCAACAACCTGGACTCCAAAGTCGGCGGCAACTACAATTACCTGTACCGGCTGTTCCGGAAGTCCAATCTGAAGCCCTTCGAGCGGGACA
TCTCCACCGAGATCTATCAGGCCGGCAGCACCCCTTGTAACGGCGTGGAAGGCTTCAACTGCTACTTCCCACTGCAGTCCTACGGCTTTCA
GCCCACAAATGGCGTGGGCTATCAGCCCTACAGAGTGGTGGTGCTGAGCTTCGAACTGCTGCATGCCCCTGCCACAGTGTGCGGCCCTAAG
AAAAGCACCAATCTCGTGAAGAACAAATGCGTGAACTTCAACTTCAACGGCCTGACCGGCACCGGCGTGCTGACAGAGAGCAACAAGAAGT
TCCTGCCATTCCAGCAGTTTGGCCGGGGATATCGCCGATACCACAGACGCCGTTAGAGATCCCCAGACACTGGAAATCCTGGACATCACCCCC
TTGCAGCTTCGGCGGAGTGTCTGTGATCACCCCTGGCACCAACACCAGCAATCAGGTGGCAGTGCTGTACCAGGACGTGAACTGTACCGAA
GTGCCCGTGGCCATTCACGCCGATCAGCTGACACCTACATGGCGGGTGTACTCCACCGGCAGCAATGTGTTTCAGACCAGAGCCGGGCTGTC
TGATCGGAGCCGAGCACGTGAACAATAGCTACGAGTGCGACATCCCCATCGGCGCTGGAATCTGCGCCAGCTACCAGACACAGACAAACAG
CCCTCGGAGAGCCAGAAGCGTGGCCAGCCAGAGCATCATTGCCTACACAATGTCTCTGGGCGCCGAGAACAGCGTGGCCTACTCCAACAAC
TCTATCGCTATCCCCACCAACTTCACCATCAGCGTGACCACAGAGATCCTGCCTGTGTCCATGACCAAGACCAGCGTGGACTGCACCATGT
ACATCTGCGGCGATTCCACCGAGTGCTCCAACCTGCTGCTGCAGTACGGCAGCTTCTGCACCCAGCTGAATAGAGCCCTGACAGGGATCGC
CGTGGAACAGGACAAGAACACCCAAGAGGTGTTCGCCCAAGTGAAGCAGATCTACAAGACCCCTCCTATCAAGGACTTCGGCGGCTTCAAT
TTCAGCCAGATTCTGCCCGATCCTAGCAAGCCCAGCAAGCGGAGCTTCATCGAGGACCTGCTGTTCAACAAAGTGACACTGGCCGACGCCG
GCTTCATCAAGCAGTATGGCGATTGTCTGGGCGACATCGCCGCCAGGGATCTGATTTGCGCCCAGAAGTTTAACGGACTGACAGTGCTGCC
TCCTCTGCTGACCGATGAGATGATCGCCCAGTACACATCTGCCCTGCTGGCCGGCACAATCACAAGCGGCTGGACATTTGGAGCAGGCGCC
GCTCTGCAGATCCCCTTTGCTATGCAGATGGCCTACCGGTTCAACGGCATGGGTGACCTGCAATGTGCTGTACGAGAACCAGAAGCTGATT
TCGCCAACCAGTTCAACAGCGCCATCGGCAAGATCCAGGACAGCCTGAGCAGCACAGCAAGCGCCCTGGGAAAGCTGCAGGACGTGGTCAA
CCAGAATGCCCAGGCACTGAACACCCTGGTCAAGCAGCTGTCCTCCAACTTCGGCGCCATCAGCTCTGTGCTGAACGATATCCTGAGCAGA
CTGGACCCTCCTGAGGCCGAGGTGCAGATCGACAGACTGATCACAGGCAGACTGCAGAGCCTCCAGACATACGTGACCCCAGCAGCTGATCA
GAGCCGCCGAGATTAGAGCCTCTGCCAATCTGGCCGCCACCAAGATGTCTGAGTGTGTGCTGGGCCAGACAAGAGAGTGGACTTTTGCGG
CAAGGGCTACCACCTGATGAGCTTCCCTCAGTCTGCCCCTCACGGCGTGGTGTTTCTGCACGTGACATATGTGCCCGCTCAAGAGAAGAAT
TTCACCACCGCTCCAGCCATCTGCCACGACGGCAAAGCCCACTTTCCTAGAGAAGGCGTGTTCGTGTCCAACGGCACCCATTGGTTCGTGA
CACAGCGGAACTTCTACGAGCCCCAGATCATCACCACCGACAACACCTTCGTGTCTGGCAACTGCGACGTCGTGATCGGCATTGTGAACAA
TACCGTGTACGACCCTCTGCAGCCCGAGCTGGACAGCTTCAAAGAGGAACTGGACAAGTACTTTAAGAACCACACAAAGCCCGACGTGGAC
CTGGGCGATATCAGCGGAATCAATGCCAGCGTCGTGAACATCCAGAAAGAGATCGACCGGCTGAACGAGGTGGCCAAGAATCTGAACGAGA
GCCTGATCGACCTGCAAGAACTGGGGAAGTACGAGCAGTACATCAAGTGGCCCTGGTACATCTGGCTGGGCTTTATCGCCGGACTGATTGC
CATCGTGATGGTCACAATCATGCTGTGTTGCATGACCAGCTGCTGTAGCTGCCTGAAGGGCTGTTGTAGCTGTGGCAGCTGCTGCAAGTTC
GACGAGGACGATTCTGAGCCCGTGCTGAAGGGCGTGAAACTGCACTACACACATGATGACTCGAGCTGGTACTGCATGACACGCAATGCTAGCT
GCCCCTTTCCCGTCCTGGGTACCCCGAGTCTCCCCCGACCTCGGGTCCCAGGTATGCTCCCACCTCCACCTGCCCCACTCACCACCTCTGC
TAGTTCCAGACACCTCCCAAGCACGCAGCAATGCAGCTCAAAACGCTTAGCCTAGCCACACCCCCACGGGAAACAGCAGTGATTAACCTTT
AGCAATAAACGAAAGTTTAACTAAGCTATACTAACCCCCAGGGTTGGTCAATTTCGTGCCAGCCACACCCTGGAGCTAGCA
```

Cyan: Putative 5′ UTR
Green: Start Codon
Yellow: Signal Peptide
Orange: Spike encoding region
Red: Stop codon(s)
Purple: 3′ UTR
Blue: Start of polyA region (incomplete)

FIGURE 4.18 Spike-encoding contig assembled from Moderna mRNA-1273 vaccine. (Source: https://tinyurl.com/mRNASeq)

Table 4.5 shows testing attributes of COVID-19 vaccines.

Table 4.6 shows a comparison of mRNA vaccines; for comparison purposes, a siRNA vaccine is added along with the three mRNA vaccines. However, the CureVac mRNA vaccine failed, as it did not modify the nucleosides that the other two vaccines did.

LNP technology is currently used in all of the major mRNA COVID-19 vaccines. The presence of lipids in the core is a crucial feature of LNPs that distinguishes them

TABLE 4.5

Assays and Attributes of mRNA vaccines

Assays	Attributes
Characterizing DNA templates and RNA transcripts	
DNA template sequencing/mRNA sequencing	Identification of mRNA
UV spectroscopy (A260 nm, A260/A280, A260/A230)	Quantiflcation—purity dependent
Fluorescence-based assays (e.g., residual DNA)	Quantiflcation—purity dependent
Agarose/acrylamide electrophoresis	Molecular mass, RNA integrity and quantification
Reverse transcriptase qPCR	Identiflcntion and quantification of mRNA
Western blot for dsRNA	Quality assessment
mRNA capping analysis	Quality assessment
mRNA polyadenylated tail analysis	Quality assessment
Chromatographic assays: RP-HPLC, SE-HPLC, IP-HPLC, and IEX-HPLC	Quantity and quality assessment
Characterizing mRNA-encoded translation products	
In vitro translation—cell free medium	Translation into target protein
Messenger RNA evaluation using various cell-based systems	Translation product analysis and potential toxicity assay
Characterizing mRNA-lipid complexes	
DLS	Particle size (distribution)
Laser Doppler electrophoresis	Zeta potential
NTA/TRPS	Particle size (distribution)
SE-HPLC(-MALS)	Particle size distribution; assessing bound/unbound mRNA
Microscopy (ciyo TEM, ESEM. AFM)	Nanopaiticle morphology, panicle size (distribution)
Gel or capillaiy electrophoresis	Assessing bound/unbound mRNA and surface charge
Chromatographic assays: RP-HPLC, SE-HPLC, IP-HPLC, and IEX-HPLC/mass spectrometiy	Quantification and integrity of lipids and/or mRNA; for some: assessing bound/unbound mRNA and molar mass
Fluorescent dyes	Encapsulation efficiency
General pharmaceutical tests	
	Appearance, pH osmolality, endotoxin concentration, sterility

Abbreviations: AF4, asymmetrical flow field-flow fractionation; AFM, atomic force microscopy; dsDNA, double-stranded DNA; DLS, dynamic light scattering; ESEM, environmental scanning electron microscopy; IEX-HPLC, ion-exchange high-performance liquid chromatography; IP-HPLC, ion-pair high-performance liquid chromatography; MALS, multi-angle light scattering; NTA, nanoparticle tracking analysis; qPCR, quantitative polymerase chain reaction; RP-HPLC, reversed-phase high-performance liquid chromatography; SE-HPLC, size-exclusion high-performance liquid chromatography; TEM, transmission electron microscopy; TRPS, tunable resistive pulse sensing.

TABLE 4.6
Comparison of mRNA Vaccines

Category	siRNA	Pfizer-BioNTech mRNA vaccine	Moderna mRNA vaccine	CureVac mRNA
Name product	Onpattro patisiran	BNT162b2; Comirnaty	mRNA-1273	CVnCoV
mRNA dose; route of administration	0.3 mg/kg, intravenous	30 μg; intramuscular	100 μg; intramuscular	12 m×; intramuscular
Lipid nanoparticle components	DLin-MC3 DMA: (6Z,9Z,28Z,31Z)-heptatriaconta-6,9,28,31-tetraen-19-yl-4-(dimethylamino) butanaate 1,2-DIstearoyl-5n-glycero-3-phosphocholinc (DSPC) PEG2000-DMG = Alpha (3'-[[1,2-di(myristyloxy) propanoxy] carbonylamino] propyl)-ω-methoxy, polyoxyethylene Cholesterol	0.43 mg ALC-0315 = (4-hydroxybutyl) azanediyl)bis(hexane-6,l-diyl)bis(2-hexyldecanoate) 0.05 mg ALC 0159 2-[(polyethylene glycol)-2000]-N,N ditetradecylacetamide 0.09 mg 1,2-Distearoyl-sn-glycero-3-phosphocholine (DSPC) 0.2 mg Cholesterol	SM-102 (heptadecan-9-yl 8-((2-hydroxyethyl) (6- oxo-6-(undecyloxy) hexyl) amino) octanoate) PEG2000-DMG =1-monomethoxypolyethyleneglycol-2,3-dimyristylglycerol with polyethylene glycol of average molecular weight 2000 1,2-Distearoyl-5n-glycero-3 phosphocholine (DSPC) Cholesterol	Cationic lipid (Acuita Therapeutics) Phcspholipid Cholesterol PEG-lipid conjugate
Molar lipid ratios (%) ionizable cationic lipid: neutral lipid: cholesterol: PEGylated lipid	50:10:38.5:1.5	46.3:9.4:42.7:1.6	50:10:38.5:1.5	50:1C:38.5:1.5
Molar N/P ratios[a]	3	6	6[b]	6[b]
Buffer	Potassium phosphate, monobasic, anhydrous Sodium phosphate, dibasic, heptahydrate pH~7	0.01 mg Potassium dihydrogen phosphate 0.07 mg Disodium hydrogen phosphate dihydrate pH 7–8	Tris (tromethamine) pH 7–8	? pH
Other excipients	Sodium chloride Water for injection	0.01 mg Potassium chloride 0.36 mg Sodium chloride 6 mg Sucrose Water for injection	Sodium acetate Sucrose Water for injection	Saline

from liposomes, spherical vesicles with at least one lipid bilayer, and an aqueous core. At the same time, data from numerous research suggests that water is also present to some level. This means that mRNA could be exposed to an aqueous environment even when encapsulated. Cryogenic transmission electron microscopy revealed this core structure type in unloaded and siRNA (small interfering RNA)-containing LNPs earlier (Table 4.2).

Although mRNA-LNPs are known for having a lipid core, the exact shape of this core and its dependence on lipid constituents (molar ratios) and mRNA localization is still being debated. The RiboGreen assay has confirmed that mRNA is present inside the LNPs. RiboGreen is a dye that fluoresces when attached to single-stranded mRNA but cannot enter LNPs. Because the fraction of accessible mRNA in mRNA-LNP formulations, such as those employed in mRNA vaccines, is relatively low, encapsulation efficiencies derived from RiboGreen experiments are often > 90%. The cryo-TEM and encapsulation findings, taken combined, reveal that mRNA-LNPs create nanoparticles with encapsulated mRNA that is protected from the external medium. The core-shell model, in which the nanoparticles have a surface layer and an amorphous, isotropic core, is the best description of the structure of mRNA encapsulated by LNPs. It has an amorphous core with water holes and inverted cationic lipids surrounding it. The lipids in the core are evenly distributed, with small water pockets interspersed.

The Pfizer-BioNTech COVID-19 vaccine mentions percentages of mRNA integrity between 70 and 75% that were found acceptable by EMA. This information was leaked in an EMA website hack. The deterioration of lipids in LNPs sensitive to hydrolysis and oxidation is chemical instability. Comirnaty and mRNA-1273 do not contain unsaturated fatty acid moieties that can undergo oxidation. Oxidation of encapsulated mRNA can also be caused by oxidative contaminants. Temperature and pH-dependent hydrolysis affect the carboxylic ester linkages in lipids like DSPC and ionizable cationic lipids.

Physical deterioration is another important feature of LNP stability. Aggregation, fusion, and leakage of the encapsulated medicinal substance are the three basic types of physical instability that might occur. LNPs clump together during storage and fusing. LNPs are frequently prepared with PEG-lipids at the surface to prevent individual LNPs from aggregating and increasing shelf stability. The other type of physical degradation, mRNA leakage, primarily affects the encapsulated product's stability. Although the release of the RNA payload from LNPs during storage is not recorded, encapsulation efficiencies are normally > 90%. Unencapsulated mRNA ("naked mRNA") is rarely taken up by cells; additionally, it degrades quickly and is thus unavailable for translation.

The PEG-lipids may be linked to hypersensitivity events, which are uncommon after intramuscular injection of the mRNA-LNP COVID-19 vaccines. Alternative lipids have thus been studied to prevent aggregation formation. Polysarcosine-modified lipids reduced the immunostimulatory response while stabilizing lipid-based systems against aggregation.

4.6.2 ANTIALLERGY mRNA VACCINE

Even though therapeutic DNA vaccines against cedar and peanut allergies have recently entered clinical trials, it is unclear whether these vaccines will meet the high safety requirements required for preventive vaccination in healthy people. Therefore, mRNA vaccines have resurfaced as a possible alternative to DNA vaccines that avoid their risks. mRNA vaccines can prevent allergy sensitization or the formation of TH2 biased immune responses marked by high levels of allergen-specific IgE and the characteristic cytokines IL-4, IL-5, and IL-13. The requirements for preventative allergy vaccination differ significantly from those for regular immunizations. Unlike vaccines for infectious diseases, which aim to induce significant titers of protective antibodies and cellular immunity, a preventive vaccine for allergies introduces an immunological bias, which is then strengthened when the allergen is naturally encountered. Even a barely detectable first immune response elicited by the vaccine is adequate to prevent allergy sensitization.

4.6.3 ANTI-INFECTIVE mRNA VACCINES

Nucleic acid-based vaccines enhance the follicular T helper and germinal B-cell immune responses by simulating infection by live pathogens. The non-replicating mRNA vaccines (modified and unmodified mRNA (NRM)) and self-amplifying mRNA (SAM) vaccines, both generated from positive-strand RNA virus, are currently in use in the prevention of the SARS-Cov-2 virus spread. The alphavirus, a positive-strand virus, is the basis for another mRNA vaccination platform that produces antibodies against the SARS-CoV-2. The structural proteins in these vaccines can be replaced with a gene of interest to produce many anti-infective vaccines. These self-amplifying mRNAs can direct RNA-dependent RNA polymerase complex self-replication and generate numerous copies of the antigen-encoding mRNA.

The immunological response to the mRNA vaccination is subject to many research projects. The RIG-I-like receptor family and TLRs are two types of RNA sensors found in humans. TLR3, TLR7, TLR8, and TLR9 are four TLRs found in dendritic cells, macrophages, and monocytes. TLR3 can distinguish between double-stranded RNA (dsRNA) and single-stranded RNA (ssRNA). TLR7 identifies both dsRNA and ssRNA, whereas TLR8 solely recognizes ssRNA. RIG-I, MDA-5, and LGP2 are all members of the RIG-I family. RIG-I increases interferon production by recognizing ssRNA and dsRNA. MDA5 is a cytosolic RNA sensor that recognizes long double-stranded RNA produced during viral RNA replication. The identification of ds RNA activates IRF-3 and NFKB, increasing IFN-I production. Interferon (IFN) induction using mRNA vaccines is dependent on the in vitro transcribed mRNA, injection route, and delivery vehicle. Pattern recognition receptors (PRRs) are activated after mRNA immunization, and type I IFN production increases. 1 IFN production can be positive or negative, depending on whether the immune response is activated or mRNA translation is blocked.

In contrast to neutralizing the virus, which is achieved by humoral immunity, a cellular immune response such as cytotoxic T lymphocytes (CTLs) directly targets virally infected cells. The amount of LNPs transported to draining lymph nodes and activating B cells determines the degree of antibody production. B cells may ingest LNPs containing mRNA, allowing the mRNA to be translated into protein. Furthermore, B cells interact with B-cell receptors that express foreign antigens. B cells in draining lymph nodes (containing LNP-mRNA) release specific low-affinity antibodies, and some of these antibodies may enter a germinal center (GC). Somatic hypermutation (SHM) and affinity maturation occur in B cells that enter GC. B cells that have developed affinity become plasma blasts and release high-affinity antibodies. They can, however, re-enter GCs that have undergone SHM and become memory B cells.

Antigens should enter the antigen processing pathway for effective CTL induction. The pathogenic antigens are then transported to the cytosol and processed by proteasomes. The transporter involved with antigen processing then delivers the peptides produced by the proteasomal pathway to the endoplasmic reticulum (ER) (TAP). These peptides bind to class I of the major histocompatibility complex in the ER (MHC). The MHC I-antigen peptide complex is then identified at the cell surface by CD8 T cells. 9 Because they may express the antigen in the cytoplasm of antigen-presenting cells, mRNA-based vaccines are particularly well suited for producing powerful CTL responses.

Self-amplification mRNA is released into the body, where it forms a complex with RdRp, which is then translated into protein, eliciting an immunological response. The protein is produced and recognized by CD4+ T helper cells, which activate CD8+ T and B cells, eliciting an immunological response. B cells make neutralizing antibodies, and memory B cells keep the infection memory for future infections. CD8+ T lymphocytes attack virus-infected cells.

4.6.4 RABIES

The rabies virus infects the central nervous system. It is a single-stranded, negative-sense enveloped RNA virus that belongs to the rhabdovirus family. The virus is spread to humans through the bite of an infected mammal (cat or dog). Humans experience flu-like symptoms after infection, followed by severe neurotropic symptoms produced by progressive encephalomyelitis. Various vaccinations against the rabies virus have been licensed; however, rabies infection still has a significant fatality rate. As a result, newer and more effective vaccination candidates are required. In addition, several clinical trials are undergoing for mRNA-based rabies vaccines.

4.6.5 INFLUENZA

Influenza viruses are members of the Orthomyxoviridae family. They are single-stranded RNA viruses with a negative sense. RNA polymerase subunits, viral glycoproteins (haemagglutinin (HA), neuraminidase (NA), nucleoprotein (NP), matrix protein (M1), membrane protein (M2), nonstructural protein (NS1), and nuclear export protein (NEP) are all components of the influenza virus (NEP). Infectious respiratory disease is caused by influenza viruses A and B in humans. In 1918, a major influenza epidemic killed over 40 million people worldwide, similar to SARS-CoV-2. There will be a need for effective influenza vaccination in the future. Three types of influenza vaccinations are currently available in the clinic: inactivated, live attenuated, and recombinant HA vaccines. The HA protein, responsible for viral entry into the host, targets these vaccinations. However, antigenic drift occurs because of the virus's fast evolution, necessitating yearly influenza vaccine modifications. As a result, alternate antigen targeting and quick vaccine manufacture are critical as soon as a new influenza strain appears. For the influenza virus, several mRNA vaccines have been created.

4.6.6 Respiratory Syncytial Virus

Respiratory Syncytial Virus (RSV) is a single-stranded, negative-sense RNA virus that belongs to the Paramyxoviridae family. M2-1 (transcription processivity factor) and M2-2 (switches transcription to DNA replication) make up RSV. There is also a lipid bilayer with fusion (F), attachment (G), and tiny hydrophobic proteins (SH). RSV infection in children causes acute bronchiolitis, associated with a high morbidity and mortality rate. Current RSV vaccine candidates target the highly conserved F protein, which prevents viral fusion; nevertheless, most failed clinical trials due to insufficient neutralizing antibody titers. mRNA-1345 has recently been created as a possible RSV mRNA-based vaccination. Compared to the prior vaccine candidate, mRNA-1777, the sequence of mRNA-1345 has been designed and codon-optimized to improve translation and immunogenicity. The mRNA encodes for a stable prefusion F glycoprotein of RSV by altering the coding sequence.

4.6.7 Human Metapneumovirus and Type 3 Parainfluenza Virus

The respiratory pathogens human metapneumovirus (HMPV) and type 3 parainfluenza virus (PIV3) are members of the Paramyxoviridae family. HMPV is a negative-strand RNA virus with three viral glycoproteins: fusion (F), attachment (G), and short hydrophobic proteins (SHP) (SH). In newborns and young children, HMPV causes respiratory tract infections. PIV3 is a negative-sense RNA virus with a single strand. The nucleoprotein (N), phosphoprotein (P), large polymerase protein (L), an accessory protein (C) encoded by the second open reading frame (ORF) in the P mRNA, an internal matrix protein (M), and two envelope-associated proteins, the fusion (F) and hemagglutinin-neuraminidase (HN) glycoproteins, are the major neutralization and protective antigens. For HMPV and PIV3, there is currently no licensed vaccination; nevertheless, various vaccine candidates have been produced and are now being investigated in preclinical research.

4.6.8 Human Cytomegalovirus

The human cytomegalovirus (HCMV) is a type 5 human herpes virus. These viruses have a protein matrix and double-stranded linear DNA in an icosahedral nucleocapsid. HCMV can be passed from one person to another via direct transmission. Several potential vaccines against HCMV infection and illness are currently being developed. No vaccine, on the other hand, has been approved for use. mRNA-1647 and mRNA-1443, two mRNA vaccine candidates, utilize envelope glycoprotein B precursor (gB) to create HCMV neutralizing antibodies.

4.6.9 ZIKA VIRUS

The Zika virus (ZIKV) is an arthropod-borne virus belonging to the Flaviviridae family that causes Zika. The Zika virus is spread by Aedes mosquito bites, followed by direct transmission from an infected person to an infected person by saliva or sexual contact. Zika is a positive-sense RNA virus with seven structural proteins and three structural proteins: capsid (C), pre membrane (prM), and envelope (E) (NS1, NS2A, NS2B, NS3, NS4A, NS4B, and NS5). ZIKV infection causes moderate influenza-like symptoms and multi-organ failure, meningitis, and encephalitis in difficult situations. The membrane and envelope protein (prM-E) is a common antigen for Zika virus mRNA vaccines because neutralizing antibodies against prM-E can impede viral fusion.

4.6.10 EPSTEIN–BARR VIRUS

The Epstein–Barr virus (EBV), which belongs to the Herpes family, causes mononucleosis. EBV comprises a torsoid-shaped protein core, envelope protein, double-stranded DNA, a 162-capsomere icosahedral capsid, a viral tegument, and a nucleocapsid. EBV is spread by direct contact with infected individuals' saliva. Efforts have been made to produce an EBV prophylactic vaccine to prevent primary infection and eventually chronic disease, but no vaccine for therapeutic use has yet been developed.

4.6.11 HIV

Human immunodeficiency virus (HIV) is a retroviral virus that causes acquired immunodeficiency syndrome (AIDS). HIV is made up of a 5′ long terminal repeat region (LTR) that codes for a promoter for viral gene transcription, the reading frame of the gag gene that codes for outer core membrane (MA), capsid protein (CA), nucleocapsid (NC), and a nucleic acid stabilizing protein. Protease (PR), reverse transcriptase (RT), RNase H, and integrase are all encoded by the pol gene, which comes after gag (IN). The env gene, located next to the pol gene, codes for the envelope glycoproteins gp120 and gp41. HIV became a pandemic, with 17 million individuals infected worldwide. Direct human-to-human transmission is how HIV is spread. Due to the antigenic variety of the envelope protein and the extensive "glycan shield" that masks the envelope protein epitopes, despite years of research, there is currently no effective vaccine against HIV. There have been efforts to develop mRNA vaccines against HIV in recent years. A self-amplifying mRNA vaccine encoding clade C envelope glycoprotein and viral replicon particle (VRP) were tested in rhesus macaques.

4.6.12 STREPTOCOCCUS

Streptococci are gram-positive coccoid bacteria. They are spore-forming and non-motile. They are responsible for a wide range of illnesses and infections. Streptococcus is divided into three groups: A, B, and C. Invasive Skin, soft tissue, and respiratory tract infections are caused by Group A Streptococcus (GAS). The majority of GAS infections are serious and, in some situations, fatal. Invasive infections caused by Group B Streptococcus can affect newborns, pregnant women, and the elderly (GBS). GBS infection causes pneumonia, meningitis, and sepsis, among other symptoms. Infection with Group C Streptococcus is zoonotic, meaning it is spread by contact with infected farm animals. Group C infection causes infections of the skin and soft tissues. There are currently no vaccinations authorized against GAS/GBS, and a vaccine is urgently needed due to the severity of the diseases.

4.6.13 EBOLA VIRUS

Ebola virus belongs to the Filoviridae family and includes negative-sense RNA, surface glycoprotein, lipid membrane envelope, and tubular helical nucleocapsid. Ebola is a zoonotic virus that spreads from vertebrates to humans and other mammals. Secondary transmission occurs when a person comes into contact with tainted blood or body fluids. The gastrointestinal system and the central nervous system are both affected by the virus. It can lead to multi-organ failure, coma, and death in severe situations. The FDA authorized VSV-based Ebola vaccine (rVSV-EBOV) has several safety concerns, including severe arthritis and skin rash at large doses. However, mRNA vaccinations against the Ebola virus may be safer than this viral-based vaccine because they do not reproduce inside the body. The EBOV envelope glycoprotein (EBOV GP) was used to develop two mRNA vaccines. To aid delivery, the mRNAs were encased in lipid nanoparticles.

4.7 CONCLUSION

More lives have been saved by vaccinations than any other modality in the history of humanity; however, the arrival of nucleoside vaccines has transformed the future of disease prevention and expanded it to a level never possible before. Now we can be confident that every immune disorder can be prevented with a proper RNA vaccine; we are also entering the era where instead of expressing antibodies ex vivo, we will have RNA to produce these therapeutic entities. While the RNA vaccines are still produced using a DNA template, they will no longer be needed as PCR techniques become more efficient. The chemical nature of RNA also makes it possible to create copies of these vaccines. This effort will boost the availability of vaccines across the globe and at a cost that would be readily affordable. The technology for RNA vaccine manufacturing is relatively cheaper than any other vaccine, and the speed of development brings us a possibility of managing future pandemics with greater efficiency and fewer deaths.

5 cGMP mRNA Vaccine Manufacturing

5.1 BACKGROUND

Commercial manufacturing of mRNA vaccines is a relatively small-scale and straightforward since the dose administered is small (30 mcg to 100 mcg). It is a chemical production process governed by the regulatory guidelines for chemical drugs (ICH Q7). The upstream process is intended to produce a DNA template, and it is considered a non-GMP step. RNA products produced for clinical trials or commercial distribution must follow the Q7 guideline in this chapter, a list of steps, and documentary proofs required to comply with the requirements. Any form of RNA, including small interfering RNA (siRNA), antisense RNA, CRISPR RNA, ribozyme, aptamer, riboswitch, immunostimulant RNA, transfer RNA (tRNA), ribosomal RNA (rRNA), small nuclear RNA (snRNA), small nucleolar RNA (snoRNA), microRNA (miRNA), or Piwi-interacting RNA (piRNA) can be created.

Technology for manufacturing RNA products is subject to many patents, both issued and pending. Therefore, the information included in this chapter is drawn from public information that is not subject to copyrights. The following US patents were reviewed to compile this chapter: the United States Patent 10017826, 10711315, 10017826; US Applications 20200308634, 20160024547, 20190083602, 20160032273; WO2014140211A1.

[Note—The developer must confirm whether any of the details provided here are protected under intellectual property rights.]

Besides finding newer uses for RNA, its manufacturing process is also evolving rapidly. For example, the standard method of producing mRNA vaccines involves a cell-free IVT process, as shown in Figure 5.1.

Newer trends include continuous processing utilized in the chemical and pharmaceutical industries to provide on-demand output. The relative ease with which mRNA is manufactured lends itself to continuous processing, particularly on a microfluidic scale. Reaction rates can be accelerated under certain conditions, expensive reagents can be avoided, and cascade reactions can be readily segregated at this size. In addition, in situ product removal (ISPR) and substrate feed and product recovery (SFPR) techniques can be used in flow to help with process control, recirculation, and compound reuse. These methodologies will allow the separation of molecules that can be recirculated, such as enzymes (if free enzymes are utilized), cofactors, or NTPs. TFF, aqueous two-phase systems (ATPS), and precipitation are examples of unit operations that could be employed for this. These could ease the pressure on downstream processing while also lowering overall processing costs. In addition, the suggested technology could be used in conjunction with a microfluidic formulation step in which the

DOI: 10.1201/9781003248156-6

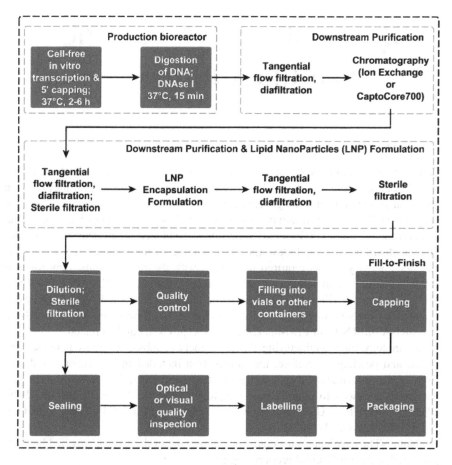

FIGURE 5.1 Process flow diagram for mRNA drug substance production and drug product manufacturing.

mRNA is encapsulated in lipid nanoparticles (LNPs). This would allow continuous mRNA processing to be established until the fill-to-finish phases (Figure 5.2).

Downstream processing and fill-to-finish are still the critical bottlenecks in mRNA vaccine production. The process continues as traditional precipitation or nuclease digesting processes. Alternative cost-effective procedures that may be used in a continuous mode, such as single-pass tangential flow filtration (SPTFF) or aqueous two-phase systems (ATPS), could enhance process time and manufacturing flexibility while lowering costs and maintaining quality. New chromatographic operation modes can also eliminate the requirement for repeated mRNA purification procedures. Multimodal chromatography, for example, has a lot of potential since the combination of interactions between the molecule and the matrix might result in an integrated and intensified purification process without the need for several chromatographic processes.

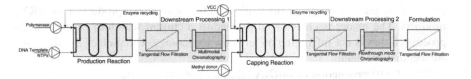

FIGURE 5.2   A conceptual architecture for a continuous manufacturing process for mRNA vaccines. The technique consists of a continuous 2-step enzymatic reaction, enzyme recycling employing tangential flow filtering strategies, and two multimodal chromatography phases, one in a bind-elute mode for intermediate purification and the other in a flowthrough mode for polishing. In addition, a third tangential flow filtration module is used for formulation.

mRNA instability and inefficient protein production make optimizing therapeutic mRNAs and vaccines difficult. PERSIST-seq is a new approach that uses an RNA sequencing technology to systematically characterize in-cell mRNA stability, ribosome load, and in-solution stability of a library of different mRNAs. Protein output is driven more by in-cell stability than by a high ribosome load. There are guidelines for preventing hydrolytic deterioration depending on sequence and structure. Highly organized "super-folder" mRNAs can be created to promote both stability and expression, with pseudo-uridine nucleoside modification providing even more benefits.

5.2   CGMP PROCESS

mRNA is a transitory copy of genetic information that acts as a model for protein synthesis in all species. Unlike DNA, it has all of the ingredients necessary for constructing a suitable vector for the transfer of foreign genetic information in vivo. Since the discovery of these properties of mRNA, many advancements in mRNA manufacturing have been made, including in vitro transcribed RNA and pharmaceutical-grade mRNA produced in vitro using a runoff transcription method in which all structural mRNA elements (save the 5' Cap and, in some methods, the 3' poly(A) tail) are contained in the template plasmid DNA (pDNA). To ensure defined transcription termination, purified plasmid DNA is linearized by sequence-specific cleavage using a restriction enzyme and then employed as a DNA template for RNA in vitro transcription. The in vitro transcription reaction mixture includes linearized template DNA, reaction buffer, recombinant RNA polymerase, nucleotides, and, in some methods, Cap analog. A second enzymatic capping step following transcription is used in other procedures. When the RNA polymerase reaches the end of the DNA template, transcription comes to a halt, releasing both the template DNA and the freshly created mRNA. Polyadenylation of the mRNA molecule is accomplished either by encoding a poly(T) sequence of about 50 nucleotides on the pDNA and adding it during the in vitro transcription reaction or by enzymatically synthesizing the poly(A) tail in a post-transcriptional step. Finally, multiple purification techniques are used to purify the mRNA product, all of which comprise a nuclease digestion phase followed by template DNA removal.

The cGMP-compliant chromatographic method improves the activity of mRNA molecules up to about five times regarding protein expression in vivo. Several recent patents filed provide details of innovations in the commercial production of mRNA products. The reader is encouraged to conduct a current search to ensure that the process chosen is not infringing on any new technology. The preface discusses this subject in more detail.

The cGMP production of mRNA takes a different path than the research-grade mRNA manufacturing, where economics require a yield of 1–10g of mRNA batch to make the process commercially feasible.

5.3   MANUFACTURING PROCESS

5.3.1   PROTOCOL 1 STEPS

1. Selection of an RNA sequence (to be produced by in vitro transcription);
2. Reverse transcription of the target RNA sequence;
3. Plasmid template DNA synthesis with a nucleic acid sequence encoding the RNA sequence;
4. Plasmid template DNA quality assurance: transformation of the plasmid template DNA into bacteria; identification of the nucleic acid sequence encoding the RNA sequence;
5. Fermentation;
6. Plasmid template DNA quality control: plasmid template DNA yield estimation and identification of the nucleic acid sequence encoding the RNA sequence; plasmid template DNA isolation (giga preparation);
7. Isolated plasmid template DNA quality control includes determining the identity of the nucleic acid sequence encoding the RNA sequence as well as the purity of the plasmid template DNA preparation.
   - Photometric determination of the plasmid template DNA content;
   - Determination of RNA contaminations; restriction analysis of the test plasmid isolation for determining the identity of the nucleic acid sequence encoding the RNA sequence; sequencing of the insert DNA sequence for determining the identity of the nucleic acid sequence encoding the RNA sequence
   - Determination of the presence and the amount of an endotoxin;
   - Determination of protein content;
   - Determination of bioburden; and
   - Determination of bacterial DNA.
8. Linearization of plasmid template DNA;
9. Quality control of linearized plasmid template DNA, such as linearization completeness, RNA yield estimation, and RNA identity determination.
   - Control of linearization;
   - Determination of RNA identity in test in vitro transcription by agarose gel electrophoresis
   - Determination of RNase contaminations in linearized plasmid template DNA;

5.3.1.1   IVT Steps

1. In vitro transcription;
2. The first purification of the in vitro transcribed RNA by precipitation is LiCl precipitation;
3. Quality control of in vitro transcribed RNA: RNA identity determination, followed by preparative RP-HPLC and precipitation of in vitro transcribed RNA
4. Quality control of in vitro produced RNA includes determining RNA identity and integrity using gel electrophoresis, which is more often known as agarose gel electrophoresis. Lyophilization of in vitro transcribed RNA, freeze-dried RNA resuspension, and sterile filtration of the resuspended RNA. The sterile filter used in step Q is tested by conducting a bubble-point test. After resuspending the RNA, the RNA yield is measured photometrically.

5.3.1.2   Final Quality Testing Steps:

1. Determination of RNA identity by RNase digestion;
2. Determination of RNA identity by RT-PCR;
3. Determination of RNA identity and RNA integrity by agarose gel electrophoresis;
4. Determination of pH;
5. Determination of osmolality;
6. Determination of bioburden;
7. Determination of endotoxins;
8. Determination of protein content;
9. Determination of plasmid template DNA;
10. Determination of bacterial DNA; and
11. Acetonitrile, chloroform, triethylammonium acetate (TEAA), isopropanol, and phenol) are used to determine the presence and quantity of an organic solvent.

5.3.2   PROTOCOL 2 STEPS

1. Selection of an RNA sequence (to be produced by in vitro transcription);
2. Reverse transcription of the target RNA sequence;
3. Quality control of the plasmid template DNA: determination of the identity of the nucleic acid sequence encoding the RNA sequence; synthesis of a plasmid template DNA containing a nucleic acid sequence encoding the RNA sequence;
   • By restriction analysis and
   • By sequencing the nucleic acid sequence encoding the RNA sequence;
4. Transformation of the plasmid template DNA into bacteria;
5. Fermentation;
6. Plasmid template DNA quality control: plasmid template DNA yield estimation and identification of the nucleic acid sequence encoding the RNA

sequence; test plasmid template photometric assessment of the plasmid template DNA content and DNA isolation (mini preparation) to estimate plasmid template DNA yield;

- Test plasmid template DNA isolation (mini preparation) and photometric determination of the plasmid template DNA content to estimate the yield of plasmid template DNA; and
- Determination of the identity of the nucleic acid sequence encoding the RNA sequence by restriction analysis of the test plasmid isolation;

7. Plasmid template DNA isolation (giga preparation);
8. Quality control of isolated plasmid template DNA: determination of the identity of the nucleic acid sequence encoding the RNA sequence and determination of the purity of the plasmid template DNA preparation:
   - Photometric determination of the plasmid template DNA content;
   - Determination of RNA contaminations;
   - Determination of the identity of the nucleic acid sequence encoding the RNA sequence by restriction analysis of the test plasmid isolation;
   - Determination of the identity of the nucleic acid sequence encoding the RNA sequence by sequencing the insert DNA sequence;
   - Determination of the presence and the amount of an endotoxin;
   - Determination of protein content;
   - Determination of bioburden; and
   - Determination of bacterial DNA.
9. Linearization of plasmid template DNA;
10. Quality control of linearized plasmid template DNA, e.g., completeness of linearization, estimation of RNA yield, and determination of RNA identity:
    - Control of linearization;
    - Determination of RNA identity in test in vitro transcription by agarose gel electrophoresis; and
    - Determination of RNase contaminations in linearized plasmid template DNA;
11. In vitro transcription;
12. The first purification of the in vitro transcribed RNA by precipitation is LiCl-precipitation;
    - Quality control of the in vitro transcribed RNA: determination of RNA identity by agarose gel electrophoresis;
13. The second purification of the in vitro transcribed RNA by preparative RP-HPLC and precipitation;
14. Quality control of the in vitro transcribed RNA: determination of RNA identity and RNA integrity determination of the RNA identity and RNA integrity by agarose gel electrophoresis;
15. Lyophilization of the in vitro transcribed RNA, resuspension of the freeze-dried RNA, and sterile filtration of the resuspended RNA;
16. Quality control: determination of the RNA yield:
    - Photometric determination of RNA content; and
    - Bubble-point-test for control of the sterile filter.

17. End-product-control: determination of RNA identity, RNA integrity, and purity of in vitro transcribed RNA:
    - Determination of RNA identity by RNase digestion;
    - Determination of RNA identity by RT-PCR;
    - Determination of RNA identity and RNA integrity by agarose gel electrophoresis;
    - Determination of pH;
    - Determination of osmolality;
    - Determination of bioburden;
    - Determination of endotoxins;
    - Determination of protein content;
    - Determination of plasmid template DNA;
    - Determination Of Bacterial DNA; and
    - Determination of the presence and the amount of an organic solvent (acetonitrile, chloroform, triethylammonium acetate (TEAA), isopropanol, and phenol).

5.3.3 FACILITY

A commercial mRNA vaccine facility is small; to produce ten billion doses per year, a facility of about 10,000 sq-ft will be sufficient. The mRNA production is a four-stage process: creating linearized DNA (upstream), in vitro transcription into mRNA (downstream), LNP (formulation), fill, and finish. Unlike the production of recombinant therapeutic proteins, the upstream area will be non-GMP, where the plasmid is made and the DNA linearized, while the downstream area should be class 10,000. Since the downstream process is smaller, this can be achieved by using laminar downdraft or standard hoods to reduce the cost. MRNA production can be established in any space available without spending millions on building a qualified facility. The manufacturing can begin in less than six months; the bulk of the cost goes into chemical materials for production. The equipment requirements are standard, including a smaller 30 L bacterial fermentation reactor to produce pDNA, single-use mixing chambers, chromatography systems, and filtration systems. Special equipment is required to formulate LNP, and these mixers are in high demand requiring early acquisition. The fill and finish part is a standard injectable facility as a clean room, and using dedicated filling heads prevents cross-contamination.

A proposed design for a cGMP-compliant manufacturing facility is shown in Figure 5.3.

The overall production involves several well-defined steps (Figure 5.4).

5.3.4 PRODUCT SELECTION

The mRNA vaccine sequence is established based on the target protein desired for translation, such as the surface protein A chosen for the two mRNA vaccines against COVID-19. Figures 5.3). The mRNA sequence of the target vaccine is analyzed first by extracting it in a phenol-chlor4form mixture using TRIzol Reagent (a complete,

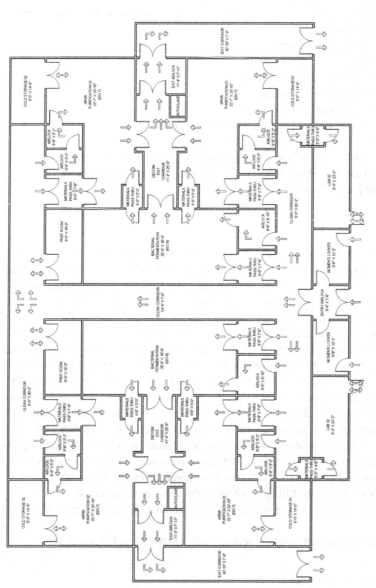

FIGURE 5.3 cGMP compliant manufacturing facility to produce 10 billion doses of mRNA vaccine. The upstream and downstream areas can be used to produce multiple batches, including plasmid DNA, the IVT, purification, and formulation steps. Manufacturing and testing starting materials for ATMPs do not require a GMP accreditation (EU designation of mRNA products). For mRNA products, this includes creating plasmid and DNA linearization. However, the FDA has not yet guided GMP compliance of plasmid and linearization, but it is understood. This means that the high cost of GMP compliance is avoided—at least in the upstream manufacturing stage of plasmid production and DNA linearization.

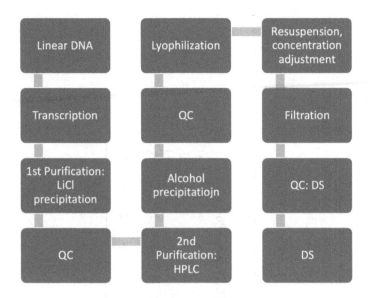

FIGURE 5.4   Flowchart of manufacturing of mRNA vaccine.

ready-to-use reagent for the isolation of total RNA). Within one hour, this monophasic solution of phenol and guanidine isothiocyanate is designed to isolate different fractions of RNA, DNA, and proteins from human, animal, plant, yeast, or bacterial cell and tissue samples, with intactness verified using a bioanalyzer before and after extraction. The RNA is then fragmented by heating to 94°C, primed with a random hexamer-tailed adaptor, amplified through a template-switch protocol, and finally sequenced using a sequencing instrument with paired-end 78-per-end sequencing such as for the COVID-19 vaccines. An RNA of known concentration and sequence (such as from bacteriophage MS2) is used as the reference for the target vaccine.

5.3.5 Reverse Transcription of the Target RNA Sequence

The target RNA sequence is reverse transcribed into a DNA sequence to provide a template DNA for RNA in vitro transcription (cDNA, complementary DNA). This cDNA is produced, e.g., by using reverse transcriptase and an RNA sequence comprising the target RNA sequence as the template (also termed as "enzymatic reverse transcription"). Alternatively, the reverse transcription is performed in silico, which means that the reverse transcription is performed virtually, e.g., by a computer.

For in vitro transcription, the template DNA has the elements in 5′–3′ orientation, as shown in Table 5.1.

When a peptide or protein is encoded, the RNA sequence is tweaked or designed to produce proteins with certain properties (optimized stability, defined localization, membrane integration, etc.). However, without modifying the encoded protein sequence, the open reading frame encoding the protein encoded by the RNA can be sequence-modified, for example, by GC-enrichment, codon optimization,

TABLE 5.1
A Promoter/Binding Site for a DNA-Dependent RNA Polymerase such as T3, T7, and SP6

																	+1					
T7	T	A	A	T	A	C	G	A	C	T	C	A	C	T	A	T	A	G	G	G	A	G	A
SP6	A	T	T	T	A	G	G	T	G	A	C	A	C	T	A	T	A	G	A	A	G	N	G
T3	A	A	T	T	A	A	C	C	C	T	C	A	C	T	A	A	A	G	G	G	A	G	A

elimination of restriction sites needed for subcloning, and elimination of instability motifs (e.g., AU-rich elements, miRNA binding sites). These AU-rich fingerprints are especially common in genes with a high turnover rate. AU-rich elements (AREs) are divided into three groups based on their sequence characteristics and functional attributes.

Class I AREs have several copies of an AUUUA pattern within U-rich locations. Class I AREs can be found in the proteins C-Myc and MyoD. Two or more UUAUUUA(U/A)(U/A) nonamers are present in Class II AREs. TNF-a and GM-CSF are two molecules that include this form of ARE. ARES of Class III has a hazy definition. There is no AUUUA pattern in these U-rich locations.

Alternatively, you might choose a wild-type nucleic acid sequence that encodes a protein of interest.

Artificial gene syntheses, such as solid-phase DNA synthesis, oligonucleotide annealing, or PCR, generate the DNA sequence encoding the target RNA sequence (unmodified (wild type) or modified).

5.3.6 SYNTHESIS OF THE TEMPLATE DNA BY PCR

Class I AREs have several copies of an AUUUA pattern within U-rich locations. Class I AREs can be found in the proteins C-Myc and MyoD. Two or more UUAUUUA(U/A)(U/A) nonamers are present in Class II AREs. TNF-a and GM-CSF are two molecules that include this form of ARE. ARES of Class III has a hazy definition. There is no AUUUA pattern in these U-rich locations.

Alternatively, you might choose a wild-type nucleic acid sequence that encodes a protein of interest.

Artificial gene syntheses, such as solid-phase DNA synthesis, oligonucleotide annealing, or PCR, generate the DNA sequence encoding the target RNA sequence (unmodified (wild type) or modified).

5.3.7 SELECTION AND DESIGN OF A PLASMID DNA VECTOR BACKBONE

Depending on the host organism, plasmid DNA vectors for the synthesis of template DNA plasmids are chosen. Bacteria, notably Escherichia coli (E. coli), are employed to produce, replicate, and amplify plasmid DNA. In genetic engineering, plasmids are widely utilized as vectors. In addition, plasmids are useful tools in genetics and biotechnology labs because they may be used to replicate (produce numerous copies) or express (convert genes into proteins). pDP (Ambion), pGEM (Promega), pBluescript (Stratagene), pCRII (Invitrogen), pUC57, pJ204 (from DNA 2.0), and pJ344 (from DNA 2.0), pUC18, pBR322, and pUC19 are only a few of the commercially available plasmids for this purpose.

Commonly, cDNA encoding or corresponding to the RNA sequence of interest (target RNA sequence) is inserted into a plasmid that typically contains several features. These include a gene that makes the bacterial cells resistant to particular antibiotics (normally kanamycin or ampicillin), an origin of replication to allow bacterial cells to replicate the plasmid DNA, and a multiple cloning site (MCS, or polylinker). A multiple cloning site is a short region containing several commonly used restriction sites allowing the easy insertion of DNA fragments at this location.

Although many host organisms and molecular cloning vectors are in use, most molecular cloning experiments begin with a laboratory strain of the bacterium Escherichia coli (E. coli) and a plasmid cloning vector. E. coli and plasmid vectors are in common use because they are technically sophisticated, versatile, widely available, and offer rapid growth of recombinant organisms with minimal equipment.

Particularly useful cloning vectors for E. coli are vectors based on pUC19 or pBR322. For the use as a template for in vitro transcription reactions, the plasmid DNA vector typically carries a binding site for a DNA-dependent RNA polymerase, T3, T7, or SP6 polymerase (T3-, T7-, or SP6 promoter). To increase the transcription, translation, and stability, further elements are included in the plasmid:

12. a 5′-UTR (particularly preferred are TOP-UTRs;
13. a Kozak sequence, or another translation initiation element (CCR(A/G) CCAUGG, where R is a purine (adenine or guanine) three bases upstream of the start codon (AUG), which is followed by another "G." 5′ UTR also have been known to form secondary structures, which are involved in elongation factor binding);
14. a 3′ UTR (particularly preferred are UTRs from stable RNAs, particularly from albumin gene, an a-globin gene, a β-globin gene, a tyrosine hydroxylase gene, a lipoxygenase gene, and a collagen alpha gene;
15. a poly(A) sequence;
16. a poly(C) sequence; and
17. a stem-loop sequences, e.g., histone stem-loop sequences according to WO2012019780.

The preferred plasmids are based on the DNA plasmid pUC19. The different variants (pCV19, pCV26, pCV32, and pCV22min) differ in restriction sites and 5′ and 3′ UTRs. Vectors are based on pCV26, as shown in Figure 5.5.

The template DNA comprising a nucleic acid sequence encoding an RNA is a plasmid DNA vector.

5.3.8 SYNTHESIS OF A TEMPLATE PLASMID DNA VECTOR BY CLONING

A restriction endonuclease is used to linearize the DNA at the place where the DNA sequence encoding the target RNA sequence (the insert DNA sequence) is introduced into a DNA plasmid vector backbone. The restriction enzyme is chosen so that the cleavage site on the vector generates a configuration that is compatible with the insert sequence ends. Typically, this is accomplished by using the same restriction enzyme(s) to cleave the plasmid DNA vector backbone and insert DNA sequence (PCR product, DNA sequence generated by artificial gene synthesis, e.g., solid-phase DNA synthesis, or insert extracted from a plasmid).

Two distinct enzymes, generating two different cleavage site configurations, are chosen to introduce an insert into a vector to allow orientated integration (one

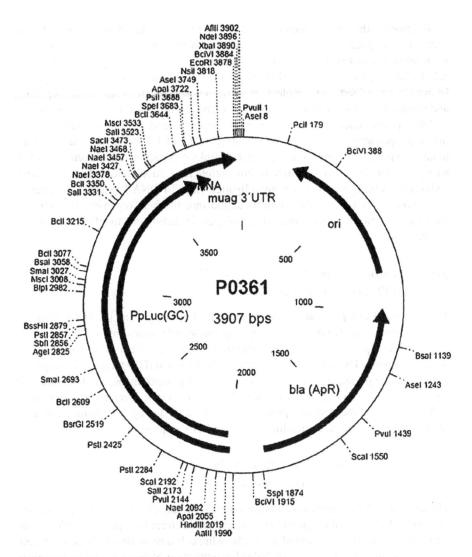

FIGURE 5.5 Synthesis of a template plasmid DNA vector:

enzyme at the 5' end and a separate enzyme at the 3' end). This prevents the vector from ligating to itself during the ligation process and guarantees that the inserts are incorporated in the proper orientation.

Vectors typically contain a variety of convenient cleavage sites accumulated in the multiple cloning site (MCS) that are unique within the vector molecule (so that the vector can only be cleaved at a single site). Optionally the MCS is located within a reporter gene (frequently beta-galactosidase) whose inactivation is used to distinguish recombinant from non-recombinant constructs at a later step in the process (colonies without insert develop a blue color in the presence of the respective substrate and an (optionally) an inducer; blue-white selection).

To improve the ratio of recombinant to non-recombinant constructs, the cleaved vector is additionally treated with an enzyme (a phosphatase, e.g., alkaline phosphatase) that removes the 5′ phosphate and therefore prevents the ligase from being able to fuse the two ends of the linearized vector, and therefore avoids self-ligation. Moreover, linearized vector molecules with dephosphorylated ends cannot replicate, and replication can only be restored if insert DNA is integrated into the cleavage site.

DNA inserts encoding the target RNA sequence and the linearized vector are mixed at appropriate concentrations (commonly 1:1 or 1:3 molar ratio) and exposed to an enzyme (DNA ligase) that covalently links compatible ends together (that is, sticky ends produced by the same or compatible restriction endonucleases, or blunt ends). This joining reaction is termed ligation (e.g., T4 DNA Ligase). The resulting DNA mixture is then ready for introduction into the host organism (Escherichia coli) using common transformation techniques, including chemical transformation or electroporation.

5.3.9   Synthesis of the Template Plasmid DNA Vector by Oligonucleotide Annealing

The template DNA plasmid vector is synthesized by integrating the DNA sequence encoding the target RNA sequence by oligonucleotide annealing. In this case, the insert DNA sequence is directly synthesized into the sequence of a plasmid DNA vector backbone. This alternative is particularly preferred if the target RNA sequence is not a wild-type sequence comprised of a naturally occurring RNA. Therefore, the reverse transcription cannot be performed by an enzymatic reverse transcription.

The quality of the template plasmid DNA is controlled by determining the identity of the DNA sequence encoding the target RNA sequence.

5.3.10   Amplification of the Template Plasmid DNA Vector: Transformation

The template DNA plasmid vector is amplified by propagation in bacteria, particularly in E. coli. Therefore, the plasmid is inserted into bacteria by a process called transformation. Particularly preferred are Escherichia coli host strains. Different methods for transforming plasmid DNA include electroporation of electro-competent cells or heat shock transformation of chemically competent cells. A preferred method is the transformation of chemically competent cells by heat shock, using strains comprising DH5alpha, DH10B, Mach1, OmniMax 2, Stbl2, Top 10, and Top 10F. In this context, 1–10 ng, is (4–5 ng) purified plasmid are mixed with 50 ml chemical competent cells, e.g., CaCl2-competent cells, is DH5 alpha. The mixture is incubated for at least 30 minutes at 0–5°C. Subsequently, the mixture is incubated for 20 s at 42°C. After the heat shock, the mixture is incubated at 0–5°C for several minutes.

For plating the cells, 900 ml LB-medium is added; incubated for 1–3 h at 37°C and plated on LB agar plates containing antibiotics, e.g., ampicillin or kanamycin, dependent on the antibiotic resistance gene encoded on the vector and incubated 12–24 h at 37°C.

The transformation efficacy is evaluated based on the number of colonies formed. E. coli cells are transformed for each production campaign. Only bacteria that take up copies of the plasmid survive since it makes them resistant (ampicillin resistance). In particular, the resistance genes are expressed (used to make a protein), and the expressed protein either breaks down the antibiotics or prevents them from inhibiting certain bacterial pathways. The antibiotics act as a filter to select only the bacteria containing the plasmid DNA. These bacteria are grown in large amounts, harvested, and lysed to isolate the plasmid of interest.

The next step is to design a plasmid DNA that contains the gene, restriction site, 3′ primer site, origin of replication, antibiotic resistance gene, a selectable marker, promoter, 5′ primer site, and restriction site. This design is readily created using online resources such as www.en.vectorbuilder.com. The gene of interest (above) is inserted into the pDNA, which is then introduced into host bacteria (typically E. coli) in transformation, usually by electroporation. The host cells are gown to produce DNA. E. coli in a small bioreactor, not more than 30L in size, to produce about 30 g of plasmid DNA in each batch. Alternately, the PCR technology can be used to produce DNA; developments in the PCR technology are coming fast, and it is anticipated to replace the current upstream process. The main reason for selecting the fermentation process is the lower cost of the product. However, the PCR-based DNA is purer, reducing the amount needed and thus the cost. In addition, the PCR-produced DNA provides about 4–5 times higher yield than the fermentation process.

When the projected cell density is achieved, cells are harvested, and pDNA extracted, typically by alkaline lysis. Next, the lysate is clarified and DNA linearized by restriction digestion using enzymes that generate blunt ends or 5′-overhangs.

No animal-derived raw materials are used to produce mRNA, which is done in a cell-free environment. As a result, there are no cell-derived contaminants or accidental contaminations, making the production of these compounds safer.

The selected RNA sequence corresponds to the target RNA molecule in the DNA template stage. The selected RNA sequence is a coding RNA, which encodes a protein sequence or a fragment or variant thereof (e.g., fusion proteins), and is selected from therapeutically active proteins or peptides, including adjuvant proteins, tumor antigens, pathogenic antigens (e.g., selected, from animal antigens, from viral antigens, from protozoal antigens, from bacterial antigens), allergenic antigens, autoimmune antigens, or further antigens from allergens, from antibodies, from immunostimulatory proteins or peptides, from antigen-specific T-cell receptors, biologics, cell-penetrating peptides, secreted proteins, plasma membrane proteins, cytoplasmic or cytoskeletal proteins, intracellular membrane-bound proteins, nuclear proteins, proteins associated with human disease, targeting moieties, or those proteins encoded by the human genome, for which no therapeutic indication has been identified but which, nonetheless, have utility in areas of research and discovery.

The cGMP process mandates in-process controls such as the concentration of the template as measured by a photometric method); nucleic acid sequence coding of the RNA by PCR, restriction analysis or sequence analysis, etc. The purity of template, endotoxin, bacteria DNA and ribonuclease is also tested. The purity of the RNA is obtained by determining the presence and the amount of protein; the presence and the amount of endotoxin; the presence and the amount of bacterial DNA; the presence and the amount of plasmid DNA; and the presence the amount of organic solvent.

The presence of a protein, an endotoxin, a bacterial DNA, a plasmid DNA, and an organic solvent is determined qualitatively, such as PCR. The presence and the amount of bacterial DNA are determined using a universal primer pair for bacterial DNA. Alternatively, a primer pair specific for E. coli DNA is used to determine the presence and the amount of E. coli DNA. The pH and the osmolality are determined, and these must fall within the acceptable ranges.

The template DNA or fragment is synthesized chemically by ligating at least two DNA fragments. Each DNA fragment is a nucleic acid sequence encoding a fragment of the selected RNA sequence. The template DNA is generally a circular DNA plasmid comprising a bacterial origin of replication and a selection marker. Such a plasmid DNA is typically produced in bacteria. The plasmid DNA is transformed into bacteria, the bacteria are cultured under selective conditions, and the plasmid DNA is isolated from the bacteria.

To control the quality of the template DNA, its concentration is monitored by photometric methods, determining the presence and the amount of RNA contamination; determining the identity of the template DNA by restriction analysis; determining the identity of the template DNA by sequence analysis; determining the presence and the amount of endotoxin; determining the presence and the amount of protein; determining the bioburden; determining the presence and the amount of bacterial DNA; and determining the presence and the amount of E. coli DNA.

The quality of the template DNA is controlled, after linearization of the template DNA, by controlling the linearization, estimating RNA yield in an in vitro transcription reaction, determining the identity of an RNA obtained in the in vitro transcription reaction, and determining any ribonuclease contamination.

A single transformed E. coli colony is taken from the agar plate and used to inoculate a liquid LB medium culture (containing antibiotics, e.g., 100 mg/ml ampicillin). The culture is grown for 4–8 h at 37°C under shaking. 5–10 ml of that culture are then used to inoculate a larger volume (e.g., 1 l LB medium containing antibiotics) in the fermenter. Standard parameters (e.g., pH, oxygen concentration, anti-foam, shaking, temperature) are precisely regulated and continuously monitored during fermentation overnight (12–20 h). In addition, the cell density is controlled by photometric determination at 600 nm. After fermentation, a culture sample is taken for quality control, and cells are harvested and centrifuged. The cell pellet is stored at £–20°C.

5.3.11 QUALITY CONTROL: ISOLATION OF PLASMID DNA AND SUBSEQUENT ANALYSIS OF THE PLASMID DNA

Plasmid DNA is isolated from 1 ml of E. coli cells using a standard plasmid preparation kit known in the art. The concentration of the isolated plasmid DNA is determined by a standard photometric method for nucleic acids via measurement of the absorption at 260 nm (OD260) to estimate the expected total plasmid DNA yield of the whole fermentation. To confirm the correct gene, the restriction pattern of the extracted plasmid DNA is analyzed and evaluated. Alternatively, a PCR uses suitable primer pairs with E. coli cells as a template. The PCR product is analyzed using agarose gel electrophorese.

5.3.12 Isolation of Plasmid DNA by Mini Preparation kit

Preparations of plasmid DNA are obtained by various methods comprising the alkaline lysis method and the boiling method; moreover, various kits for preparation of plasmid DNA are commercially available (e.g., NucleoSpin Plasmid Kit; Macherey Nagel; QIAprep Miniprep kit; QIAGEN) which commonly use a silica membrane that binds DNA in the presence of a high concentration of chaotropic salt, and allows elution in a small volume of low-salt buffer. This technology eliminates time-consuming phenol-chloroform extraction and alcohol precipitation. The concentration of the isolated plasmid DNA is determined by a standard photometric method for nucleic acids via measurement of the absorption at 260 nm (OD260).

The identity of the DNA sequence encoding the target RNA sequence is confirmed using restriction analysis.

5.3.13 Plasmid Preparation

Plasmid DNA was isolated from the frozen E. coli cell culture pellet by chromatography using an endotoxin-free Giga preparation kit (e.g., EndoFree Plasmid Giga Kit of Qiagen, or Endotoxin-free plasmid DNA purification of Macherey Nagel). It is important to minimize the endotoxin level during the production process. The concentration of the isolated plasmid DNA is determined by a standard photometric method for nucleic acids via measurement of the absorption at 260 nm (OD260). Finally, the yield of the isolated plasmid DNA is calculated.

Quality control of the plasmid DNA:

- Determination of the identity of the DNA sequence encoding the target RNA sequence
- Determination of purity of template DNA plasmid by restriction analysis
- Sequencing of the insert DNA sequence.

In addition, the purity of the plasmid preparation is determined by the determination of RNA contaminations, determination of endotoxins, determination of protein content, determination of bioburden, and determination of residual E. coli DNA.

5.3.14 Linearization

The isolated plasmid DNA is linearized by a specific, singular, enzymatic restriction to provide a defined linear template for the following RNA in vitro transcription process. This ensures a defined termination of the in vitro RNA transcription procedure by avoiding transcriptional read-through. The linearized DNA template is purified, and the content and yield of the linear DNA are determined. Preferred endonucleases for linearizing the pDNA template include BciVI, XbaI, SpeI, HindIll, NotI, EcoRI, NdeI, AflII, HindIll, and SapI. The most preferred restriction enzyme is EcoRI. Composition of one reaction:

1. 1 mg plasmid DNA
2. 0.5 ml reaction buffer
3. 3 units restriction enzyme
4. Add 5 ml water for injection (WFI)

The composition is calculated according to the plasmid DNA used for linearization (at least 1000 reactions, is 10,000 reactions). The reaction is incubated for 4–5 h at 37°C.

5.3.15 PURIFICATION OF THE LINEARIZED TEMPLATE PLASMID DNA:

The linearized template DNA is purified by phenol/chloroform extraction with subsequent alcohol precipitation, chromatographic methods, filtration methods, or silica-based DNA capture methods. [These methods are described in Sambrook et al., Molecular Cloning, Second Edition, 1989, Cold Spring Harbor Laboratory Press).] This step also ensures the reduction of impurities (e.g., proteins) from the previous manufacturing steps, including E. coli proteins, restriction enzymes and BSA (contained in reaction buffers).

The phenol/chloroform/isoamyl alcohol precipitation with subsequent isopropanol precipitation is preferred. After precipitation, the plasmid DNA is resuspended in a suitable buffer, which is water for injection.

Quality control of linearized template plasmid DNA vector: determination of the completeness of linearization, estimation of RNA yield, and determination of the identity of RNA.

Determination of completeness of linearization Linear template plasmid DNA is analyzed for successful/complete linearization. The band uniqueness and band size of the linear plasmid DNA are analyzed via agarose gel electrophoresis. Alternatively, any other method for determining DNA fragments can be used.

5.3.16 TEST TRANSCRIPTION

A small-scale transcription test with linear template DNA into RNA via a polymerization reaction by RNA polymerase is performed to estimate the expected yield of in vitro transcribed RNA and analyze the identity of the in vitro transcribed RNA. An in vitro transcription reaction commonly contains a DNA template, a suitable buffer (HEPES, Tris-HCI pH 7.5), DNA dependent RNA polymerase (e.g., T7, T3, SP6), a suitable nucleotide mixture (natural and modified nucleotides), DTT, spermidine, NaCl, MgCl2, RNase inhibitor and pyrophosphatase Subsequently, the in vitro transcribed RNA is purified. Different methods for RNA purification include phenol/chloroform/isoamyl alcohol extraction with subsequent ethanol or isopropanol precipitation, precipitation with alcohol and a monovalent cation such as sodium or ammonium ion, LiCI precipitation, chromatographic methods, or filtration methods. The LiCI precipitation is particularly preferred and performed by adding 50% of the volume of 8 M LiCI. The reaction is mixed and incubated at room temperature. Subsequently, the reaction is centrifuged, the supernatant discarded, and the RNA pellet washed with 75% ethanol. After drying, the RNA is resuspended in water.

Estimation of RNA yield is made by photometric analysis.

Determination of RNA identity in test in vitro transcription: the RNA identity in the test in vitro transcription is determined by agarose gel electrophoresis. It is used to estimate the yield of in vitro transcribed RNA and to analyze the identity of the in vitro transcribed RNA.

5.4   RNA TRANSCRIPTION

RNA is produced "in vitro," for example, from a PCR-based or plasmid linearized DNA template using DNA-dependent RNA polymerases. A preferred method is in vitro transcription of RNA using a linearized plasmid DNA template. The linearized template DNA plasmid produced in the previous steps is transcribed using DNA-dependent RNA in vitro transcription. That reaction typically is a transcription buffer, nucleotide triphosphates (NTPs), an RNase inhibitor, and a DNA-dependent RNA polymerase. The NTPs are selected from but are not limited to those described herein, including naturally occurring and modified NTPs. The DNA-dependent RNA polymerase is selected from, but is not limited to, T7 RNA polymerase, T3 RNA polymerase, SP6 RNA polymerase, and mutant polymerases such as, but not limited to, polymerases able to incorporate modified nucleic acids. Preferred is T7 RNA polymerase as an enzyme for RNA in vitro transcription. During polymerization, the mRNA is co-transcriptionally capped at the 5' end with a standard cap analog as defined herein (e.g., N7-MeGpppG). The following buffers are preferred as transcription buffers: 40 mM Tris pH 7.5 or 80 mM HEPES. 80 mM HEPES is particularly preferred.

Template DNA: 10–500 mg/ml, particularly preferred are 50 mg/ml

Nucleotide triphosphates of the desired chemistry are used, including naturally occurring nucleotides (e.g., at least one of the nucleotides ATP, CTP, UTP, and GTP) and modified nucleotides, modified nucleotides, or a combination of them.

ATP, CTP, UTP, and GTP are used in a concentration of 0.5–10 mM, 3–5 mM, and most in a concentration of 4 mM. Useful guanine analogs include, but are not limited to, N7-MeGpppG (=m7G(5')ppp(5')G), m7G(5')ppp(5')A, ARCA (anti-reverse CAP analog, modified ARCA (e.g., phosphothioate modified ARCA), inosine, N1-methyl-guanosine, 2'-fluoro-guanosine, 7-deaza-guanosine, 8-oxo-guanosine, 2-amino-guanosine, LNA-guanosine, and 2-azido-guanosine. If 5'-CAP (cap analog) is used, the concentration of GTP is decreased compared to the other used nucleotides. 10 to 50% of GTP is used compared to the concentration of ATP, CTP, and UTP. Most are 20–30% of 5 GTP is used.

Furthermore, the cap analog is used in a concentration that is at least the same as the concentration of ATP, CTP, and UTP.

The ratio of cap analog: GTP is varied from 10:1 to 1:1 to balance the percentage of capped products with the efficiency of the transcription reaction, is a ratio of cap analog: GTP of 4:1–5:1 is used. In this context, it is preferred to use 5.8 mM Cap analog and 1.45 mM GTP if ATP, UTP, and CTP are used in a concentration of 4 mM. MgCl2 can optionally be added to transcription reaction. Preferred is a concentration of 1–100 mM. Particularly preferred is a concentration of 5–30 mM, and most are 24 mM MgCl2 is used. Spermidine can optionally be added to the transcription reaction, which is 1–10 mM, and most are 2 mM spermidine. Dithiothreitol (DTT) can optionally be added to the transcription reaction at a concentration of 1–100mM, more is 10–100 mM, and most are 40 mM. An RNase inhibitor can optionally be added to the transcription reaction, 0.1–1 U/ml, at 0.2 U/ml. E. coli pyrophosphatase can optionally be added to the transcription reaction, is in a concentration of 1–10 U/mg template DNA, and most is in a concentration of 5 U/mg template DNA. This ensures that magnesium, essential for transcription, remains in the solution and does not precipitate as magnesium pyrophosphate.

The following viral DNA-dependent RNA polymerases are used: T3, T7, and Sp6 polymerases. 1–1000 Units/mg DNA is used. It is in a concentration of 100 U/mg DNA.

BSA can optionally be used, is in a concentration of 1–1000 mg/ml, and most are in a concentration of 100 mg/ml. Most are, BSA is not present in the transcription reaction. the in vitro transcription reaction is the following components:

1. 1 mg linearized plasmid DNA
2. 4 mM ATP, CTP, and UTP
3. 1.45 mM GTP,
4. 5.8 mM CAP analog 80 mM HEPES
5. 24 mM MgCl2
6. 2 mM Spermidine 40 mM DTT
7. 5 u pyrophosphatase 4 u RNase inhibitor
8. 100 u T7 RNA polymerase

The in vitro transcription reaction is incubated at 37 °C; more is for at least 4 hours. Purification of the in vitro transcribed RNA:

5.4.1 REMOVAL OF TEMPLATE DNA

The template DNA is removed from the in vitro transcription, e.g., the DNA template is separated from the RNA transcript. In one embodiment, the RNA transcript is removed chromatographically using a polyA capture, e.g., oligo dT, based affinity purification step. The RNA transcript binds the affinity substrate while the DNA template flows through and is removed. The polyA capture-based affinity purification is oligo dT purification. For example, a poly-thymidine ligand is immobilized to a derivatized chromatography resin. The purification mechanism involves the hybridization of the polyA tail of the RNA transcript to the oligonucleotide ligand. The DNA template will not bind. In addition, RNA transcripts that do not contain PolyA stretches (short aborts and other truncates formed during in vitro transcription) will not bind to the resin and will not form a duplex with the affinity ligand. Polyadenylated RNA can then be eluted from the resin utilizing a low ionic strength buffer or a competitive binding oligonucleotide solution. A one-pot purification method can yield highly purified poly(A) containing RNA with recoveries >80% actively removes endotoxin, DNA template, and enzymes utilized in the production of RNA using a simple capture and elute methodology with no subsequent fraction of captured poly(A) containing RNA. This purification increases mRNA product purity and, in turn, significantly increases target protein expression. Particularly preferred is the enzymatic removal of DNA template using DNAse I. Following transcription, the DNA template is removed using DNase I digestion. Such a step additionally removes residual bacterial genomic DNA. Adding 6 ml DNAse l (1 mg/ml) and 0.2 ml CaCl2 solution (0.1 M) / mg DNA template to the transcription reaction and incubate it for at least 3 h at 37°C.

5.4.2 Enzymatic Capping

The RNA obtained is further capped. The RNA is capped enzymatically as an alternative to co-transcriptional capping using CAP analogs. Capping is performed either before or after purification of the RNA transcript. For large-scale manufacturing, 5' capping of RNA transcripts is typically performed using a chemical cap analog. This was performed co-transcriptionally where the reaction's cap analog: GTP molar ratio is £4: 1. This typically results in 80% capping efficiency and reduced RNA transcript yields due to consumption of GTP. This high abundance of uncapped species is undesirable when developing therapeutic RNA. Since only capped mRNA is translated into protein, the presence of a high abundance of uncapped species (i.e., 20%) is problematic as efficacy (protein production/ mg RNA) is reduced by 20%> and 20%> of the final drug substance is an inert impurity, decreasing process productivity. Following RNA purification (e.g., LiCI precipitation), a 5' Cap can enzymatically be added to the RNA transcript (if no Cap analog has been used in the in vitro transcription mix). The recombinant Vaccinia Virus Capping Enzyme and recombinant 2'-O-methyltransferase enzyme can create a canonical 5'-5'-triphosphate linkage between the 5'-terminal nucleotide of an RNA and the guanine cap nucleotide wherein the cap guanine contains N7 methylation, and the 5'-terminal nucleotide of the RNA contains a 2'-O-methyl. Such a structure is termed the Cap1 structure. A natural CapO /Cap1 structure is post-transcriptionally added to the RNA using vaccinia virus capping enzyme (and potentially 2'-O-Methyltransferase) GTP and the Methyl donor SAM in suitable buffer conditions. Kits comprising capping enzymes are commercially available (e.g., ScriptCapTM Capping Enzyme and Script-CapTM 2'-O-Methyltransferase (both from CellScript)). Therefore, the RNA transcript is treated according to the manufacturer's instructions. Preferably, RNA is dissolved in WFI, denatured at 65°C for 10 minutes, and then placed on ice. A capping reaction mixture is then prepared containing 0.6 g/l RNA, 1 mM GTP, 0.5 mM S-adenosyl-methionine (SAM), 0.4 units/ml Capping Enzyme, 4 units/ml 2'-O-Methyltransferase, 0.05 M Tris-HCI (pH 8.0), 6 mM KCI and 1.25 35 mM MgCl2 and added to the RNA. The capping reaction mixture is incubated at 37°C for

60 min, adding a Cap1 to the RNA transcript. Alternatively, only Capping Enzyme (without 2'-O-Methyltransferase) is used to generate Cap0 structures. The capping reaction is followed by precipitation or purification of the RNA transcript.

5.4.2.1 Enzymatic polyadenylation

The RNA obtained is further polyadenylated. Enzymatic Polyadenylation is performed before or after further purification of the RNA transcript. First, the RNA transcript is incubated with a bacterial poly (A) polymerase (polynucleotide adenylyltransferase), e.g., from E. coli, together with ATP in the respective buffers. The poly (A) polymerase catalyzes the template-independent addition of AMP from ATP to the 3' end of RNA. Preferably, the RNA transcript is reacted with E. coli poly(A) polymerase (e.g., from Cellscript) using 1 mM ATP at 37°C for at least 30 min. Immediately afterward, the RNA is purified according to the purification methods described above (e.g., LiCI purification). Finally, RNA is run on an agarose gel to assess RNA extension.

5.4.3 QUALITY CONTROL: SIZE DETERMINATION OF POLY(A)-TAIL VIA POLY(A) BINDING PROTEIN ASSAY

The poly(A) length is determined in units of or as a function of polyA binding protein binding. In this embodiment, the polyA tail is long enough to bind at least 4 monomers of polyA binding protein. PolyA binding protein monomers bind to stretches of approximately 38 nucleotides. It has been observed that polyA tails of about 80 nucleotides and 160 nucleotides are functional.

Three methods for measuring the length of a poly(A) tail include the poly(A) length assay, the ligation-mediated poly(A) test (LM-PAT), and the RNase H assay. The first two methods are PCR-based assays involving cDNA synthesis from an oligo(dT) primer. The third method involves removing the poly(A) tail from the mRNA of interest. A major obstacle to studying the enzymatic step of mammalian mRNA decay has been the inability to capture mRNA decay intermediates with structural impediments such as the poly(G) tract used in yeast. To overcome this, combine a standard kinetic analysis of mRNA decay with a tetracycline repressor-controlled reporter with an Invader RNA assay. The Invader RNA assay is a simple, elegant assay for quantifying mRNA. It is based on signal amplification, not target amplification, so it is less prone to artifacts than other methods for nucleic acid quantification. It is also very sensitive, able to detect at molar levels of target mRNA. Finally, it requires only a short sequence for target recognition and quantitation. Therefore, it is applied to determining the decay polarity of an mRNA by measuring the decay rates of different portions of that mRNA.

5.4.4 TRANSCRIPTION

LiCI precipitation is the preferred method to precipitate the RNA transcript. First, high-molar LiCI solution is added to precipitate the RNA transcript specifically. Following precipitation, the RNA transcript is re-suspended in water for injection.

LiCl precipitation is performed by adding 50% of the volume 8M LiCl. The reaction is mixed and incubated at room temperature. Subsequently, the reaction is centrifuged, the supernatant discarded, and the RNA pellet washed with 75% ethanol. After drying, the RNA is resuspended in water. This step also ensures the removal of proteins from previous manufacturing steps, including E. coli proteins, restriction enzymes, RNA polymerase, RNase inhibitor, DNase I, and BSA. Moreover, the RNA-specific precipitation also removes residual plasmid DNA and bacterial (genomic) DNA contamination.

The in vitro transcription (IVT) enzymatic reaction used to generate mRNA relies on T7, SP6, or T3 RNA polymerases to catalyze the synthesis of the target mRNA from the corresponding DNA template. This template must be produced in advance, usually by linearizing a purified plasmid or amplifying the region of interest using PCR. Apart from the linear DNA template, the IVT components must include an RNA polymerase, nucleotide triphosphates (NTPs) substrates, the polymerase cofactor $MgCl2$, and a pH buffer containing polyamine and antioxidants. The reaction only takes a few hours, in contrast with the time-consuming processes used to manufacture conventional vaccines. Furthermore, this reduced time lowers the probability of contamination occurring. In general, milligrams of mRNA per mL of reaction can be obtained. Additionally, the production process can be standardized as it does not depend on the template's antigen encoded.

5.4.4.1   Capping

As for mRNA capping can be performed during the IVT reaction by substituting a part of the guanosine triphosphate (GTP) substrate for a cap analog (Figure 5.6). Alternatively, mRNA can be capped in a second enzymatic reaction using the vaccinia capping enzyme (VCC) and a methyl donor as a substrate. Although the capping efficiency of this method is higher (100% compared to 60–80% obtained with the use of a cap analog), the process with cap analogs is faster as it does not require the setup of a second enzymatic reaction. However, due to their price, cap analogs can impact production costs, especially if large-scale manufacturing is considered.

Nevertheless, a cost analysis should be performed to compare the costs of the one-step and two-step production options. Alternatively, co-transcriptional capping can be performed using CleanCap Reagent A. Although this method does not compete with GTP and delivers a Cap 1 construct, it requires the use of templates with a modified T7 promoter.

The IVT reaction mixture in a rocking bioreactor contains ribonucleotides, a viral RNA polymerase (e.g., T7 RNA polymerase), and the linearized DNA. The cap analog is also added to the reaction mixture that additionally includes a source of magnesium ions (e.g., $MgCl2$) and a polyamine, such as spermidine; magnesium is required for RNA polymerases to work, and polyamines help enhance transcription. After transcription, a deoxyribonuclease (DNase) is added to break down the DNA template and facilitate its subsequent removal. By the end of IVT, the reaction mixture contains a variety of impurities: buffer components, enzymes, unused nucleotides, cap analogs, truncated RNA/RNA fragments, dsRNA, DNA template, $Mg2+$, spermidine, etc. CleanCap AG; Deoxyribonuclease I (DNase I); RNase enzyme

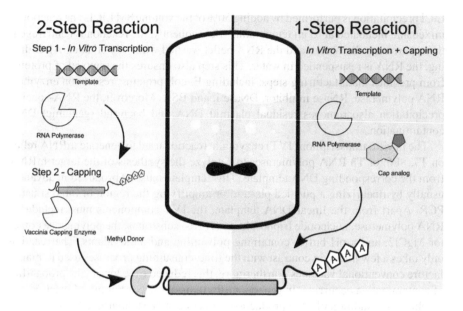

FIGURE 5.6   Schematic representation of an mRNA vaccine manufacturing process's production and purification steps. mRNA production can be performed in a one-step enzymatic reaction, where a capping analog is used, or in a two-step reaction, where the capping is performed using a vaccinia capping enzyme.

inhibitor; T7 RNA polymerase; linear template DNA; 1-methylpseudouridine-5′-triphosphate (mod-UTP).

Although commercial kits are available to produce mRNA for preclinical studies at a laboratory scale, their costs are high. In addition, the generation of mRNA by IVT at a large scale and under current good manufacturing practice (cGMP) conditions is also challenging. For example, the specialized components of the IVT reaction must be acquired from certified suppliers that guarantee that all the material is animal component-free and GMP-grade.

5.4.4.2   In Vitro Synthesis

The technology used to synthesize in vitro-transcribed RNAs, predominantly using phage RNA polymerases (RNAPs), is well established. However, transcripts synthesized with RNAPs are known to display an undesirable immune-stimulatory activity in vivo. The double-stranded RNA (dsRNA), a major by-product of the in vitro transcription (IVT) process, triggers cellular immune responses and should be removed. One method to achieve this goal is to use a high-temperature IVT process using thermostable T7 RNAPs to synthesize functional mRNAs that demonstrate reduced immunogenicity without a post-synthesis purification step. Combining high-temperature IVT with template-encoded poly(A) tailing prevents the formation of both kinds of dsRNA by-products generating functional mRNAs with reduced immunogenicity.

The dsRNA products in the IVT reactions show that high-temperature transcription results in the reduction of 3′-extended RNA, but not antisense RNA by-products. A template-encoded poly(A) tail has a beneficial effect on the formation of antisense by-products but not on 3′-extended by-products. The RNAs synthesized with thermostable RNAPs at higher temperatures are functional and have reduced immunogenicity in vivo. The TsT7 RNAPs are transcriptionally active at temperatures greater than 45°C, where the activity of wild-type T7 RNAP is compromised. However, the reactions can be conducted at 60°C as TsT7-1 remains active, the temperature at 50°C allows a better outcome.

The RNAs synthesized with the thermostable RNAPs are functional in vivo and demonstrate a reduced immune response in dendritic cells due to a reduction in 3′-extended byproducts. Furthermore, the combination of template-encoded poly(A) tailing and high-temperature IVT reduces the formation of two types of dsRNA by-products, improves the purity of RNA, and could potentially alleviate the need for extensive post-synthesis purification (Figure 5.7).

The RNA obtained in IVT, such as the purified RNA, is dried by lyophilization.

5.4.5 Purification

The RNA obtained is purified by any suitable purification step consisting of a precipitation step and a chromatographic step. The precipitation step is an alcoholic precipitation step or a LiCI precipitation step. The chromatographic step is selected from the group consisting of HPLC, RP-HPLC, anion exchange chromatography, affinity chromatography, hydroxyapatite chromatography, and core bead chromatography. The first purification step is a precipitation step, and the one-second purification step is a chromatographic step. The first purification step is an alcohol precipitation step or a LiCI precipitation step and the second purification step is a chromatographic step: HPLC, which is RP-HPLC, anion exchange chromatography, affinity chromatography, hydroxyapatite chromatography, and core bead chromatography.

Purification starts with a crossflow filter to remove small impurities and condition the mRNA in an appropriate buffer for the subsequent affinity (oligo-dT) chromatography step that is operated in a capture mode, removing most of the remaining impurities. Another step of hydrophobic chromatography does the final polishing. A second crossflow filtration allows the exchange of the buffer and the adjustment of the mRNA concentration, followed by formulation in a lipid nanoparticle.

Once the mRNA is generated by IVT, it is isolated and purified from the reaction mixture using multiple purification steps to achieve clinical purity standards. The reaction mixture contains the desired product and several impurities, including enzymes, residual NTPs and DNA template, and aberrant mRNAs formed during the IVT. Traditional lab-scale purification methods are based on DNA removal by DNAse digestion followed by lithium chloride (LiCl) precipitation. However, these methods do not allow the removal of aberrant mRNA species such as dsRNA and truncated RNA fragments. Removing these product-related impurities is crucial for mRNA performance, as they lower translation efficiency and modify the immunostimulatory profile. For example, a 10–1000-fold increase in protein production can

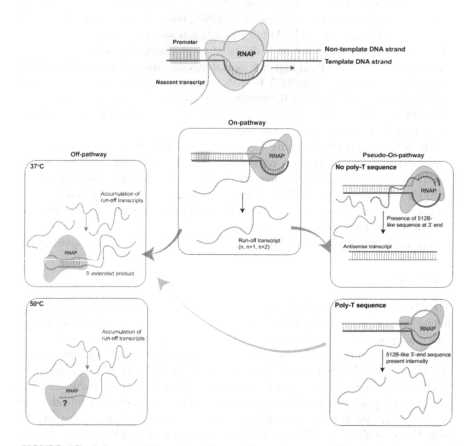

FIGURE 5.7 Schematic illustration of competing pathways resulting in the formation of dsRNA by-products during IVT. The canonical "on-pathway" results in promoter-dependent transcription initiation and synthesis of the runoff products. Accumulation of the runoff transcripts in the reaction results in a competing "off-pathway" wherein the RNAP rebinds the runoff product and results in self-extension of the runoff transcript. At temperatures higher than 48°C, the 3'-extension of the runoff products is reduced (due to either reduced rebinding of the RNAP to the runoff product or the folding of the runoff product). In the presence of a sequence at the 3' end of the template (similar to the 512-B 3'-end sequence), the RNAP initiates transcription of the antisense RNA product in a "pseudo-on-pathway." The presence of poly(T) sequences prevents the formation of the antisense RNA products. A poly(A) sequence at the 3'-end of the runoff transcript does not affect the "off-pathway" at 37°C and can lead to the synthesis of longer products if reactions are performed under standard conditions.

be achieved when nucleoside-modified mRNA is purified by reverse phase HPLC before delivery to primary DC.

The purification of the RNA transcript by HPLC is preferred. HPLC is an established method of separating mixtures of substances widely used in biochemistry, analytical chemistry, and clinical chemistry. An HPLC apparatus consists in the simplest case of a pump with an eluent reservoir containing the mobile phase, a sample application system, a separation column containing the stationary phase, and the detector. In addition, a fraction collector is also provided, with which the individual fractions are separately collected after separation and are thus available for further applications.

Chromatography is a mainstream purification process that selectively offers versatility, scalability, and cost-effectiveness. The size exclusion chromatography (SEC) allows a preparative scale purification process, achieving high purity and yields. However, SEC presents limitations, as it cannot remove similar size impurities, such as dsDNA.

5.4.5.1 Reversed-Phase Chromatography

Reversed-phase HPLC consists of a nonpolar stationary phase and a moderately polar mobile phase. One common stationary phase is, e.g., silica, which has been treated with RMe2SiCl, where R is a straight-chain alkyl group such as $C_{18}H_{37}$ or C_8H_17. Therefore, the retention time is longer for more nonpolar molecules, allowing polar molecules to elute more readily. Retention time is increased by adding polar solvent to the mobile phase and decreased by adding more hydrophobic solvent.

The product RNA is purified from various contaminations from previous manufacturing steps. These include buffer contaminations, protein impurities (Escherichia coli proteins, Restriction enzymes, T7-RNA-Polymerase, RNase-Inhibitor, DNase I, and BSA), impurities from RNA–RNA hybrids, from DNA–RNA hybrids or their fragments, from pDNA contaminations and bacterial genomic DNA contaminations, and solvent contaminations (Acetonitrile, Chloroform, TEAA, 2-Propanol, and Phenol) and free nucleotides. Moreover, size exclusion occurs during that procedure (smaller and larger RNAs are excluded).

5.4.5.2 TFF

Small-size impurities can also be removed while concentrating or diafiltrating solutions by tangential flow filtration (TFF). Core bead chromatography can also be used for this purpose. In this case, small impurities are trapped inside the beads, and the product will be in the flowthrough. However, both techniques rely on DNase digestion or denaturing agents to remove high-size molecules such as the DNA template or the polymerase. DNA removal can also be achieved using hydroxyapatite chromatography without a DNase. Finally, as a polishing step, hydrophobic interaction chromatography (HIC) can be applied using connective interaction media monolith (CIM) containing OH or SO3 ligands.

Large-scale adaptations of the traditional laboratory-scale mRNA purification methods include mRNA precipitation combined with the TFF technique. During TFF, the membrane captures the precipitated mRNA product while other impurities are removed by diafiltration. The product is then eluted by re-solubilizing the mRNA. Furthermore, DNA template removal can be achieved by performing the digestion with immobilized DNase. Another approach is to use a tagged DNA template that can then be removed after IVT using affinity chromatography. However, despite being scalable, these methods present limited effectiveness since they only focus on removing some specific impurities and hence must be coupled with other purification steps.

5.4.5.3 Ion Exchange Chromatography

An alternative for (common) HPLC is ion/anion-exchange HPLC, which leverages ionic interaction between positively charged sorbents and negatively charged molecules. AEX sorbents typically include a charged functional group cross-linked to solid-phase media. Ion exchange chromatography for preparative RNA transcript also provides a solution that allows for separations of longer RNA transcripts, including lengths of up to at least 10,000 nucleotides. In addition, the methods allow for the separations of chemically modified RNA transcripts.

A sample comprising the RNA transcript is contacted with an ion exchange sorbent comprising a positively charged functional group linked to solid-phase media. The sample is delivered with at least one mobile phase, where the RNA transcript in the sample binds the positively charged functional group of the ion exchange sorbent. The sample is delivered under denaturing conditions; for example, the sample is contacted with urea. Or else, the mobile phase is a Tris-EDTA-acetonitrile buffered mobile phase, or there are two mobile phases made of Tris-EDTA-acetonitrile. The mobile phase may also be a chaotropic salt, such as sodium perchlorate. The ion exchange sorbent elutes a portion of the sample comprising the RNA transcript and one or more separate portions of the sample comprising any impurities. RNA transcript and the separate portions of the sample comprising the impurities are then analyzed. The aspect is charge heterogeneity of the RNA transcript, mass heterogeneity of the RNA transcript, process intermediates, impurities, or degradation products. The RNA transcript is then characterized by using the analysis to determine the charge heterogeneity of the RNA transcript.

Ion exchange chromatography (IEC) is used to purify mRNA on a large scale. This technique explores the charge difference between the target mRNA species and the different impurities. For example, weak anion exchange chromatography helps separate mRNA from IVT impurities. IEC presents several advantages: it is scalable and cost-effective; it allows the separation of longer RNA transcripts, and it presents higher binding capacities (when compared with IPC). Nevertheless, this chromatography must be performed under denaturing conditions. This makes the process more complex as it requires a mobile phase heater and tight control of the temperature during chromatography.

5.4.5.4 Ion Pair Reverse Phase Chromatography

The use of ion-pair reverse-phase chromatography (IPC) is good for mRNA purification. In IPC, the negatively charged sugar-phosphate backbone of the oligonucleotides will pair with quaternary ammonium compounds present in the mobile phase (in this case, triethylammonium acetate) to become lipophilic and then interact with the stationary phase of a reverse-phase chromatography column. Elution is then performed with a gradient of an adequate solvent, e.g., acetonitrile. This approach effectively removes dsRNA impurities while maintaining the process's high yield. However, IPC is challenging and costly to scale, and the use of toxic reagents, such as acetonitrile, is not desirable. Therefore, a new cellulose-based chromatography process for the removal of dsRNA has been described that leverages the ability of dsRNA to bind to cellulose in the presence of ethanol. This method creates an mRNA yield greater than 65% with a dsRNA removal of over 90%. Still, the removal of other impurities requires other pre-purification steps.

5.4.5.5 Affinity Purification (oligo-dT)

Affinity-based separation is another mRNA purification approach. A single-stranded sequence of deoxythymidine (dT) Oligo dT is routinely used to capture mRNA in laboratory applications. This sequence binds to the poly(A) tails present in the mRNA. Chromatographic beads with immobilized oligo dT are used for the process scale purification using affinity chromatography: the poly(A) tails of the single-stranded mRNA produced during IVT would bind to the stationary phase while impurities are washed out. This way, IVT unconsumed reagents, the DNA template, and dsRNA could be efficiently removed. While high purity products can be obtained using affinity chromatography, several drawbacks include low binding capacities and a less cost-effective process.

The poly(A) capture-based affinity purification is oligo dT purification. For example, a poly-thymidine ligand is immobilized to a derivatized chromatography resin. The purification mechanism involves the hybridization of the poly(A) tail of the RNA transcript to the oligonucleotide ligand. As a result, the DNA template will not bind. In addition, RNA transcripts that do not contain Poly A stretches (short aborts and other truncates formed during in vitro transcription) will not bind to the resin and will not form a duplex with the affinity ligand. Poly adenylated RNA can then be eluted from the resin utilizing a low ionic strength buffer or a competitive binding oligonucleotide solution. A one-pot purification method can yield highly purified poly(A) containing RNA with recoveries >80% actively removes endotoxin, DNA template, and enzymes utilized in the production of RNA using a simple capture and elute methodology with no subsequent fraction of captured poly(A) containing RNA. This purification increases mRNA product purity and, in turn, significantly increases target protein expression.

5.4.5.6 Hydroxyapatite Chromatography

Purification of an RNA transcript described in WO2014140211 involves hydroxyapatite as a stationary phase. Hydroxyapatite is calcium phosphate with the chemical formula $Ca_5(PO_4)_3(OH)$. Hydroxyapatite chromatography of nucleic acids is believed to exploit the charge interaction between their negatively charged phosphate backbone and the positively charged calcium ions on the surface of the hydroxyapatite medium. Differential elution {e.g., to separate protein, DNA, and undesired RNA species from desired RNA species) is accomplished by the application of an increasing phosphate gradient. Phosphate ions in the buffer compete with the phosphate groups of the retained nucleic acid species for calcium on the hydroxyapatite medium, thus allowing separation by selective elution of molecules. In this mixed-mode chromatography, the binding is a balance of attraction of the RNA phosphate backbone to the calcium ions of the hydroxyapatite medium and repulsion of the RNA phosphate backbone from the phosphate of the hydroxyapatite medium. Compared to ion-exchange chromatography, the binding strength on a hydroxyapatite medium depends on charge density rather than total charge. This important difference allows for the separation of molecules upon their charge density (e.g., RNA vs. DNA vs. proteins) and the binding and elution of RNA regardless of its total charge and length. Therefore, this method is used to purify RNA molecules of any length.

5.4.5.7 Core Bead Chromatography (does not require prior DNA digest)

RNA is selectively recovered from the column in the flow-through. Proteins and short nucleic acids are retained in the beads. Flow-through fractions containing RNA are identified by measuring UV absorption at 260nm. The composition comprising the RNA of interest collected in the flow-through is highly purified relative to the preparation before the core bead chromatography step. Multiple eluted fractions containing the RNA of interest are combined before further treatment. An exemplary core bead flow-through chromatography medium is Capto Core 700 beads from GE Healthcare. Suitable chromatography setups are known in the art, for example, liquid chromatography systems such as the AKTA liquid chromatography systems from GE Healthcare (now Cytiva). Parameters are set so that pDNA and proteins are captured in the beads, and RNA products flow through. Afterward, HPLC purification is conducted to eliminate RNA fragments, etc.

Alternatively, or additionally, the RNA is recovered by other purification methods (e.g., affinity chromatography, size exclusion chromatography, anion exchange chromatography, etc.). In one method, purification of the RNA transcript by LiCI precipitation, RP-HPLC using a crosslinked macroporous poly(styrene/divinylbenzene) reversed phase and subsequent isopropanol precipitation using Na+ as monovalent cation is particularly preferred.

5.4.5.8 Lyophilization of the Purified RNA Transcript

The RNA transcript is lyophilized after purification by any lyophilization method known in the art. Lyophilization of the RNA transcript particularly increases the half-life of the RNA.

5.4.5.9 Resuspension of Lyophilized RNA and Adjustment of the RNA Concentration

The resuspension is performed using the respective amount of water for injection (WFI) or pyrogen-free water at RT. The final concentration is set, and the medicament is sterile-filtered, is through a pore size of 0.22 mm, for bioburden reduction. A sample of the produced RNA solution is used for photometric determination of the RNA content. Eventually, the RNA solution is sterile-filtered. For long-term storage, the sterile-filtered, concentration-adjusted RNA solution is stored at −80°C. The RNA solution is resuspended in a concentration of 0.1–50 g/l; more is in a concentration of 1–20 g/l, more is in a concentration of 1–10 g/l, and most are in a concentration of 5 g/l.

The following chemicals are required for the downstream IVT process: 1-methyl-pseudouridine-5′-triphosphate (mod-UTP); Acetic acid; Adenosine-5′-triphosphate

(ATP); Calcium chloride (CaCl2); Cholesterol; Citric acid; CleanCap AG; cytidine-5'-triphosphate (CTP); Deoxyribonuclease I (DNase I); Disodium phosphate (Na2HPO4); Dithiothreitol (DTT); Ethyl alcohol (ethanol); Guanosine-5'-triphosphate (GTP); Ionizable lipid; Linear template DNA; Magnesium chloride (MfgCl2); Monopotassium phosphate (KH2PO4); Phospholipid; Polyethylene glycol (PEG) lipid; Potassium chloride (KCl); Pyrophosphatase; RNase enzyme inhibitor; Sodium acetate; Sodium chloride (NaCl); Sodium citrate; Sodium hydroxide (NaOH); Spermidine; Sucrose; T7 RNA polymerase; Tris hydrochloride (Tris HCl); Water for injection (WFI), RNase free.

5.4.6 Formulation

The mRNA's LNPs serve as a vector, entering the cells without destroying the mRNA by the body's abundance of RNA polymerases. Instead, LNPs are engulfed by cells through a process called endocytosis, forming vesicles inside the cell called endosomes. LNPs are self-assembled spherical structures typically composed of four different lipids (a cationic/ionizable lipid; a PEGylated lipid; a phospholipid; and cholesterol) capable of encapsulating mRNA molecules. The encapsulation starts by mixing the aqueous (acidic) solution containing the mRNA molecules with an ethanol solution containing the lipids using microfluidic mixers. The final step is another crossflow filtration step to replace the ethanol/water mixture with an appropriate formulation buffer. Following mRNA encapsulation, ethanol is removed, and the final buffer formulation is introduced by ultrafiltration that allows concentration increase; the product is kept frozen at −20 °C to −80°C for long-term stability.

5.4.7 Release Testing

The quality of the RNA obtained or the quality of the purified RNA is controlled by digesting the RNA with a ribonuclease; determining the identity of the RNA by using RT or RT-PCR; determining the identity and the integrity of the RNA by gel electrophoresis; determining the pH of a sample comprising the RNA; determining the osmolality of a sample comprising the RNA; determining the bioburden; determining the presence and the amount of endotoxin; determining the presence and amount of protein; determining the presence and amount of the template DNA; determining the presence and the amount of bacterial DNA; and determining the presence and the amounts of organic solvent. Ideally, the quality of the RNA is controlled by combining all of the above steps.

The identity of the RNA is established by digesting the RNA with a ribonuclease; determining the identity of the RNA by using RT or RT-PCR; determining the identity and the integrity of the RNA by gel electrophoresis; determining the pH of an RNA sample; determining the osmolality of a sample comprising the RNA; determining the bioburden; determining the presence and the amount of endotoxin; determining the presence and amount of protein; determining the presence and amount of the template DNA; determining the presence and the amount of bacterial DNA; and determining the presence and the amounts of organic solvent.

The vaccine is tested for nanoparticle characteristics, encapsulation, transfection efficiencies, in vitro cytotoxicity, and stability and storability. The vaccine's safety is assessed in Balb/c mice injected with the vaccine containing ten µg of spike-encoding mRNA. The vaccine efficacy is tested by inducing an immune response against SARS-CoV-2 in Balb/c and C57BL/6 mice (receiving 1 or 10 µg of mRNA) and rhesus macaque monkeys (infused with the vaccine containing 30–100 µg of mRNA). The ELISA and virus-neutralizing test (VNT) results will show a significant augmentation in the level of neutralizing antibodies against SARS-CoV-2. Moreover, the ELISA assay will show virus-specific IFN-γ secretion in immunized mice as a TH1 cell-based immune response marker. In contrast, favorably, no change in the production of IL-4 is detected. GLP guidelines are followed.

5.4.8 FILL AND FINISH

After passing through a sterilizing filter, the vaccine is filled in vials or pre-filled syringes.

5.5 QUALITY CONTROL

This section describes steps for controlling the quality of the template DNA comprising a nucleic acid sequence encoding the RNA. In particular, this section relates to steps for determining the template DNA content, determining the identity of the DNA sequence encoding the target RNA sequence, and determining the purity of the template DNA.

5.5.1 DETERMINATION OF TEMPLATE PLASMID DNA CONTENT

The concentration of the isolated template plasmid DNA (dsDNA) is determined by a standard photometric method for nucleic acids via measurement of the absorption. Moreover, the OD 260/280 value is determined which measures the purity of a nucleic acid sample. For pure DNA, A260/280 is approximately 1.8.

5.5.2 DETERMINATION OF THE IDENTITY OF THE DNA SEQUENCE ENCODING THE TARGET RNA SEQUENCE

5.5.2.1 Determination of the identity of the DNA sequence encoding the target RNA sequence by PCR

To confirm that the obtained template DNA is the nucleic acid sequence encoding the RNA sequence, PCR with appropriate primers is performed. Primers located in the nucleic acid sequence encoding the target RNA sequence or primers located outside of the nucleic acid sequence encoding the target RNA sequence are used for PCR. Suppose a plasmid DNA vector is used as a template for the in vitro transcription. In that case, primers located on the backbone of the plasmid DNA vector are used, e.g., standard primers such as M13, Sp6, or T7 primers flanking the insert

DNA sequence encoding the target RNA sequence. The resulting PCR-amplified products are analyzed by gel electrophoresis, e.g., agarose gel electrophoresis, DNA sequencing, or chromatography, e.g., HPLC). Particularly preferred is the analysis by agarose gel electrophoresis or HPLC.

PCR is used as a method for analysis of template DNA, controlling the identity of the DNA sequence encoding the target RNA sequence. In addition, this method is used as quality control for the production of template DNA in a method for producing RNA, which is in the production process of in vitro transcribed RNA.

5.5.2.2 Determination of the identity of the DNA sequence encoding the target RNA sequence by restriction analysis

Alternatively, or additionally to other methods, such as PCR, restriction analysis of the template plasmid DNA vector comprising the insert DNA sequence encoding the target RNA sequence is conducted, and the resulting fragments of the plasmid DNA vector are analyzed to confirm that the template plasmid DNA vector contains the insert DNA sequence encoding the target RNA sequence.

5.5.3 RESTRICTION REACTION

Restriction enzymes specifically bind to and cleave double-stranded DNA at specific sites within or adjacent to a particular sequence known as the recognition site. Most of the restriction enzymes recognize a specific sequence of nucleotides that are four, five, or six nucleotides in length and display twofold symmetry. Some cleave both strands exactly at the axis of symmetry, generating fragments of DNA that carry blunt ends; others cleave each strand at similar locations on opposite sides of the axis of symmetry, creating fragments of DNA that carry single-stranded termini (See Glossary).

The reaction conditions used for the restriction digestion are dependent on the used restriction enzymes. Particularly, the salt concentration differs depending on the used restriction enzyme. Therefore, the manufacturer of restriction enzymes optimized buffers for their restriction enzymes.

Suggested conditions for a restriction reaction with one restriction enzyme are:

1. 0.5 mg plasmid DNA (0.2–2 mg plasmid DNA)
2. 1.5 ml 10 x reaction buffer
3. 1 ml restriction enzyme (1 ml normally is 1 u). Add. 15 ml WFI (water for injection)
4. Suggested conditions for a restriction reaction with two restriction enzymes are: 0.5 mg plasmid DNA (0.2–2 mg plasmid DNA) 1,5 ml 10 x reaction buffer
5. 1 ml restriction enzyme 1 (1 ml normally is 1 u) 1 ml restriction enzyme 2 (1 ml normally is 1 u). Add. 15 ml WFI (water for injection)

The restriction reaction is typically mixed and incubated for 1–4 hours at 37°C. It is suggested that restriction enzymes are combined, which cut 5′ and 3′ of the insert

DNA sequence. Alternatively, a specific combination of restriction enzymes is chosen dependent on the insert DNA sequence. In this case, it is preferred to choose a restriction enzyme, which cuts only once in the DNA plasmid backbone, and a restriction enzyme, which cuts once in the insert DNA sequence. It is preferred to perform at least one, 2, 3, 4 or 5 different restriction reactions using different restriction enzyme(s) (combinations) to control the identity of the insert DNA sequence comprising the nucleic acid sequence encoding the target RNA sequence.

The identity of the insert DNA sequence contained in the template plasmid DNA vector is controlled by enzymatic restriction and subsequently analyzed via agarose gel electrophoresis. For this purpose, template plasmid DNA is incubated with a certain number of specific restriction enzymes (in at least five independent reactions), leading to a specific fragmentation of the template plasmid DNA vector. Subsequently, the restricted DNA samples are analyzed by separating the obtained fragments of different sizes, e.g., on an agarose gel or, e.g., by HPLC. Finally, the received fragmentation pattern of the DNA is compared to the theoretically expected restriction pattern.

5.5.4 ANALYSIS OF THE DNA FRAGMENTS RESULTING FROM RESTRICTION REACTION

Exemplary methods for analyzing DNA fragments are, for instance, agarose gel electrophoresis, polyacrylamide gel electrophoresis, chip gel electrophoresis, capillary electrophoresis, fluorescence-based automatic DNA-fragment analysis, and HPLC (e.g., WAVE™ DNA Fragment Analysis System).

Electrophoresis through agarose gels is a method to separate DNA fragments. The DNA is determined in the agarose gel by adding the fluorescent intercalating dye ethidium bromide or other commercially available DNA dyes (SybrSafe DNA stain, Cybr Green, Orange DNA loading dye). Different running buffers is used, e.g., TBE (Tris-borate) or TAE (Tris-acetate) buffer: 1xTBE (Tris-borate):

1. 89 mM Tris base 89 mM boric acid 2 mM EDTA
2. 1xTAE (Tris-acetate)
3. 40mM Tris 20mM acetic acid 1mM EDTA

For the preparation of the agarose gel 0.3–5% (w/v) agarose or more is 0.8% (w/v) agarose is melted in 1 x running buffer, is 1xTBE buffer. Ethidium bromide is added to the solution, is 1–5 ml per 100 ml agarose gel solution. The solution is poured into a mold and allowed to harden. When an electric field is applied across the gel, DNA, which is negatively charged, migrates to the anode. As a running buffer, the same buffer used to prepare the agarose gel is used.

Loading buffer (e.g., 63 Orange DNA Loading Dye) is added to the sample and loaded onto the agarose gel. In this context, the whole reaction (15 ml) is mixed with an appropriate volume of loading buffer, e.g., 3 ml 6 Orange DNA Loading Dye. After gel running, the DNA fragments are determined by ultraviolet light. The pattern of fragments is compared to the predicted restriction pattern and therefore allows the determination of the correct DNA sequence encoding the target RNA sequence integrated into the plasmid.

5.5.4.1 Determination of the Identity of the DNA Sequence Encoding the Target RNA Sequence by DNA Sequencing

Automated DNA sequencing of the insert DNA sequence of the plasmid DNA or the PCR product encoding the target RNA sequence is performed to confirm the identity of the DNA sequence encoding the target RNA sequence. The DNA sequencing is performed by selection of appropriate primers for DNA sequencing that ensures that the complete length of the DNA sequence encoding the target RNA sequence is completely covered for both complementary strands of the DNA primers (primers flanking the DNA sequence encoding the target RNA sequence, e.g., the insert DNA sequence, located on the backbone of the plasmid, e.g., M13 forward, and M13 reverse). The received sequence information is compared to the expected sequence of the DNA sequence encoding the target RNA sequence. Therefore, it is particularly preferred to confirm or control the identity of the DNA sequence encoding the target RNA sequence. by using primers that lay 5' and 3' of the DNA sequence encoding the target RNA sequence, e.g., comprised in the template plasmid DNA vector or the template PCR product.

The following primer is particularly preferred: M13-universal Primer: 5'-CGC CAGGGTTTTCCCAGTCACGAC.

5.5.4.2 Determination of Purity of Template Plasmid DNA Preparation

5.5.4.2.1 Determination of RNA Contaminations in the Template DNA Preparation Using RNase Treatment

Template DNA is further controlled concerning RNA contamination. The template DNA e.g., plasmid DNA is incubated with RNase A. Afterwards the concentration of the purified template DNA is determined again and the difference before and after RNase treatment is calculated.

The following reaction is particularly preferred: 1–20 mg template DNA, is 10–15 mg template DNA are incubated with 1 ml RNase A (1 g/l) for 1h at 37°C. Nucleotides are separated, e.g., by alcohol precipitation, and chromatography is on Sephadex columns. The concentration of the isolated template DNA after RNase A digestion is determined by the photometric method for nucleic acids via measurement of the absorption at 260 nm (OD260)

5.5.4.2.2 Determination of Endotoxins in Template DNA Preparation

A test for bacterial endotoxins is carried out to determine the presence and the amount of endotoxins in the template DNA preparation. The endotoxins of gram-negative bacterial origin are detected and quantified by using amoebocyte lysate from the horseshoe crab (Limulus polyphemus or Tachypleus tridentatus).

In general, there are at least three techniques for performing this test: the gel-clot technique, which is based on gel formation; the turbidimetric technique, based on the development of turbidity after cleavage of an endogenous substrate; and the chromogenic technique, based on the development of color after cleavage of a synthetic peptide-chromogen complex. However, the preferred method is the LAL-test. According to pH, the amount of endotoxins per volume of plasmid DNA is determined and evaluated via kinetic-turbidometric LAL (Limulus-Amoebocyte-Lysate) test. Eur. 2.6.14.

5.5.4.2.3 A.3.3 Determination of Protein Concentration in Template DNA Preparation

The total protein content per volume of template plasmid DNA is calculated, including UV absorbance measurements at 280 nm (due to aromatic amino acids), the Lowry assay, the Biuret assay, and the Bradford and the BCA (Bicinchoninic Acid) assay. The BCA assay, a colorimetric detection method, is based on the complexation of proteins with copper and BCA. The total protein concentration contained in the RNA is measured via absorption at 562 nm compared to a protein standard (bovine serum albumin, BSA). The bicinchoninic acid (BCA) assay principle is similar to the Lowry procedure. Both rely on forming a Cu2+ protein complex under alkaline conditions, followed by a reduction of the Cu2+ to Cu+. The amount of reduction is proportional to the protein present. It has been shown that cysteine, cystine, tryptophan, tyrosine, and the peptide bond are able to reduce Cu2+ to Cu+. BCA forms a purple-blue complex with Cu+ in alkaline environments, thus providing a basis to monitor the reduction of alkaline Cu2+ by proteins at absorbance maximum 562 nm.

Another method that is used for the determination of protein is the Bradford method. The Bradford assay, a colorimetric protein assay, is based on an absorbance shift of the Coomassie Brilliant Blue G-250 dye. Under acidic conditions, the red form of the dye is converted into its bluer form to bind to the protein being assayed. The (bound) form of the dye has an absorption spectrum maximum historically held at 595 nm. The cationic (unbound) forms are green or red. The binding of the dye to the protein stabilizes the blue anionic form. The increase of absorbance at 595 nm is proportional to the amount of bound dye, and thus to the amount (concentration) of protein present in the sample. Particularly preferred is the BCA assay. For performing a BCA assay, several commercially available kits are used.

5.5.4.2.4 Determination of the Bioburden in Template DNA Preparation

To determine sterility of the template DNA preparation, a PCR using universal bacterial primers (detecting universal occurring genes in bacteria) is performed. Moreover, a plating assay is conducted. Particularly preferred is a plating assay according to PhEur 2.6.12. To determine the bioburden, the presence/absence of bacteria is tested under aerobe and anaerobe conditions after plating the plasmid DNA on agar and glucose plates and incubation for several days (e.g., 5 and 7 days, respectively). The bioburden is assessed by counting the bacteria clones grown on bacteria plates. For this purpose, different media for plating is used. Tryptic Soy Agar (TSA) (Soybean Casein Digest Agar (CSA)) and Sabouraud Glucose (2%) agar plates are preferred.

5.5.4.2.5 Determination of Residual Bacterial DNA

In case E. coli is used for amplification of the template plasmid DNA, the residual E. coli DNA is determined. Residual E coli DNA is detected via PCR, is via quantitative PCR (qPCR) using primers and probes specific for E. coli genes. In this context, primers and probes specific for any genomic sequence or gene comprised in the respective bacterial strain (e.g., E. coli strain) are useful to perform a PCR or qPCR to determine residual bacterial DNA. Particularly preferred are primers and probes specific for the E. coli gene uidA.

Plasmid DNA is checked for residual E. coli DNA. For this purpose, quantitative PCR (qPCR) is performed with the plasmid DNA sample together with a positive, and a negative control and the calculated number of copies of genomic E. coli DNA is assessed. For this purpose, the E. coli specific gene uidA is amplified and quantified. The Light Cycler from Roche is used in combination with FastStart DNA MasterPlus Hybridization Probes.

The following primers and probes are used for the quantitative PCR detecting the uidA gene:

Primer EC 679U: GGACAAGGCACTAGCG Primer EC 973 L: ATGCGAGGTACGGTAGGA

robe EC1 FL: CATCCGGTCAGTGGCAGT-FL

Probe EC1 LC: LC640-AAGGGCGAACAGTTCCTGA-ph

Alternatively, any other gene of the respective bacterial strain (particularly E. coli strain) used for fermentation is used for the PCR or quantitative PCR.

5.5.4.2.6 A.3.6 Determination of RNase Contaminations in Template DNA

The template DNA (e.g., the linear template plasmid DNA) is analyzed for RNase contamination using commercially available RNase detection kits, including RNaseAlert (Applied Biosystems), RNase contamination assay (New England Biolabs), or an assay where the incubation of the template DNA with a reference RNA serves as a readout for RNase contamination.

The template DNA is analyzed for RNase contamination by using the RNaseAlert kit, which utilizes an RNA substrate tagged with a fluorescent reporter molecule (fluor) on one end and a quencher of that reporter on the other. In the absence of RNases, the physical proximity of the quencher dampens fluorescence from the fluor. In the presence of RNases, the RNA substrate is cleaved, and the fluor and quencher are spatially separated in solution. This causes the fluor to emit a bright green signal when excited by light of the appropriate wavelength. Fluorescence is readily detected with a filter-based or monochromator-based fluorometer.

The template DNA is alternatively analyzed for RNase contamination by using an RNase Contamination Assay Kit (New England Biolabs) which detects general RNase activities including non-enzyme-based RNA degradation due to heavy metal contamination in samples and high pH. The assay probe is a fluorescein-labeled RNA transcript (300-mer). After incubation with a pDNA sample, the integrity of the RNA probe is analyzed on denaturing PAGE followed by SYBR Gold staining or by scanning with a FAM/Fluorescein capable imaging system.

The template DNA is analyzed for RNase contamination by incubation of the template DNA (the linear template plasmid DNA) with a reference RNA and subsequent analysis via RNA agarose gel electrophoresis. In case of the absence of RNase, both the linear DNA and the reference RNA are detected on the agarose gel; in case of RNase contamination, only the DNA band is detected.

mRNA purification process at lab scale consists of Dnase I digestion followed by LiCl precipitation. Purification at a larger scale is obtained using well-established chromatographic strategies coupled with tangential flow filtration. Alternatively, new types of chromatography can be used to complement the standard purification.

5.5.5 DETERMINATION OF THE RNA CONCENTRATION/ RNA CONTENT/RNA AMOUNT

The RNA content is determined by spectrometric analysis. Spectrophotometric analysis based on the principles that nucleic acids absorb ultraviolet light in a specific pattern. In the case of DNA and RNA, a sample that is exposed to ultraviolet light at a wavelength of 260 nanometers (nm) will absorb that ultraviolet light. The resulting effect is that less light will strike the photodetector and this will produce a higher optical density (OD). An optical density of 1 measured at 260 nm corresponds to a 40 mg/ml single-stranded RNA concentration. The yield of the test transcription is evaluated by measurement of the absorption at 260 nm (OD260).

5.5.5.1 Determination of RNA Identity

5.5.5.1.1 Determination of Transcript Length and Transcript Uniqueness

The correct transcript length and transcript uniqueness is confirmed to verify the identity and purity of the RNA obtained by the method disclosed herein. The band uniqueness and band size of mRNA is analyzed by agarose gel electrophoresis, capillary gel electrophoresis, polyacrylamide gel electrophoresis, or HPLC. Particularly preferred is agarose gel electrophoresis. Electrophoresis through agarose gels is a method to separate RNA. The RNA is determined in the agarose gel by addition of the fluorescent intercalating dye ethidium bromide or other commercially available dyes (SybrSafe DNA stain, Cybr Green, Orange DNA loading dye). As running usually 1xMOPS buffer is used (MOPS, 0.74 % Formaldehyde, in ultra-pure water). For the preparation of the agarose gel, 0.5–3% (w/v) agarose or more is 1.2% (w/v) agarose is melted in 1 x running buffer. The solution is poured into a mold and allowed to harden. When an electric field is applied across the gel, RNA, which is negatively charged, migrates to the anode. As a running buffer, the same buffer used to prepare the agarose gel is used. Loading buffer (e.g., gel loading buffer with ethidium bromide (10mg/l)) is added to the sample and loaded on the agarose gel. After gel running, the RNA is determined, for example, by ultraviolet light. The RNA length is compared to the predicted length and therefore allows the determination of the correct DNA sequence encoding the target RNA sequence integrated into the plasmid.

Alternatively, polyacrylamide gel electrophoresis, capillary gel electrophoresis, or HPLC is used.

5.5.5.1.2   Determination of RNA Identity by RNase Treatment with Subsequent Analysis of the Degraded Product

RNA identity is confirmed by a test, which uses RNase A digestion of a sample of the RNA obtained of the method disclosed herein. The digested RNA is compared with an untreated sample on an RNA gel electrophoresis. It is preferred to digest 1 mg RNA transcript with 10 mg RNase A.

5.5.5.1.3   Determination of RNA Identity by RT-PCR with Subsequent Analysis of the Product via Agarose Gel Electrophoresis

In a first step, the RNA is converted into complementary DNA (cDNA) using the enzyme reverse transcriptase. In a second step, the resulting cDNA is amplified via PCR (polymerase chain reaction) using appropriate primers to provide a PCR product of a certain size. Finally, the PCR product is analyzed via agarose gel electrophoresis for correct band size.

RT-PCR using the RNA as a template is used to determine the size of the RNA product. For reverse transcription, kits are commercially available. Afterward, produced cDNA is amplified with target-specific primers, and product band sizes are analyzed in a conventional DNA agarose gel electrophoresis, as described above.

5.5.5.2   Determination of RNA Identity by Reverse Transcription Sequencing:

The RNA transcript is characterized by reverse transcription sequencing. First, the RNA product is incubated with a common reverse transcriptase, a set of primers, and dNTPs to obtain cDNA samples. The cDNA serve as a template for PCR to amplify the cDNA. The PCR product is then characterized by analysis using a sequencing procedure as defined herein such as Sanger sequencing or bidirectional sequencing.

5.5.5.3   Determination of RNA Identity by Oligonucleotide Mapping

The RNA obtained is incubated with various nucleotide probes under conditions sufficient to allow hybridization of the probes to the RNA to form duplexes, where each of the nucleotide probes includes a sequence complementary to a different region of the RNA transcript. The formed duplexes are then contacted with an RNase (such as RNase H or RNase TI) under conditions sufficient to allow RNase digestion of the duplexes to form reaction products.

Next, the reaction products are analyzed, for example, by using a procedure such as reversed-phase high-performance liquid chromatography (RP-HPLC), anion exchange (AEX) HPLC, or RP-HPLC coupled to mass spectrometry (MS). Finally, the RNA is characterized by using the analysis of the reaction products to determine the RNA sequence.

5.5.5.4 Determination of RNA Identity by RNA Sequencing

The identity of the RNA is determined by RNA sequencing.

5.5.5.5 Determination of RNA Integrity

The relative integrity of the RNA is determined as the percentage of full-length RNA (i.e., non-degraded RNA) concerning the total amount of RNA (i.e., full-length RNA and degraded RNA fragments (which appear as smears in gel electrophoresis)).

5.5.5.6 Determination of pH

Potentiometric determination of the pH content using a conventional voltmeter, according to the European Pharmacopeia (PhEur) 2.2.3, is used to determine the pH value in the RNA preparation.

5.5.5.7 Determination of Osmolality

The osmolality of the RNA is determined using a conventional osmometry device, according to PhEur 2.2.35.

5.5.5.8 Determination of Bioburden/Microbial Content

To determine the sterility of the RNA preparation, an RT-PCR using universal bacterial primers (detecting universal, occurring genes in bacteria) is performed. Moreover, a plating assay is conducted. The preferred method is a plating assay, according to PhEur 2.6.12. To determine the bioburden, the presence/absence of bacteria is tested under aerobic and anaerobic conditions after plating the RNA on agar and glucose plates and incubation for several days (e.g., 5 and 7 days, respectively). Then, the bioburden is assessed by counting the bacteria clones grown on bacteria plates. For this purpose, different media for plating is used. Tryptic Soy Agar (TSA) (Soybean Casein Digest Agar (CSA)) and Sabouraud Glucose (2%) Agar plates are particularly preferred.

5.5.5.9 Determination of Endotoxin Contamination

A test for bacterial endotoxins is used to detect or quantify endotoxins of gram-negative bacterial origin by using amoebocyte lysate from horseshoe crab (Limulus polyphemus or Tachypleus tridentatus). In general, there are three techniques for performing this test: the gel-clot technique, which is based on gel formation; the turbidimetric technique, based on the development of turbidity after cleavage of an endogenous substrate; and the chromogenic technique, based on the development of color after cleavage of a synthetic peptide-chromogen complex. However, preferred is the LAL test. According to pH, the amount of endotoxins per volume of RNA is determined and evaluated via kinetic-turbidimetric LAL (Limulus-Amoebocyte-Lysate) test. Eur. 2.6.14 (Pharmacopoeia Europaea).

5.5.5.10 Determination of Protein Contamination

The total protein content per volume of RNA is calculated using UV absorbance measurements at 280 nm (due to the presence of aromatic amino acids), the Lowry assay, the Biuret assay, the Bradford assay, and the Bicinchoninic Acid (BCA) assay, a colorimetric method of detection based on the complexation of proteins with copper and BCA. The total protein concentration contained in the RNA is measured via absorption at 562 nm compared to a protein standard (BSA). The bicinchoninic acid (BCA) assay principle is similar to the Lowry procedure. Both rely on forming a Cu2+ protein complex under alkaline conditions, followed by a reduction of the Cu2+ to Cu+. The amount of reduction is proportional to the protein present. It has been shown that cysteine, cystine, tryptophan, tyrosine, and the peptide bond are able to reduce Cu2+ to Cu+. BCA forms a purple-blue complex with Cu+ in alkaline environments, thus providing a basis to monitor the reduction of alkaline Cu2+ by proteins at absorbance maximum 562 nm.

Another method that could be used to determine protein is the Bradford method. The Bradford assay, a colorimetric protein assay, is based on an absorbance shift of the dye Coomassie Brilliant Blue G-250 in which under acidic conditions the red form of the dye is converted into its bluer form to bind to the protein being assayed. The (bound) form of the dye has an absorption spectrum maximum historically held at 595 nm. The cationic (unbound) forms are green or red. The binding of the dye to the protein stabilizes the blue anionic form. The increase of absorbance at 595 nm is proportional to the amount of bound dye, and thus to the amount (concentration) of protein present in the sample.

Particularly preferred is the BCA assay. For performing a BCA assay, several commercially available kits are used.

5.5.5.11   Determination of Plasmid DNA Contamination

Residual plasmid DNA is optionally detected by PCR or quantitative PCR, using specific primers and probes for DNA plasmid used for in vitro transcription. Particularly preferred is detecting residual plasmid DNA via quantitative PCR as described herein, using specific primers and probes for the ampicillin gene hosted in the production vector. The probes are used as positive control and thus for calculating the plasmid DNA concentration.

The use of the following primers and probes are particularly preferred:
Sense-Primer bla13U: GATACCGCGAGACCCAC Antisense-Primer bla355L: GGAACCGGAGCTGAATG Probe BL04FL: GCCAGCCGGAAGGGCC-FL
Probe BL04LC: LC Red640-GCGCAGAAGTGGTCCTGCA-Ph

5.5.5.12   Determination of Bacterial DNA Contamination

Residual bacterial DNA is optionally detected, e.g., by PCR or quantitative PCR using specific primers and probes for bacterial genomic sequences. Particularly preferred is the detection of residual bacterial DNA via quantitative PCR using specific primers and probes for the E. coli gene uidA. The probes are used as positive control and thus calculate the bacterial DNA concentration.

The following primers and probes are used for the quantitative PCR:
Primer EC 679U: GGACAAGGCACTAGCG
Primer EC 973 L: ATGCGAGGTACGGTAGGA Probe EC1 FL: CATCCGGTCAGTGGCAGT-FL

Probe EC1 LC: LC640-AAGGGCGAACAGTTCCTGA-pH
Determination of residual solvent contamination
Using the standard addition method, residual solvents are analyzed based on the PhEur 2.2.28 method via headspace gas chromatography. Samples are heated to 80°C, equilibrated, and the gas phase is injected and analyzed using flame ionization detection (FID). The analysis includes acetonitrile, chloroform, triethylammonium acetate (TEAA), isopropanol, and phenol.

5.6 CONCLUSION

The cGMP manufacturing of mRNA vaccines is a complex process; however, the process is validated, and it should result in consistent product. Therefore, of great importance are the in-process control QC checks.

6 Regulatory Guidance

6.1 BACKGROUND

The RNA molecules are singular chain nucleosides that can be fully confirmed for their structure, just like chemical drugs. Does it mean RNA products can be classified as generic drugs? These are broad questions, and the regulatory agencies have dealt with them in diverse manners. The US Food and Drug Administration (FDA) does not have any specific classification. Still, if it is a vaccine, it will fall under the Biological License Application, not because it is biological but because all vaccines have been biologics. Hence, the filing process remains under the CBER. The US government was required to provide licenses to oversee vaccine safety and regulation.

In the European Union (EU), the Advanced Therapies Medicinal Products (ATMP) centralized filing is required for RNA-based products that are intended for gene therapy; however, for RNA against infectious diseases, it is no longer an ATMP. However, if recombinant DNA technology is used, mRNA-based vaccinations for infectious diseases will also need to be approved through the centralized process. Suppose the centralized procedure's conditions are not met. In that case, mRNA medicines for infectious diseases may be routed through the national system, while the applicant can still request access to the centralized method. These guidelines are undergoing revisions both in the US and EU with the expansion of RNA therapies and vaccines, and it is anticipated that soon, both agencies will form unified criteria for approval.

The RNA product copies can be viewed as biosimilars since their critical quality attributes can be tested and compared to assure high similarity. While the legal definition of these products will keep RNA vaccines out of this route, the current regulatory guidelines suggest reduced testing of therapeutics or vaccines that are similar to the approved product.

The terms "RNA therapies" and "small interfering RNA (siRNA)" are used interchangeably in this chapter. The European Medicines Agency (EMA) and the prophylactic and therapeutic vaccines against infectious diseases have yet to be designated as "gene therapy medical goods" or "gene therapy products" by the FDA.

6.2 REGULATORY BACKGROUND

Characterization of harmful effects concerning target organs, dose dependence, relationship to exposure, and when appropriate, potential reversibility, are all goals of nonclinical safety evaluations. These data are used to determine an initial safe starting dose, dose range for human trials, and parameters for clinical monitoring of potential side effects. Although frequently limited at the start of clinical research,

DOI: 10.1201/9781003248156-7

nonclinical safety studies should be sufficient to identify any adverse effects in the clinical trial settings to be justified.

6.2.1 Requirements for Safety/Toxicity Testing

A checklist of some general basic requirements for starting toxicity studies of a *New Chemical Entity* (NCE) include:

- Information on dosage and pharmacokinetics (PK)
- Information about the test species
- Sufficient quantity and quality of the test item (e.g., drug substance or vehicle) available
- Suitable formulation
- Guarantee that the test item used in clinical trials will not have a different impurity pattern than the test item used in toxicity testing
- Planned and tested points for the handling, storage, and logistics of the test item in drug substance
- Information on the adherence of preclinical and clinical trials materials and any particular materials required
- Package units have been determined and are available
- Suitable drug substance concentrations are available to ensure the lowest and maximum application volumes
- Formulation and dilution analysis procedure has been validated
- Confirm analytical approach for bioanalytic in various matrices and ascertain the method's validation status
- Available stability statistics for the stored test item: formulation stability and serum/plasma stability (including freeze/thaw cycles)

For *New Biologic Entities* (NBE), there are additional requirements:

- In an ideal world, the therapeutic ingredient is in its (nearly) final formulation for use in clinical trials; the formulation appears to have little effect on immunogenicity modulation.
- Is it necessary to use activity assays? Are they established and validated?
- The material should be derived from the clinical testing material's manufacturing procedure. It should come from a GMP or pre-GMP batch (often referred to as the "tox-batch"), with the material and the method adequately defined.
- Is it possible to establish and evaluate bioactivity assays (batch release tests)?

The GLP-compliant study protocol includes:

- The item that will be put to the test
- The test, which is based on regulatory procedures

- The setting where the testing takes place (facility, people involved)
- All of the activities that were scheduled
- The information that will be recorded and reported
- Record-keeping (what and where)

The following is an example of a toxicological in vivo study procedure that summarizes the essential points.

6.2.2 STUDY REPORT (GLP COMPLIANT)

All of the findings must be clearly described in the study report. However, it is not the place to make any scientific interpretations or statements on the implications of the test results for the drug's administration to humans. A report, like a study protocol, offers extensive information about:

- The item used
- The regulatory processes that exam was based on
- The conditions of facilities and training of people involved in the testing
- All completed activities
- All observable findings and endpoints
- The evaluation of the findings of toxicity testing (both summary and in-detail appendices)
- Archiving
- A toxicological animal study report is summarized in the following example.

6.3 TESTING METHODS

Specific regulatory requirements for new RNA vaccines may not be available. In the absence of specific guidance, the safety testing strategy and the study design are developed case-by-case. The protocols will be based on more general principles applying to safety testing of the vaccine, adjuvants, DNA vaccines, and combination vaccines of gene therapy products, all based on the risk assessment's scientific rationale.

The anticipated risks include: Local reactions (e.g., pain, redness, swelling, granuloma formation, abscess, necrosis, and regional lymphadenopathy) as well as typical systemic reactions (e.g., anaphylaxis, pyrogenicity, organ-specific toxicity, nausea/diarrhea/malaise); immunological-mediated toxicity (cytokine release, immune suppression, autoimmune illness); teratology; and carcinogenicity—all are examples of immune-mediated toxicity. Following the stated basic toxicity assessment described in the WHO guideline on the nonclinical evaluation of vaccines is advised for assessing these subjects and including the question of unanticipated toxicity. Additional toxicity testing may be required in some circumstances. This is followed by immuno-stimulation/inflammatory activation, which can have negative consequences for the host, such as the production of fever or flu-like symptoms and increased inflammation expression of autoantigens.

6.3.1 Prerequisites

Before starting the nonclinical assessment of the RNA vaccine, information on the following of the vaccine formulation should be available: Mass, Identity, Purity, Sterility, Stability, and Potency.

The purpose of nonclinical studies is to support the intended clinical use of the vaccine, and it is thus necessary to know:

- The patient population and the planned clinical application (clinical indication)
- The clinical route/device of administration that will be used
- This is the formulation
- The dosage level that is expected
- The timetable for immunizations

Although a GMP lot is preferred, a pre-GMP (validation) lot equivalent to the proposed clinical lot can be used to ensure that nonclinical and clinical data are comparable. In addition, control formulations should be available to treat the control groups.

In smaller animals, administering a full human dose (FHD) can be problematic because the total amount used in humans is difficult to achieve. However, this issue can be overcome, or partially overcome, by employing multiple administrative sites per animal.

6.4 ANIMAL TESTING

For vaccines, safety testing in a single, relevant species is sufficient. Ideally, the selected species should fulfill a series of criteria:

- To discover toxicities linked to the vaccine's pharmacodynamic action, the selected species must have an immunological response to the vaccine and adjuvants following inoculation that is similar to the predicted response in humans.
- If vaccines are directed against a pathogen, the chosen species must be vulnerable to that infection.

Furthermore, prior familiarity with a certain model may be a solid justification for adopting that model for safety investigations. The model's feasibility is based on the route and the volume of vaccine to be given, the volume of biological samples required for analysis, and the availability of serological kits and reagents for that animal species.

6.4.1 Testing Strategy for the Safety Assessment

Mice, rats, rabbits, and, occasionally, minipigs (or non-human primates) are a commonly employed species. It's possible to find species that are not as well-known.

To paraphrase the WHO guideline on the nonclinical evaluation of vaccines, the following guidance should be followed to create a study design:

"The preclinical toxicity study should be adequate to identify and characterize potential toxic effects of a vaccine to allow investigators to conclude that it is reasonably safe to proceed to clinical investigation. The parameters to be considered in designing animal toxicology studies are the relevant animal species and strain, dosing schedule, method of vaccine administration, and the timing of evaluation of endpoints (e.g., sampling for clinical chemistry, antibody evaluation, and necropsy). The route of administration should correspond to that intended for use in clinical trials. When the vaccine is to be administered in human clinical trials using a particular device, the same device should be used in the animal study where feasible (e.g., measles aerosol vaccine in the monkey model). Potential toxic effects of the product should be evaluated with regard to target organs, dose, route(s) of exposure, duration, and frequency of exposure, and potential reversibility. The toxicity assessment of the vaccine formulation can be done either in dedicated stand-alone toxicity studies or in combination with studies of safety and activity that have toxicity endpoints incorporated into the design. The study should also include an assessment of local tolerance."

(www.who.int/teams/health-product-policy-and-standards/standards-and -specifications/vaccine-standardization/non-clinical-evaluation-of-vaccines)

In addition to the WHO's standards, the Guideline on the Non-Clinical Studies Required Before First Clinical Use of Gene Therapy Medicinal Products applies to RNA vaccines. According to EMEA/CHMP/GTWP/125459/2006, investigations should be devised and carried out with the goal of determining the following:

- Pharmacodynamic "proof of concept" in a nonclinical model(s)
- The GTMP's biodistribution
- Recommendation for the proposed clinical trial's initial dose and dose escalation method
- Identification of possible toxicity target organs
- Identification of putative biological activity target organs
- Identification of the indicators that will be tracked in the clinical experiment
- Specific patient qualifying requirements must be identified

In general, consulting with regulatory agencies to evaluate the suitability of a proposed testing approach for a specific RNA vaccination is highly recommended and encouraged. Then, a testing program can be finalized and launched based on the topics mentioned during such a meeting.

6.4.2 SINGLE DOSE TOXICITY

A sample nonclinical safety evaluation program for an RNA vaccine might look like this:

- Toxicity from a single dose
- Toxicity from repeated doses (if feasible, including local tolerance, immunological, and safety pharmacology endpoints)

- Adsorption by tissues and removal from the organism are all part of biodistribution
- Pharmacology of safety (In single or repeated dosage toxicity investigations, safety pharmacology evaluations should be included if possible)
- Tolerance in the community (acute and chronic inflammation)
- Studies on immunogenicity (induction of hypersensitivity, anaphylaxis, immune suppression, autoimmunity)

Vaccines do not generally require toxicity testing. However, in vitro tests for mutation and chromosomal damage should be undertaken prior to the first human exposure if the vaccine formulation's components require such studies. Vaccines are not usually subjected to carcinogenicity tests. However, it is necessary to assess whether certain components of the vaccine formulation may necessitate such research.

Developmental toxicity studies are usually not required for vaccines intended for childhood immunization. Development and Reproductive Toxicology (DART) studies should be considered if women of reproductive age are included in the intended clinical research/target population unless good evidence suggests that DART studies are not required.

Single-dose toxicity trials give preliminary data on the vaccine's acute safety and acceptability. They follow the standard protocol for rodent acute toxicity studies, including administering the full human dose (FHD) or more. Single-dose toxicity studies are rarely conducted when this information is already available from repeated dose toxicity studies. However, single-dose studies may be necessary if no in vivo data is available before initiating a repeated dosage trial or if the immune response elicited by the first injection alters the response to a subsequent administration.

6.4.3 Repeated Dose Toxicity

Repeated dosage toxicity testing has a wide range of applications. Its objectives are to determine the toxicological profile and toxicological targets and learn as much as possible about the causes of discovered toxicities (and if wisely designed, it is also possible to assess pharmacological parameters and exaggerated pharmacological effects).

The dose to be evaluated for vaccinations must be the full human dose (FHD) and the formulation designed for clinical trials. If the FHD isn't possible, the maximum feasible dosage (MFD) must be used. Higher (just tiny multiples of the FHD to avoid any irrelevant immunological effects) or lower (if unacceptable toxicities are expected, and a NOAEL needs to be calculated) doses may be preferable to have flexibility in determining the clinical dose. Include appropriate control groups in the study (placebo, vehicle, adjuvant-only or antigen-only, etc.). The vaccine's routes and doses (how, how much, and how often it is given) are determined by the vaccine's intended clinical usage. The time plan can be compressed if the dose intervals are largely consistent with the underlying immunological events. In particular, successive doses in animals should be separated by sufficient time to avoid interfering with each other's immunological responses. A two-to-three-week interval between

Animal species:	Mouse
Duration in-life:	28 days to 3 months
Administration:	Repeated, route as close as possible to the clinical one
Test item:	RNA vaccine clinical formulation, lyophilized as ready to dissolve
Dose level:	1
Groups:	6 groups:
	1. saline control group, main
	2. saline control group, recovery
	3. dose group, main
	4. dose group, recovery
	5. saline control, satellite
	6. dose group, satellite
Group size:	20 (10 m + 10 f)
Total animals:	120

Monitoring:	Mortality
	Body weight
	Clinical observation
	Food consumption
	Local reaction
	Body temperature
	FOB (mod. Irwin)
	Hematology
	Clinical chemistry
	Urinalysis*
	Bone marrow smear
	Blood coagulation parameters
	Cytokines: TNF-α, IFN-g, IL-6, IL-10, etc...
Post mortem:	Necropsy and weight of selected organs
	Full histopathological evaluation of all animals including recovery animals
	RNA biodistribution in satellite animals (administration site, lymph nodes, liver, lung, gonads)
Duration:	Study plan to report: 6 to 8 months

FIGURE 6.1   Repeated dose toxicity: a sample case study.

administrations is thought to be sufficient. To ensure the safety of the human dosage schedule, the number of administrations in the toxicity research should surpass the number scheduled for human administration (at least one more administration should be given than in the proposed clinical scheme).

A sample case study for a repeated dosage study, encompassing biodistribution, CNS safety pharmacology, and local tolerance evaluation, is provided to understand what a safety testing study can entail (Figure 6.1).

Blood collection is required for various monitoring purposes (including clinical chemistry, blood coagulation, hematology, and toxicokinetic). There are species-specific restrictions on how much blood can be taken without endangering the animals. The WHO and EMA guidelines set the tissue list for histopathology.

If possible, ophthalmological examinations should be included in the clinical observations to monitor uveitis as a possible indicator of autoimmune responses.

GLP must be followed in terms of testing, reporting, and archiving.

6.5   SAFETY PHARMACOLOGY

If pharmacological safety studies are required, they must be reviewed on a product-by-product basis. In so-called safety pharmacology investigations, the acute effect of the test chemical on important organ systems when delivered at doses in the therapeutic range or higher is evaluated. The core battery studies consist of a standard series of assays that measure cardiovascular, central nervous system, and pulmonary effects.

In telemetered non-rodents (guinea pigs, rats, and mice), an in vivo cardiovascular safety investigation is routinely conducted. Animals are given a low, medium, and high dose of the test drug, with washout periods in between. After administration, cardiovascular parameters (e.g., arterial pressure, heart rate, ECG, and body temperature) are monitored and analyzed. Drugs that prolong the QT interval block the activation of the human hERG gene channel in cardiomyocytes. This could result in torsades des pointes, a potentially fatal tachyarrhythmia. As a result, electrophysiological recordings in cells stably transfected with the hERG clone are used to perform in vitro monitoring for QT prolongation (hERG channel test).

After delivery of the test drug, respiratory safety is evaluated by recording and analyzing respiratory parameters in vivo.

Safety testing of the central nervous system (CNS) (e.g., Irwin test) can be done as a stand-alone test in rats or as part of a more extensive toxicity study (e.g., repeated dose studies; see case study). It is based on assessing a collection of behavioral parameters at predetermined time intervals following the injection of the test material.

6.5.1 IMMUNOGENICITY

The first screen for immunotoxicity comes from general toxicity studies, where special attention should be paid to hematological changes, changes in immune system organs (weight and histopathology), changes in serum albumins without plausible explanation, increased infection incidence, increased body temperature, Increased tumor occurrence in the lack of reasonable genotoxic factors, immunological biomarker levels that are outside the normal range or when compared to controls. Further immunotoxicity testing is required if immunotoxicity is a concern, either as a result due to the literature search and substance attributes or because of the intended therapeutic usage (i.e., immunocompromised patients).

Immune reactions are a major part of the pharmacological activity of RNA vaccines, hence testing for undesired hematological changes, changes in immune system organs (weight and histopathology), changes in serum albumins without plausible explanation, increased infection incidence, increased body temperature, increased tumor occurrence in the absence of plausible genotoxic, immunological biomarker values outside the normal range, or when compared to controls.

Factually, there are no standards for immunogenicity testing GLP status. Despite this, a functioning validated immunological test is ideal due to the complexity of the immune response.

6.6   ENVIRONMENTAL RISK ASSESSMENT (ERA)

Contrary to popular belief, toxicity testing is not limited to human health research. This becomes evident as a lot of therapeutic goods are disposed of. As a result, a request for an Environmental Risk Assessment (ERA) similar to that required for chemicals is reasonable. The Regulation on the Registration, Evaluation, and Authorization of Chemicals (REACH) governs the latter in the EU; an ERA of novel drug compounds is required under Article 8(3) (ca) and (g) of Directive 2001/83/EC as amended. In addition, all new marketing authorization applications must include an ERA.

The evaluation of potential environmental threats is a two-phase, step-by-step process. The first part (Phase I) assesses the drug substance's exposure to the environment, and the second phase (Phase II) examines the drug substance's environmental fate and effect. The EMA's Guideline on environmental risk assessment of pharmaceutical products for human use contains more information.

6.7 NONCLINICAL DATA

Nonclinical examinations of a vaccine candidate establish its immunogenicity and safety features through in vitro and in vivo testing. In addition, nonclinical research in animal models aid in the identification of potential vaccine-related safety hazards and selecting the dose, dosing regimen, and method of administration for clinical trials. The amount of nonclinical evidence needed to support moving on with first-in-human (FIH) clinical trials is determined by the vaccine architecture, available supportive data, and data from closely related vaccines.

Any investigational product's preclinical program should be tailored to its specific breadth, complexity, and overall design. We support the "3Rs" principles of reducing, refining, and replacing animal experimentation when possible. Proposals should be submitted during early communication sessions with the FDA, along with justification for any potential alternative methodologies (e.g., in vitro or in silico testing). We'll look at whether such an alternative method could be utilized instead of animal testing.

Nonclinical safety studies may not be required before FIH clinical trials in some circumstances since sufficient information to characterize product safety may be available from other sources. For example, if the vaccine candidate is sufficiently characterized and made using the same platform technology as a licensed vaccine or other previously studied investigational vaccines, toxicology data (e.g., data from repeat-dose toxicity studies, biodistribution studies) and clinical data from other products made using the same platform may be used to support FIH clinical trials for that virus vaccine candidate. If vaccine producers consider utilizing these data instead of nonclinical safety studies, they should explain the findings and provide a reason.

Nonclinical safety evaluations, such as toxicity and local tolerance studies, must be done per regulations dictating good laboratory practices (GLP) for conducting nonclinical laboratory studies as needed to support continuing FIH clinical trials (21 CFR Part 58). Before FIH clinical trials, such research should be done and analyzed. Additional safety testing should be done if toxicology studies do not adequately identify danger.

If the vaccine design is novel and there is no previous biodistribution data from the platform technology, biodistribution studies in an animal species should be explored. If there is a chance of changing infectivity and tissue tropism, or if a new method of administration and formulation will be utilized, these investigations should be done.

To evaluate the vaccine candidate's immunologic features and assist FIH clinical trials, immunogenicity studies in animal models sensitive to the selected virus vaccine antigen should be done. In addition, measurements of immunogenicity should be appropriate for the vaccine design and mechanism of action.

As appropriate to each virus antigens included in the study, humoral, cellular, and functional immune responses should be assessed. To define the humoral response, antigen-specific enzyme-linked immunosorbent tests (ELISA) should be investigated. CD8+ and CD4+ T cell responses should be examined utilizing sensitive and specific assays for cellular response evaluation. Immune responses' functional activity should be assessed in vitro in neutralization tests employing either wild-type or pseudovirion virus. The assays used to assess immunogenicity should be proven appropriate for their intended use.

Animal models (e.g., rats and nonhuman primates) are needed to investigate the possibility of vaccine-associated enhanced respiratory disease (ERD). To assess the vaccine's risk of causing vaccine-associated ERD in people, post-vaccination animal challenge experiments and characterization of the sort of nonclinical and clinical immune response generated by the vaccine candidate can be used.

Sponsors should conduct studies defining the vaccine-induced immune response in animal models and evaluating immunological markers of probable ERD outcomes to support moving forward with FIH human trials. In animals inoculated with clinically relevant dosages of the COVID-19 vaccine candidate, these should include assessments of functional immune responses (e.g., neutralizing antibody) against total antibody responses and Th1/Th2 balance.

In determining whether Phase 3 studies can proceed in the absence of post-vaccination challenge data to address the risk of ERD, the totality of data for a specific vaccine candidate, including data from post-vaccination challenge studies in small animal models and data from FIH clinical trials characterizing the type of immune responses induced by the vaccine, will be considered.

6.8 ANALYTICAL TESTING

An essential vaccine release assay is the potency assay. Potency tests are available to ensure that the vaccine has the required immunologic effect according to the manufacturer's instructions. Animals are generally used in most potency tests, but novel vaccinations are now being tested in vitro. The following are some examples of potency assay approaches:

- Immunization-challenge test: immunological specificity, immune activity, and the potential for immune toxicity
- Serological analyses: antibody concentration, antibody avidity (a surrogate marker for memory), cellular immune responses (T-cell proliferation and cytokine quantification), functional antibody assays (e.g., pathogen or toxin neutralizing)
- Cell-based assays: cellular immune responses in T cells (e.g., cytotoxic CD8þ and CD4þ)
- Titration assays: measure potency indirectly

The animal challenge test is the gold standard for determining vaccination effectiveness. Inoculate the same type of animal with the recommended immunological dose to the same day of age after the optimal immune response period and, at the same time, induce the infection that can cause pathogenesis in the animal, measure the vaccine's ability, and reduce disease incidence after a certain time based on the immunized animal's protection.

Experimental animal substitution and serological substitution are two further options. The first way is to substitute other animals with identical clinical signs as the original animals, so indirectly testing the vaccine's efficacy. In the case of the serological approach, the vaccine's efficacy is determined by measuring the antibody titer level after inoculation. It entails virus neutralization experiments as well as several ELISA tests (Figure 6.2).

6.8.1 CAPABILITY AND CAPACITY

The mRNA QC facility should be capable of conducting the following analyses:

- Sequencing system for RNA analysis
- DNA synthesizer [https://kilobaser.com/]
- RP-HPLC purity
- Concentration: UV spectrometry
- Immunization-challenge test: immunological specificity, immune activity, and the potential for immune toxicity [https://www.fda.gov/regulatory-information/search-fda-guidance-documents/immunotoxicity-testing-guidance; https://www.fda.gov/media/135312/download]

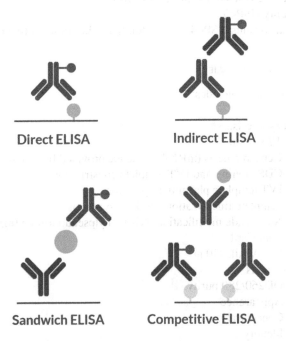

FIGURE 6.2   Potency testing methods: assays ranging from animal challenge test, PD_{50} test, PGP test, ELISA to PCR.

- Serological analyses: antibody concentration, antibody avidity (a surrogate marker for memory), cellular immune responses (T-cell proliferation and cytokine quantification), functional antibody assays (e.g., pathogen or toxin neutralizing)
- Cell-based assays: cellular immune responses in T cells (e.g., cytotoxic CD8þ and CD4þ)
- DNA Detection: detect region(s) of plasmid using qPCR; Primers and Tm Probe specific for 3'UTR, Kan-R, or Amp-R
- RNase digestion: in vitro translation; RT-PCR for a specific amplicon; RT-PCR followed by PCR followed by Sanger Sequencing
- Capping efficiency: LCMS
- Integrity and purity: Bioanalyzer
- Poly(A) tail length: LCMS
- Residual protein
- Residual plasmid DNA
- Double-stranded RNA
- Purity
- pH USP<791>
- Endotoxin USP<85>
- Bioburden USP<61>
- Sterility USP<71>
- Appearance USP<631> and USP<790>
- Osmolality USP<785>
- Residual solvents USP<467>: acetonitrile, chloroform, ethanol

6.8.2 TECHNICAL DOSSIER

The technical dossier includes:

1.1. mRNA synthesis:
    1.1.1. T7 system
    1.1.2. Gene synthesis (mRNA sequence provided by Client)
    1.1.3. CDS cloning and IVT template construction
    1.1.4. IVT template plasmid preparation
    1.1.5. Template linearization and IVT synthesis
    1.1.6. Nucleoside modification: N1-methylpseudouridine (m1Ψ)
    1.1.7. Cap: Cap1
    1.1.8. PolyA tail: 110 nt
1.2. QC tests mRNA:
    1.2.1. OD260/280 purity
    1.2.2. Appearance
    1.2.3. Concentration
    1.2.4. Identity
    1.2.5. Endotoxin
    1.2.6. Residual dsRNA

1.2.7. Residual template
1.2.8. Residual host protein
1.3. Deliverables:
  1.3.1. CoA
  1.3.2. mRNA stock (if available after LNP encapsulation)
  1.3.3. Template plasmid
  1.3.4. E. coli stock of template plasmid: 20 vials
  1.3.5. Sample report of GMP-grade manufacture
  1.3.6. Project report
  1.3.7. STMs for testing, validated, or suitable
1.4. LNP encapsulation and test:
  1.4.1. mRNA sample size: X mg
  1.4.2. QC tests formulated product:
    1.4.2.1. CopA
    1.4.2.2. Concentration
    1.4.2.3. Size
    1.4.2.4. Zeta potential
    1.4.2.5. Encapsulation efficiency
    1.4.2.6. Stability tests
  1.4.3. Deliverables:
    1.4.3.1. mRNA-LNP stock (if available after animal study)
    1.4.3.2. Project report
    1.4.3.3. In vitro expression test
  1.4.4. Dose escalation study:
    1.4.4.1. Strain: BALB/c mouse
    1.4.4.2. Administration route: im
    1.4.4.3. Single-dose
    1.4.4.4. Grouping:
      1.4.4.4.1. Group 1: 0.01 mg/kg (n=6, 3M/3F)
      1.4.4.4.2. Group 2: 0.05 mg/kg (n=6, 3M/3F)
      1.4.4.4.3. Group 3: 0.1 mg/kg (n=6, 3M/3F)
      1.4.4.4.4. Group 4: 0.5 mg/kg (n=6, 3M/3F)
      1.4.4.4.5. Group 5: 1 mg/kg (n=6, 3M/3F)
    1.4.4.5. Clinical observation (mortality, weight, food consumption, other abnormal clinical signs)
    1.4.4.6. Deliverables: Study report, STM
  1.4.5. Potency study
    1.4.5.1. Strain: BALB/c mouse
    1.4.5.2. Administration route: im
    1.4.5.3. Single dose
    1.4.5.4. Grouping:
      1.4.5.4.1. Group 1: mRNA-LNP, dose (n=10, 5M/5F)
      1.4.5.4.2. Group 2: Vehicle control (n = 4, 2M/2F)
    1.4.5.5. Serum collection
    1.4.5.6. Measurement of binding antibody by ELISA

1.5. mRNA-LNP Stability and Storability
   1.5.1. Size, zeta potential, and pH after stored for 30 days at refrigerator
           temperature (5±3 oC), followed by periodic sampling at 0, 1, 2, 4,
           24, and 48 h storage at room temperature (24±2 oC)
   1.5.2. Leakage of encapsulated mRNA outside the nanoparticles
   1.5.3. In vitro cytotoxicity of mRNA-LNPs
           1.5.3.1. KG-1 and HEK 293T cell lines were cultured as suspen-
           sion and adherent cells
           1.5.3.2. Cell viability is determined using an XTT assay
   1.5.4. Animal studies
           1.5.4.1. Spike-encoding mRNA potency in inducing a humoral
                     immune response
           1.5.4.2. Two groups of Balb/c mice were given 100 L of
                     Lipofectamine (diluted in sterile PBS) containing either
                     10 or 20 g of Spike-encoding mRNA intramuscularly
                     (IM) (eight mice in each mRNA receiving group and
                     six mice in the control group). Blood is drawn on days
                     21, 28, and 84 after the injection and evaluated after the
                     serum has been separated
           1.5.4.3. Vaccine efficiency is evaluated in the two types of mice:
                     Balb/c (6–8 weeks) and C57BL/6 (6–8 weeks) and in
                     rhesus macaque monkeys (4–6 years) as a non-human
                     primates (NHPs) model
   1.5.5. Humoral immune response
           1.5.5.1. Survey the humoral immune response generated by
                     administration of Spike-encoding mRNA-LNPs, the
                     indirect configuration of ELISA method is used
   1.5.6. Virus neutralization test (VNT)
           1.5.6.1. The humoral immune response induced by mRNA-
                     LNPs, Twofold serial dilutions of C57BL/6, and Balb/c
                     mouse sera are produced in 2% DMEM for the viral neu-
                     tralization test
           1.5.6.2. Cell-mediated immune response
                     1.5.6.2.1. On day 28 after the booster immunization,
                                 spleen tissues from Balb/c mice received
                                 mRNA-LNPs containing either 1 or 10 g of
                                 Spike-encoding mRNA
   1.5.7. Spleen tissues from Balb/c mice that had received mRNA-LNPs
           containing either 1 or 10 μg of Spike-encoding mRNA at day 28
           post booster immunization

6.9 THE EUROPEAN REGULATORY FRAMEWORK

mRNA-based therapies are well-integrated into the existing EU regulatory system from a regulatory standpoint. Depending on the categorization, marketing

authorization applications are examined by the EMA's CAT (gene therapy) or the CHMP. Since ATMPs/gene therapy products and medicines made utilizing recombinant DNA technology require the centralized EMA approval procedure, most, if not all, mRNA-based medicinal goods must be approved through the EMA centralized system. As a result, full market access to the European Union is now possible. ATMPs/gene therapy products can be approved at the national level provided certain criteria are met, such as non-routine manufacture. Regulatory organizations in EU member states, on the other hand, are currently solely responsible for clinical development. After the new clinical trials law takes effect, this will remain the case in theory, but clinical trial applications will have to be submitted through the new EMA portal. However, it is advised that inventors of mRNA-based medicines seek scientific help from the European Medicines Agency before beginning important clinical trials (EMA). As a result, the European Medicines Agency's quality, preclinical, and clinical standards for obtaining a marketing authorization will be clarified (EMA).

Like any other pharmaceutical product, mRNA-based therapies are regulated in the EU at both the national and EU or central levels, depending on their stage of development. While clinical trials and the manufacture of experimental medicinal items are regulated at the national level, certain products are switched to the EU level when a marketing license is sought. Depending on the product class, an mRNA drug can get marketing permission in all EU member states by following the so-called centralized method. The Committee for Human Medicinal Products (CHMP) at the European Medicines Agency evaluates marketing authorization applications (EMA). The European Commission receives the CHMP's view on the approvability of a pharmaceutical product. As a result, the European Commission is the final authority that decides whether a marketing permission application is approved or denied.

Individual EU member state regulatory bodies can act as Rapporteurs or Co-rapporteurs in EMA centralized procedures. In addition, national delegations can serve on EMA committees such as the CHMP, the Pharmacovigilance Risk Assessment Committee (PRAC), and the Committee for Orphan Drugs.

National delegates can also participate in EMA working groups, such as the Biologics Working Party (BWP), the central EMA platform for discussing quality issues related to biological medicinal products, such as those arising during centralized marketing authorization or scientific advice procedures. As of this writing, clinical trial applications must be submitted to the respective member state authorities where the clinical trial will be conducted. With the implementation the new clinical trials rule, this procedure is expected to change. The EMA-centralized method applies if an mRNA-based treatment is intended to be marketed via a single license across the entire EU market. A "regular" marketing authorization, a conditional marketing authorization, or an authorization under extraordinary circumstances can be issued depending on the disease to be treated, and the evidence presented. However, if an mRNA-based drug is to be utilized in a clinical study, a separate application must be submitted to the relevant member state regulatory agencies.

6.9.1 ADVANCED THERAPIES FOR THE APPROVAL OF mRNA-BASED MEDICINES

The centralized EMA approach is required for RNA-based medications that are gene therapy medicinal products. For example, according to the legislation, if mRNA is utilized for the goal of a vaccine against infectious disease, it is no longer an ATMP. However, if recombinant DNA technology is used, mRNA-based vaccinations for infectious diseases will also need to be approved through the centralized process. Suppose the centralized procedure's conditions are not met. In that case, mRNA medicines for infectious diseases may be routed through the national system, while the applicant can still request access to the centralized method.

The CAT is the European Medicines Agency's Committee for Advanced Therapies. The CAT is in charge of evaluating marketing authorization applications for Advanced Therapy Medicinal Products on a scientific basis (ATMP). Those mentioned above consolidated procedural schedule also applies to ATMPs. Gene therapy medicinal goods, somatic cell treatment products, and tissue engineering products are defined as ATMPs.

6.9.1.1 Classification of Medicinal Products by the CAT

A gene therapy medicinal product contains or consists of a recombinant nucleic acid used in or administered to humans to regulate, repair, replace, add, or delete a genetic sequence. Its therapeutic, prophylactic, or diagnostic effect is directly related to the recombinant nucleic acid sequence it contains or the product of gene expression of this sequence. Vaccines against infectious diseases are not permitted in gene therapy medicinal goods.

This definition leads to the following essential conclusions:

- Given that the typical manufacturing procedure for mRNAs involves in vitro transcription using plasmid templates produced from bacteria, such mRNAs must probably be classified as a biological pharmaceutical product.
- Furthermore, codon optimization, modified CAP structures, the introduction of acceptable 5' and 3' noncoding sequences, defined poly(A) tails, and other alterations cause mRNAs to be recombinant.
- Gene therapy medical products are defined as mRNAs that meet the criteria of being a recombinant biological product that is utilized to add or replace a genetic sequence and whose therapeutic, preventive, or diagnostic impact is directly mediated by the nucleic acid it contains.
- If an RNA molecule, like many RNAi molecules, is created using pure chemicals, it is no longer a biological product and cannot be regarded as a gene therapy product.

Notably, even if all of the other parameters are met, an mRNA is not a gene therapy product in the case of treating or preventing infectious disease (recombinant, biological). As a result, an mRNA molecule used for preventative immunization against, say, influenza is not considered a gene therapy product, yet it is when used for cancer treatment. As a result, when it comes to EMA marketing permission, mRNA for infectious disease vaccination is considered by the CHMP. In contrast, mRNAs that meet the criteria of an ATMP are evaluated by the CAT.

Genetically engineered T cells express an exogenous thymidine kinase (TK) gene. They are categorized using the CAT classification method based on the therapeutic, prophylactic, or diagnostic function of the recombinant nucleic acid sequence they contain and the product of gene expression of that sequence. Because the T cells were designed for immunological reconstitution after hematopoietic stem cell transplantation, they were not classed as a gene therapy pharmaceutical product. The goal of the newly introduced TK gene was to treat graft vs. host disease if it appeared in particular patients. As a result, the genetic sequence implanted in the patient (the TK gene) had no direct link to the anticipated therapeutic outcome, namely immune reconstitution. As a result, the cells were labeled as a somatic cell therapy product. For T cells transfected with mRNA encoding, for example, a novel T-cell receptor (TCR), the newly introduced TCR has a clear relationship with the targeted therapeutic impact, the death of cancer cells expressing the target antigen recognized by such a TCR. The pharmaceutical substance would most likely be categorized as an ATMP in this case. Due to the temporary nature of the genetic change, such techniques may be appealing for developing adoptive cellular treatments against novel targets for which safety data is lacking but offer an acceptable risk/benefit profile.

Vaccines against infectious diseases are not included in gene therapy pharmaceutical products. However, according to the CAT reflection article, a gene therapy-based vaccine can still be classed as gene therapy if used to cure or prevent infection-related illnesses (e.g., malignancies). A gene therapy product is, for example, an mRNA-based vaccine for the treatment or prevention of HPV16-induced cancers (if the criteria for gene therapy are fulfilled). Therefore, using the same mRNA for HPV16 vaccination will result in the virus being classified as a vaccine.

6.9.2 Quality Regulatory Requirements

In the EU, the information to be supplied to regulatory authorities for clinical study approval has been unified. On the European Commission's homepage (http://ec.europa.eu/health/documents/eudralex/vol-10/index en.htm), a detailed form with guidance on the specific information to be provided, such as the manufacturer, description, the manufacturing process, control of materials, control of drug substance/drug product, and so on, can be found. Additional information, such as how to apply for a significant change to an existing clinical trial can be found on that homepage. In addition, the EMA has published a detailed guidance document on the quality documentation of biological investigational medicinal products. Because the quality data set for experimental medicinal products is typically limited, especially in the early stages of development, investigational medicines are unlikely to be validated to the same extent as a routinely manufactured/marketed product.

Nonetheless, sterilization techniques should be evaluated as well as the premises and equipment. Virus inactivation/removal and the removal of other biological contaminants should be shown as necessary. In general, clinical trials should be conducted following good clinical practice guidelines.

The information to be provided for centralized marketing authorization applications is defined in the Common Technical Document (CTD), which includes administrative information (Module 1); quality, preclinical, and clinical data summaries (Module 2); quality data (Module 3); and preclinical and clinical information (Modules 4 and 5). Before filing a marketing permission application, it is strongly advised that applicants meet with EMA for pre-submission meetings. It is worth noting that the risk-based method can be used for ATMPs to tailor the content of applicants' marketing permission applications to a specific product. Even though the main technical requirements, i.e., the data to be supplied for ATMPs, are established in Part IV of the Annex to Directive 2001/83/ EC, modifications are permissible if justified by the risk-based approach. The risk-based approach is based on creating a risk profile by identifying hazards and variables. This enables applicants to justify the amount of information provided in various sections of the marketing permission application.

The EMA has yet to issue explicit recommendations for developing mRNA-based medicines. As a result, overarching guidance documents' general concepts must be followed. Though mRNA-based vaccines for the prevention or treatment of infectious disease are not considered gene therapy products, the concepts established in the European Medicines Agency's (EMA) guidance for gene therapy medical products take quality, nonclinical, and clinical issues into account. The latter guideline is only accessible as a draft version at the time of authoring this manuscript, and it may be updated after taking into account public feedback. In addition, the EMA recommendations on "human cell-based medical products" and the guidance on genetically modified cells should be examined if mRNA is transfected into somatic cells to obtain a cell-based product. As with all medicines, an appropriate manufacturing method must be designed to ensure a consistent quality medicinal output. Critical process steps, intermediates, drug substance, and final drug product standards must all be established. It is also necessary to establish and manage the quality of raw and beginning materials. The European Pharmacopoeia will shortly issue chapter 5.2.12 on "Raw materials of biological origin for manufacturing cell-based and gene therapy medical products" (Ph. Eur.). It includes biological materials such as sera, medium, recombinant proteins, and proteins derived from biological components like enzymes.

Appearance, identity (and, in the case of nucleic acids, integrity), content, potency, product, process-related contaminants, sterility, endotoxin, and physicochemical testing such as pH and osmolality are all quality criteria to be regulated. If mRNA molecules are complexed with poly-cationic molecules or liposomes, particle size distribution assays and requirements should be devised. A constant amount of complex ingredients should be established either as part of the therapeutic product release or validation investigations. If the complexing materials and medication product are admixed right before patient administration, the latter alternative is required. In some circumstances, particularly during the early stages of clinical development, regulatory authorities may view the final preparation of a liposomal formulation or an emulsion as manufacturing (rather than reconstitution) that must be appropriately controlled, i.e., through appropriate release testing. Whether the final formulation is defined as manufacture or reconstitution, it is reasonable to delegate this process to certified pharmacies whenever possible. During product development, in addition to release testing, additional characterization studies with complexed nucleic acids should be conducted, addressing properties such as shape, surface charge, and stability.

6.9.3 PRECLINICAL REGULATORY REQUIREMENTS FOR mRNA MEDICINAL PRODUCTS

While it is apparent that experimental drug substances and drug products must be manufactured according to GMP in the EU, it is less clear from which manufacturing stage onwards GMP must be implemented in the case of mRNA manufacture. Part II of the GMP guidelines includes examples of various drug compounds (basic requirements for active substances used as starting materials). In general, drug substance manufacturing begins with the raw components for the drug substance. The plasmid, the host bacteria, and the master cell bank of the recombinant microbial cells are the beginning materials for plasmids or nonviral vectors (such as mRNA). However, the latter reference does not define when GMP is required for plasmids and nonviral vectors. However, in the case of viral vectors used to make genetically modified cells, GMP must be followed from the cell bank system to the final product. GMP extends to medicinal compounds, such as those obtained from fermentation/ cell culture, as long as the operational cell bank is maintained. A bacterial cell bank is used as a starting material for several mRNA medicinal compounds. On the other hand, these microbial banks are employed to make a different beginning material (plasmid template) rather than the mRNA medicinal ingredient. While incorporating microbial cell banks into the GMP system may be helpful, there is currently no definite necessity. On the other hand, the published guidance does not require GMP for the recombinant method employed for the initial plasmid/template construction. However, there is no dispute that in vitro transcription is a form of drug material manufacturing that requires GMP compliance. However, while the development and testing of numerous forms of viral and nonviral vectors are covered in Ph. Eur. General chapter 5.14, mRNA is not yet included.

There is currently no specialized guideline for the preclinical evaluation of mRNA vaccines. The preclinical pharmacological and toxicological evaluation of mRNA is heavily influenced by the condition being treated and the route of administration. The following example may show this fact. Vaccines are typically given locally via intradermal or intramuscular injection. As a result, pharmacokinetic investigations are rarely required.

On the other hand, the guidelines for intravenous administration of mRNAs intended for therapeutic cancer vaccination is sometimes used. The study of pharmacokinetic parameters after a single or repeated systemic treatment appears significant from a safety and efficacy standpoint. In the event of systemic delivery, exposure, clearance, and accumulation are important plasma PK parameters to consider. mRNA may accumulate or stay in plasma after repeated treatment due to improved stability gained by complexing with appropriate molecules. This could be problematic because mRNA is immunostimulatory and can cause the release of pro-inflammatory cytokines.

6.9.4 CLINICAL REGULATORY REQUIREMENTS FOR mRNA MEDICINES

Biodistribution studies are considered essential because many gene therapy pharmaceutical items can integrate into the recipients' genomes. Studies like these appear to be less critical than, for example, studies on retroviral vector systems used for therapeutic vaccination because genome integration is not an issue with mRNA therapy. Metabolism investigations are frequently overlooked since it is assumed that mRNA medicines are processed similarly to endogenous mRNA molecules. This could be different if chemically modified nucleosides are used.

The goal of biodistribution studies is to learn more about where injected medications end up. This information is then applied to interpret the drug's pharmacological or toxicological interactions. Because mRNA therapies have several components and are processed at multiple levels, interpret all of these interactions. PEGylated LNPs, for example, can elicit immune responses; LNPs can temporarily saturate the liver's scavenging systems; impurities like dsRNA can cause pro-inflammatory cytokines and antiviral states in cells; therapeutic mRNA can act as miRNA sponges; and the expressed therapeutic protein can have local or even distant effects in the body. Furthermore, current standards for preclinical biodistribution data of (m)RNA treatments are ambiguous and ill-defined, with no thresholds for sensitivity. A more comprehensive regulatory framework would increase clinical applications and public acceptance of this extremely promising platform technology. As the number of (m)RNA treatments seeking clinical approval proliferates, shifting from a per-product approach to more universal criteria may become necessary.

Regulatory agencies do not currently consider mRNA vaccinations against infectious diseases to be gene therapies. Although they have the same composition and manufacturing procedure as mRNA therapies for protein replacement, they are classified as vaccinations. Indeed, for in vitro transcription template creation, many mRNA-based therapies (including mRNA vaccines) rely on recombinant DNA technology. Therefore, almost all mRNA-based therapies should be categorized as "gene therapy medical products," as defined by the EMA (of note, this does not apply to siRNA-based therapeutics, as these molecules are typically chemically manufactured). Furthermore, mRNA vaccines for noninfectious disorders such as cancer are classified as gene therapy products rather than mRNA vaccines. Surprisingly, an mRNA vaccine for HPV-related cancers is categorized as gene therapy, whereas utilizing the same mRNA for HPV immunization is classified as a vaccine. This distinction (and its implications) is unclear. However, it could be due to adjuvants' additional effect and the antigenic character of mRNA vaccines' translated foreign proteins. Even though these exogenous proteins are unlikely to have any physiological function in the body, these vaccines are designed to induce strong, long-lasting immune responses and are thus not physiologically inactive.

Furthermore, the non-mRNA components of mRNA vaccines have the same tissue biodistribution and off-target interactions as other (m)RNA treatments. Finally, viral-based RNA platforms like self-amplifying or trans-amplifying mRNA encode a replicase complex of viral non-structural proteins and a therapeutic protein of choice. The former can be both exogenous and endogenous in future applications to induce a vaccine-like immune response, while the latter can be exogenous.

Biodistribution studies are deemed less critical because mRNA vaccines are delivered locally in the skin or muscle. Luciferase mRNA administered intramuscularly, on the other hand, produces light in the liver. As a result, either the mRNA-LNPs or their protein product is systemically dispersed, necessitating pharmacokinetic and biodistribution studies. Biodistribution studies are not required for (non-vaccine) mRNA therapies, either. This viewpoint should be revisited in light of the development of mRNA-based CRISPR/Cas9 treatments. Furthermore, preclinical biodistribution studies can save time, money, and animals (e.g., toxicology).

Most RNA biodistribution investigations now use quantitative whole-body autoradiography as the method of choice. While maintaining tissue-level resolution, this approach provides a valuable whole-body perspective of the drug's distribution. However, the radioactive compounds utilized necessitate specific equipment and personnel. Furthermore, a significant constraint is the inability to distinguish between parent substances and their metabolites/degradation products, especially for unstable molecules like RNA. Finally, most labeled RNA will never reach the cytoplasm; therefore, it isn't always crucial in interpreting toxicological results, a major distinction between new RNA therapies and small compounds. Multi-modal imaging and quantification approaches are recommended to analyze the biodistribution of RNA therapies properly. For example, using the mRNA coding sequence of luciferase or a fluorescent protein, the distribution, and translation of cytosolic mRNA can be investigated. With hybridization techniques, tissue slices from the same animals can be used to determine subcellular RNA localization, and (single-cell) RT-qPCR can detect minute amounts of mRNA. These findings can also be correlated with immunohistochemistry results. Alternatively, RNA molecules can be seen by directly tagging them with fluorescent cytosine, and transgenic Ai14 reporter mice can be used to monitor cytosolic mRNA transport. In situ ionization techniques (e.g., MALDI-FT-ICR-MS) link this information to distribution data. Mass spectrometry is a powerful approach for assessing intact and degraded siRNA. To fully understand the biodistribution and in vivo properties of this new and rapidly growing class of drugs, we conclude that a multilayered approach is required.

The EMA's anticancer guideline provides preclinical regulatory guidelines for therapeutic cancer vaccines in Chapter 6.3.2. It is widely recognized that a feasible animal model for therapeutic cancer vaccines is sometimes unattainable due to the human-specific nature imparted by the display of antigens on human HLA molecules. Although HLA transgenic animals may be available in some cases, they may be of limited utility since they lack the human components of the complex antigen processing machinery. In the lack of a suitable animal model, proof-of-concept can be demonstrated via in vitro research. For example, therapeutic cancer vaccines could be tested in an in vitro assay to show that following repeated antigen stimulation, specific human T cells can be generated or activated (s). Preclinical pharmacological studies aim to show proof-of-concept and determine the beginning dose and timeframe.

The clinical requirements for vaccination approval are outlined in a separate EMA document, covering DNA vaccines expressing foreign antigens. Although mRNA is not covered, the concepts can certainly be used in mRNA vaccines. Although nucleic acids are listed, the recommendation does not call for pharmacokinetic investigations. On the other hand, pharmacokinetic studies are planned for gene therapy pharmaceutical drugs. This would be the case with a recombinant mRNA-based therapeutic cancer vaccination (which meets the gene therapy medical product threshold).

6.9.5 CLINICAL BATCH RECORDS

The appropriate authorities must approve clinical trials, which involve extensive quality documentation on the new drug for trial participants. In the EU, quality data is referred to as an Investigational Medicinal Product Dossier (IMPD) (IND in the US). To accomplish this, several production, quality control, and assurance preconditions must be met. In addition, specific mRNA vaccination requirements are met here in compliance with European legislation.

A competent local authority manufacturing permit for investigational medical products (IMPs) is required for a clinical trial application in the EU. All production and testing steps must follow the GMP principles established in Directive 2003/94/EC to receive a manufacturing permit. As described in Eudralex Volume 4—"Guidelines for good manufacturing procedures for medical goods for human and veterinary use," this includes GMP-compliant facilities and equipment, quality assurance, documentation, and appropriate personnel and processes.

mRNA vaccines are categorized as biotechnological/biological medicinal goods since they are frequently created using recombinant DNA technology, whereas RNAs made only chemically are classified as chemical compounds.

6.9.5.1 Substance Used to Make Drugs (2.2.1.S)

The IMPD's section "General information" (2.1.S.1.1) comprises information about the drug names, laboratory codes, and, if available, a proposed INN name for the substance's nomenclature (messenger ribonucleic acid/mRNA) (International Nonproprietary Name). The structure, sequence, and molecular weight of mRNA are also given (cap, open reading frame, UTRs, Poly(A), and so on). Physicochemical factors like pKa, osmolality, and solubility (which may affect pharmacological or toxicological safety) round out this area.

The manufacturing of the drug substance (2.2.1.S.2) begins with a list of all manufacturers, contractors, and manufacturing facilities involved in the product's development, and testing is provided. Second, the manufacturing process is described, including crucial process controls and a flow chart that includes critical beginning materials and intermediates. All relevant actions must be documented in authorized standard operating procedures to ensure reproducible processes. Third, the template is synthesized via plasmid-DNA amplification and linearization in a typical mRNA production process, followed by in vitro transcription, DNase treatment, and mRNA purification. Plasmid linearity testing is critical process control.

On the one hand, DNA electrophoresis could be used to investigate this; on the other hand, a small-scale in vitro transcription process with subsequent RNA quantification and analysis could be used to predict that the desired (amounts of) pharmacological ingredient would be produced on a large scale. Additional process controls would focus on mRNA identity and integrity after large-scale in vitro transcription and mRNA purification. Finally, information on the quality and control of all raw materials (such as RNA polymerase), reagents (such as transcription buffer), and solvents used to synthesize medicinal compounds is compiled. If certificates of analysis and origin are available, these are provided. Third, if materials of animal or human origin are employed, an adventitious agent must be used to ensure that the materials are safe. Fourth, control methods must be specified if crucial processes in the manufacture of the drug ingredient have been identified (via a risk analysis). Finally, differences should be shown if the manufacturing process has changed significantly from nonclinical to clinical batches.

Characterization (2.1.2.S.3) includes deciphering the structure of mRNA and potential impurities. The cornerstone for the correctness of the mRNA structure is the identity of the plasmid DNA template, which is checked by fully automated GMP-certified DNA sequencing. Because direct RNA sequencing has a read length restriction and mRNA to complementary DNA (cDNA) conversion has defects (e.g., failure rate), sequencing the starting material plasmid DNA remains the best approach for confirming mRNA sequence correctness.

All potential contaminants of the pharmaceutical material include residual DNA, enzymes/proteins, solvents from the manufacturing process, and breakdown products. Plasmid DNA, enzymes, and proteins can be broken down and extracted using DNase treatment paired with RNA-specific purification (precipitation and chromatography) (e.g., RNA polymerase). Solvents can be removed from the drug substance by freezing it, allowing it to dissolve in the right buffer. The value is enhanced by further remarks on the efficacy of downstream processing processes. Protein reduction by RNA-specific precipitation, for example, is one of the removal factors for identified pollutants. The potential degradation products can be found via RNA integrity studies, such as RNA electrophoresis.

6.9.5.2 Investigational Medicinal Product Under Test (2.2.1.P)

Following that, the Chapter "Control of the Drug Substance" (2.2.1.S.4) requires a drug addressing mRNA identification, assay, and contaminants and information on analytical processes and their acceptance requirements and addressing mRNA identification, assay, and impurities. Further down, more details can be found under Subheading 3 ("Control of the Drug Substance/IMP"). All analytical processes necessitate validation. Validation is sufficient for phase I clinical trials if the parameters are provided together with acceptability limits. This requires a detailed understanding of the analytical approaches. A tabular summary of the validation data is required for phase II and III clinical trials.

Batch analysis data for all batches used in the clinical trial and nonclinical investigations must be provided as a critical element, including the "batch number, batch size, production site, manufacture date, control processes, acceptability criteria, and test findings." Furthermore, any factors that may be critical for future therapeutic product performance must be specified with explanations. When possible, Ph. Eur. Limitations, such as residual solvents, should be used (see Ph. Eur. 5.4). For analytical procedures not based on a Ph. Eur. Specification, justifications should be based on a full characterization of the method.

Characterization parameters are provided if reference standards or materials (2.2.1.S.5) are used. For example, reference standards could help electrophoresis (RNA ladder), qRT-PCR, and photometry.

Furthermore, the primary packaging material (2.2.1.S.6) for storing the pharmaceutical ingredient must be stated.

Finally, statistics on essential parameters for mRNA stability (2.2.1.S.7) are presented in a tabular style. MRNA's most important stability markers are RNA integrity, content, potency, pH, appearance, and microbiological status. According to the circumstances outlined in ICH guideline Q1A(R2)—"Stability testing of novel drug substances and products," stability testing should be performed on representative batches held in container closure systems identical to those used in clinical batches. Stress testing and storage under accelerated conditions are also carried out, and studies represent the appropriate long-term storage temperature. Both are interested in degradation kinetics and patterns and can provide estimates of worst-case scenarios while maintaining RNA integrity and useful ideas for analytical tool development. For example, in stress testing, temperature, pH, photostability, humidity (for freeze-dried RNA), and several freeze-thaw cycles could all be used (when stored frozen).

In the IMP section 2.2.1.P.1, the sterile mRNA vaccination administered in clinical trial participants (e.g., intradermally) is presented. In addition, the dosage form, excipients' role, and container quantities/doses should be included.

Following that, the pharmaceutical development of the drug product (2.2.1.P.2) is discussed. This is especially true in clinical stages II and III, when modifications to the IMP's manufacture, composition, or dosing form could have a clinical impact. When preparing extemporaneously, include information on solvent compatibility (for freeze-dried IMPs), diluents, and admixtures (if applicable) and a description of the preparation technique. Testing in-use stability following reconstitution, dilution, or the addition of admixtures is very important in this setting to recreate the worst-case situations during clinical usage (For example, between reconstitution and injection by the physician, there could be a several-hour delay at room temperature.) A description of the container closure system and an explanation for the primary packing material employed are required. The container closure system must be fully functional throughout the shelf life of the sterile mRNA vaccine to prevent it from microbial contamination.

All producers, contractors, testing locations, and their separate duties must be identified, precisely like the medicine itself. The manufacturing process, any relevant process controls, and the batch formula for clinical batches should be briefly described. Because mRNA vaccines cannot be sterilized permanently by wet heat, IMP formulation, filling, and finishing (including freeze-drying) are all done in an aseptic environment (EU GMP cleanroom class A). Crucial step controls do not need to be addressed until phase III, except for procedures to ensure vaccine sterility. The results of media fill, which is a validation of aseptic operations using a microbiological growth medium instead of the IMP, should be reported here.

When it comes to excipients (2.2.1.P.4), it all boils down to whether they refer to pharmacopeia or not. If not, analytical procedures must be described, and a risk evaluation of adventitious agents should be undertaken. In addition, more detailed information on the manufacturing process, controls, and characteristics of novel excipients are required.

IMP requirements suited to the present stage of development are required by CIMP (2.2.1.P.5). The specs, parameters, test procedures, and acceptance criteria should all be justified. More information can be found in subheading 3 "Control of the Drug Substance/IMP." Analytical technique validation follows the same guidelines as drug substance validation. The requirements incorporate quality control findings from typical IMP batches. All required data includes "batch number, batch size, manufacturing site, manufacture date, control methodologies, acceptance criteria, and test results." Additional information should be provided if contaminants are discovered in the IMP but not in the drug component. There are unlikely any IMP-specific reference standards or supplies required (2.2.1.P.6).

The container closing system (2.2.1.P.7) used for the IMP in the clinical investigation must be defined. The relevant pharmacopeia reference for the primary packing material is supplied where applicable. Specifications and material certificates and a detailed description should be provided in all other cases.

Finally, the stability (2.2.1.P.8) and shelf life of the IMP are discussed. Data from development studies can be used to justify a phase I trial's preliminary shelf-life. Stability testing on sample batches starts before clinical trials begin and continues in parallel, allowing for extension of extrapolation and shelf life. To collect data, long-term and expedited research must be used. When it's acceptable, it's critical not to ignore upside-down storage. This is crucial for liquid IMPs in vials with rubber stoppers, as it allows researchers to examine the stopper's impact on RNA vaccine durability. Last but not least, in-use stability should be addressed by simulating the clinical condition following IMP creation, as previously stated (reconstitution, etc.). The ICH Q1A-1F guidelines provide more information on stability studies.

The IMPD contains an overall risk and benefit assessment, as well as additional information on nonclinical pharmacology, toxicology, and relevant clinical data, which is usually summarized in the Investigator's Brochure (IB)—a guide for the investigator—in addition to the information about the quality of the drug substance and the IMP given above. In addition to the requirements of the IMPD, the guideline lists additional elements to consider when developing mRNA vaccines for clinical trials.

6.9.5.3 Control of Drug Substances/Impact Factors

A product specification based on the current level of product development, research, and technology is crucial in ensuring the quality of the drug substance and IMP.

The ICH guideline Q6A, "Test procedures and acceptance criteria for new drug substances and new drug products: chemical substances," lays the groundwork.

Above and beyond biological activity, the parameters listed in ICH guideline Q6B "Test procedures and acceptance criteria for biotechnological/biological products," which applies to proteins and polypeptides, should be considered.

For determining the quality of a product's identification, assay/quantity, purity/ impurities, and potency/bioactivity, the specification defines a set of tests (test parameters) and references to analytical procedures and appropriate acceptance criteria. In addition, specific product information should also be mentioned in specifications, such as the product name, content, dosage form, primary packaging, storage conditions, and shelf life (see German AMWHV).

A possible specification for an mRNA-based product is shown in Table 6.1.

Proteins, plasmid DNA, host DNA, and residual solvents are purity features that may be overlooked since they are (potential) contaminants unique to the pharmaceutical production process. According to ICH Q6A, Chapter 3.3.2.3, further testing for parenteral drugs, such as mRNA-based IMPs, is required. These include sterility and endotoxin testing, osmolality, particle matter tests, water content, reconstitution time, and uniformity of dose units. Furthermore, potency and biological activity should be taken into account (see Notes 29 and 30 in the EMA guidelines). An example specification for a lyophilized mRNA-based IMP is shown in Table 6.2.

[NOTE—Please note that no responsibility is assumed for the accuracy of this information.]

Furthermore, data extractable from container closure systems may have an impact on the stability of mRNA vaccines.

6.10 FDA REGULATORY GUIDANCE FOR MRNA VACCINES

MRNA vaccine is a new category of products for all regulatory agencies. While the development of vaccines for which an alternative exists or vaccines claiming a further indication that it is a pandemic, the course of approval will be the same. However, in the case of a pandemic, like the spread of the SARS-CoV-2 virus, additional considerations apply.

6.10.1 CMC CONSIDERATIONS

- Considerations in general for vaccines must meet statutory and regulatory standards in the United States for vaccine development and licensing, including quality, development, manufacture, and control (section 351(a) of the PHS, 42 U.S.C. 262). The vaccination product must be appropriately described and manufactured following all applicable regulations, including current good manufacturing practices (cGMP). Vaccine production methods must be properly specified and appropriately managed for each vaccine to maintain consistency in manufacturing.
- To the extent legally and scientifically permissible, vaccine development could be hastened based on knowledge gathered from similar products created using the same well-characterized platform technology. Similarly, given sufficient reason, some parts of vaccine manufacture and control may

TABLE 6.1
Exemplary Specification of a Liquid mRNA-Based Drug Substance

Product information

Product name:	RNA123
Reference code:	R01-00123
Application:	The active substance, drug substance
Condition:	Liquid
Manufacturer reference:	SOP XY
Concentration:	XX g/l
Other ingredients:	e.g., water for injection (WFI)
Primary packaging material:	e.g., polypropylene containers e.g., polypropylene screw cap
Storage temperature:	−80°C
Stability/retest period:	See ongoing stability testing
RNA sequence:	GG…
Length in bases:	XX b

Specification of test parameters

Description

Parameter	Analytical procedure	Acceptance criterion
Appearance: clarity and opalescence	Clarity and opalescence of solutions (Ph. Eur. 2.2.1)	e.g., clear liquid
Appearance: coloration	The coloration of solutions (Ph. Eur. 2.2.2)	e.g., colorless to yellowish liquid

Identity

Parameter	Analytical procedure	Acceptance criterion
DNA sequence plasmid	Automated DNA sequencing according to SOP XY	Identical to theoretical DNA template XY sequence
RNA length	RNA electrophoresis and determination of run length according to SOP XY	XX ±XX
RNA sequence segment	Reverse transcription, PCR, and DNA electrophoresis according to SOP XY	Theoretical band size ±XX

Assay/quantity

Parameter	Analytical procedure	Acceptance criterion
RNA content	UV absorption, OD260 according to SOP XY	XX g/l±XX%
pH value	pH value (Ph. Eur. 2.2.3)	XX–XX
Osmolality	Osmolality (Ph. Eur. 2.2.35)	≤XX mOsm/kg

(Continued)

TABLE 6.1 (CONTINUED)

Exemplary Specification of a Liquid mRNA-Based Drug Substance

Purity/impurities

Parameter	Analytical procedure	Acceptance criterion
Bacterial count/ Bioburden	Microbial enumeration test (Ph. Eur. 2.6.12)	≤XX CFU/ml
Endotoxins	Bacterial endotoxins (Ph. Eur. 2.6.12)	≤XX EU/ml
RNA integrity	RNA electrophoresis and determination of integrity according to SOP XY	≥XX%
Proteins	Total protein (Ph. Eur. 2.5.33)	≤XX μg/ml
Plasmid DNA	qPCR according to SOP XY	≤XX copies/ml
Host DNA	qPCR according to SOP XY	≤XX copies/ml
Residual solvents	Gas chromatography (Ph. Eur. 2.2.28)	≤XX ppm (see Ph. Eur. 5.4)

Potency/biological activity

Parameter	Analytical procedure	Acceptance criterion
Translatability	In vitro translation according to SOP XY	100 % ±XX%

be based on the vaccine platform, reducing the requirement for product-specific data in some cases.

6.10.1.1 Manufacture of Drug Substances and Drug Products

- All source materials used in manufacturing should be adequately controlled, such as cell bank history and qualification, virus bank history and qualification, and identification of all animal-derived materials used for cell culture and virus growth, among other things.
- To support the licensure of a vaccine, complete information on the manufacturing process must be submitted in a Biologics License Application (BLA). Sponsors should submit data and information indicating important process parameters, critical quality attributes, batch records, defined hold durations, and the in-process testing methodology, among others. Each critical parameter should have its own set of specifications. Validation data from the manufacturing of platform-related items can help identify important parameters.
- Quality must be checked for each lot at all stages of production, and, when applicable, in-process control tests must be established.
- Process validation methods and study reports, data from engineering lots, and drug substance process performance qualifications should all be provided to ensure the consistency of the manufacturing process.
- The production process must be thoroughly validated and, if necessary, modified. Validation would require a sufficient number of commercial-scale batches that could be produced regularly that met prescribed in-process controls, critical process parameters, and lot release conditions. In most

TABLE 6.2
Exemplary Specification of a Lyophilized mRNA-Based IMP

Product information

Product name:	IMP234
Reference code:	R02-00234
Application:	Investigational medicinal product for intradermal injection
Dosage form:	Freeze-dried powder for reconstitution in, e.g., water for injection (WFI)
Manufacturer reference:	SOP XY
Dose per container:	XX mg
API:	RNA123 manufactured according to SOP XY
API concentration after reconstitution:	XX g/l
Other ingredients:	XX% buffer XY after reconstitution in XX ml, e.g., water for injection (WFI) XX g/ml excipient XY after reconstitution in XX ml, e.g., water for injection (WFI)
Primary packaging material:	e.g., glass vial 2R, type 1 bromobutyl rubber stopper, 13 mm, grey Aluminum cap, 20 mm, clear lacquered
Storage temperature:	XX°C
Stability/shelf life:	See ongoing stability testing
RNA sequence:	GG…
Length in bases:	XX b

Specification of test parameters

Description

Parameter	Analytical procedure	Acceptance criterion
Appearance, coloration	Visual analysis	e.g., colorless to yellowish powder
Appearance after reconstitution: clarity and opalescence	Reconstitution and clarity and opalescence of solutions (Ph. Eur. 2.2.1)	e.g., clear liquid
Appearance after reconstitution: coloration	Reconstitution and coloration of solutions (Ph. Eur. 2.2.2)	e.g., colorless to yellowish liquid

Identity

Parameter	Analytical procedure	Acceptance criterion
RNA length	Reconstitution, RNA electrophoresis, and determination of run length according to SOP XY	XX ±XX
Drug substance identity	Reconstitution, reverse transcription, PCR, and DNA electrophoresis according to SOP XY	Theoretical band size ±XX

(Continued)

TABLE 6.2 (CONTINUED)
Exemplary Specification of a Lyophilized mRNA-Based IMP

Assay/quantity

Parameter	Analytical procedure	Acceptance criterion
RNA content	Reconstitution and UV absorption, OD260 according to SOP XY	XX g/l±XX%
Uniformity of dosage units or mass	Uniformity of dosage units after reconstitution (Ph. Eur. 2.9.40) or uniformity of mass for powder (Ph. Eur. 2.9.5)	Conforms to Ph. Eur.
pH value	Reconstitution and pH value (Ph. Eur. 2.2.3)	XX–XX
Osmolality	Reconstitution and osmolality (Ph. Eur. 2.2.35)	XX–XX mOsm/kg
Reconstitution time	Reconstitution time in WFI	≤XX s

Purity/impurities

Parameter	Analytical procedure	Acceptance criterion
Sterility	Sterility test (Ph. Eur. 2.6.1)	Sterile
Endotoxins	Reconstitution and bacterial endotoxins (Ph. Eur. 2.6.12)	≤XX EU/ml
RNA integrity	Reconstitution, RNA electrophoresis, and determination of integrity according to SOP XY	≥XX%
Residual moisture	Water content (Ph. Eur. 2.5.12 or Ph. Eur. 2.2.32)	≤XX%
Visible particles	Visible particles (Ph. Eur. 2.9.20)	Visually free of particles
Non-visible particles	Reconstitution and sub-visible particles (Ph. Eur. 2.9.19)	Conforms to Ph. Eur.

Potency/biological activity

Parameter	Analytical procedure	Acceptance criterion
Translatability	Reconstitution, in vitro translation according to SOP XY	100 % ±XX%
Immunostimulation	Reconstitution, cytokine release according to SOP XY	100 % ±XX%

cases, data from the production of at least three commercial-scale batches are required to validate the manufacturing process.

- A quality control system should be in place at all manufacturing stages, including a well-defined testing program to assure product quality while in process/intermediate and throughout the formulation and filling process. This system should also contain a well-defined testing program to confirm the drug substance and product quality profiles before release. Data on qualification/validation for all quality indicating tests should be supplied to the BLA to support licensure.
- All quality-control release tests, including critical testing for vaccination purity, identity, and potency, should be validated and shown appropriately for the intended purpose. Release parameters are unique to each product and will be reviewed with the sponsor during the BLA review.

- If the influence on product quality is not compromised, final validation of formulation and filling procedures may be conducted after product approval if appropriately justified. Any data submitted after product approval must be agreed upon before licensure and submitted as a post-marketing commitment under the relevant submission category.
- For vaccine licensure, the vaccine's stability and expiry date in its final container should be proven using final containers from at least three final lots made from distinct vaccine bulks when stored at the prescribed temperature.
- Validation of storage conditions, including container closure integrity, is required.
- The vaccine's potency must be demonstrated for a period equivalent to the time between its release and its expiration date. However, post-marketing agreements to give full shelf life data may be permissible with proper reason.
- A product-specific stability program should ensure that licensed products maintain their quality during their stated shelf life.

6.10.2 FACILITIES AND INSPECTIONS

- Facilities must be the right size and construction to support activities, and they must be well-designed to avoid contamination, cross-contamination, and mix-ups. These must be validated, and HVAC systems must provide adequate control over air pressure, microorganisms, dust, humidity, temperature, and proper protection or containment. Cleaning and maintenance protocols for facilities and equipment must be established and validated.
- Sterile filtration and sterilization methods should be validated, and manufacturing equipment. In addition, personnel should be trained and qualified for their specific roles, and aseptic processes should be fully tested using media simulations.
- A quality control unit must be established, with responsibilities for manufacturing oversight and the review and release of components, containers and closures, labeling, in-process material, and finished goods. In addition, the quality control unit is in charge of approving validation methods and reports, investigating deviations, and implementing remedial and preventive actions.
- Pre-license inspections of manufacturing sites are part of the BLA review process and are usually undertaken once a BLA file is accepted. In addition, the FDA uses all available tools and sources of information to assist regulatory determinations on applications that involve sites impacted by the FDA's power to inspect according to a public health emergency.

6.10.3 NONCLINICAL TESTING

6.10.3.1 General Considerations

- In vitro and in vivo testing, nonclinical studies of a vaccine candidate are used to determine its immunogenicity and safety properties. In addition, nonclinical research in animal models aid in the identification of potential vaccine-related safety hazards and selecting the dose, dosing regimen, and method of administration for clinical trials. The amount of nonclinical evidence needed to support moving on with first-in-human (FIH) clinical trials is determined by the vaccine architecture, available supportive data, and data from closely related vaccines.

- Animal investigations using particular vaccine designs against other viruses have raised concerns about a potential risk of vaccine-associated enhanced respiratory illness (ERD). In these experiments, animal models were given vaccine constructs against various coronavirus and then challenged with the wild-type virus. These studies found evidence of immunopathologic lung reactions characteristic of a Th-2 type hypersensitivity, similar to ERD, in infants and animals who received formalin-inactivated respiratory syncytial virus (RSV) vaccine and were then challenged with RSV virus in the laboratory or through natural exposure. As indicated, vaccine candidates should be evaluated in light of this research.
- To support continuing FIH clinical trials and subsequent clinical development, FDA recommends that vaccine makers communicate with FDA early to discuss the type and degree of nonclinical testing required for the specific vaccine candidate.

6.10.3.2 Toxicity Studies

- Nonclinical safety studies will be necessary before advancing to FIH clinical trials for a vaccine candidate with a novel product type. No prior nonclinical and clinical data are available (312.23(a) of the 21 CFR (8)).
- In other cases, nonclinical safety studies may not be required before FIH clinical trials since adequate evidence to assess product safety may already be available. For example, toxicology data (e.g., data from repeat-dose toxicity studies, biodistribution studies) and clinical data from other products made with the same platform could be used to support FIH clinical trials for the vaccine candidate if it is made with the same platform technology as a licensed vaccine or other previously studied investigational vaccines and is sufficiently characterized. However, if vaccine manufacturers intend to use this data instead of nonclinical safety trials, they must explain and justify their decision.
- Nonclinical safety evaluations, such as toxicity and local tolerance studies, must be done following regulations dictating good laboratory practices for conducting nonclinical laboratory studies (GLP) as needed to support continuing FIH clinical trials (21 CFR Part 58). Before the start of FIH clinical trials, such research should be done and analyzed. Additional safety testing should be done if toxicology studies do not adequately identify danger.
- To expedite the start of FIH clinical trials with vaccine candidates, data from toxicity tests may be submitted as unaudited final draft toxicologic reports. Within 120 days of the initiation of the FIH clinical trial, FDA should have the final, quality-assured reports.

- The use of preventive vaccinations during pregnancy and in women of reproductive age will be a significant factor in vaccination efforts. As a result, the FDA recommends that sponsors conduct developmental and reproductive toxicity (DART) studies with their vaccine candidates before enrolling pregnant women and women of childbearing potential who are not actively avoiding pregnancy in clinical trials. Sponsors may also submit data from DART trials with a similar product using comparable platform technology. The FDA considers that the data are scientifically sufficient following consultation with the agency.
- If the vaccine design is novel and there is no previous biodistribution data from the platform technology, biodistribution studies in an animal species should be explored. If there is a chance of changing infectivity and tissue tropism, or if a new method of administration and formulation will be utilized, these investigations should be done.

6.10.3.3   Characterization of the Immune Response in Animal Models

- To evaluate the vaccine candidate's immunologic features and assist FIH clinical trials, immunogenicity studies in animal models sensitive to the selected vaccine antigen should be done. In addition, measurements of immunogenicity should be appropriate for the vaccine design and mechanism of action.
- Each of the antigens included in the study should be evaluated for humoral, cellular, and functional immune responses. To define the humoral response, antigen-specific enzyme-linked immunosorbent tests (ELISA) should be investigated. CD8+ and CD4+ T-cell responses should be examined utilizing sensitive and specific assays for cellular response evaluation. Immune responses' functional activity should be assessed in vitro in neutralization tests employing either wild-type or pseudovirion virus. The assays used to assess immunogenicity should be proven appropriate for their intended use.

6.10.3.4   Vaccine-associated Enhanced Respiratory Disease

- Current knowledge and understanding of the potential risk of vaccine-associated understanding of the efficacy of available animal models in predicting the possibility of such an occurrence in humans are limited, as is ERD. Nonetheless, animal models (e.g., rodents and nonhuman primates) are needed to investigate the possibility of vaccine-associated ERD.
- To determine the likelihood of the vaccine causing vaccine-associated ERD in people, post-vaccination animal challenge experiments and characterization of the sort of nonclinical and clinical immune response generated by the specific vaccine candidate can be used.
- Sponsors should conduct studies defining the vaccine-induced immune response in animal models and evaluating immunological markers of probable ERD outcomes to support moving forward with FIH human trials. In animals inoculated with clinically relevant dosages of the vaccine candidate,

including assessments of functional immune responses (e.g., neutralizing antibody) against total antibody responses and Th1/Th2 balance.

- Vaccine candidates with immunogenicity data showing high neutralizing antibody titers and Th1-type T-cell polarization may be allowed to move forward to FIH trials without first completing post-vaccination challenge studies in appropriate animal models, assuming adequate risk mitigation strategies are implemented in the FIH trials. Post-vaccination challenge studies are likely to be done in parallel with FIH trials in similar settings to verify that the risk of vaccine-associated ERD is addressed before enrolling large numbers of human subjects in Phase II and III clinical trials. Before progressing to FIH clinical trials, post-vaccination animal challenge data and/or animal immunopathology investigations are necessary to assess vaccine candidates' protection and/or ERD. Other results suggest heightened concerns regarding ERD.

- In determining whether Phase III studies can proceed in the absence of post-vaccination challenge data to address the risk of ERD, the totality of data for a specific vaccine candidate, including data from post-vaccination challenge studies in small animal models and data from FIH clinical trials characterizing the type of immune responses induced by the vaccine, will be considered.

6.10.4 CLINICAL TRIALS

6.10.4.1 General Considerations

- The immunology of the infecting entity would likely not be known and changing. While immunogenicity testing is a crucial part of vaccine research, development programs should focus on obtaining conventional licensure through direct demonstration of vaccine efficacy in protecting humans from virus infection and sickness at this time.

- Adaptive and seamless clinical trial designs that allow for the selection of vaccination candidates and dose regimens and a faster progression through the standard phases of clinical development could speed up the development of vaccines.

- Whether clinical development programs are carried out in discrete phases with separate studies or in a more integrated manner, a good body of data, including data on the risk of vaccine-associated ERD, will be required as clinical development progresses to support the safety of vaccinating the proposed study populations and the number of participants, and, for later-stage development, to ensure that the study design is adequate to meet its objectives.

- For expedited/seamless clinical development, the FDA provides early advice and possibly consent in principle. Therefore, sponsors should aim to submit summaries of data available at each development milestone to the FDA for assessment and approval before moving on to the next step.

- Clinical trials amid a public health emergency pose many logistical problems. However, compliance with good clinical practice (GCP) and reducing threats to trial integrity is not waived.

6.10.4.2 Trial Design

- Once sufficient preclinical evidence is available, healthy adult volunteers at low risk of infection should be enrolled in FIH and other early phase trials (which typically expose 10–100 individuals to each vaccine candidate being investigated). Excluding participants at higher risk of severe infection from early phase studies is necessary to mitigate the potential risk of vaccine-associated ERD until additional data to inform that potential risk becomes available through ongoing product development.
- Exclusion criteria should be based on current knowledge of risk factors for more severe illnesses, such as the CDC's recommendations.
- Adults over 55 may be enrolled in FIH and other early phase studies if they do not have medical comorbidities linked to a higher risk of severe infection. However, before adding older adult participants, some early safety data in younger people (e.g., seven days after a single immunization) should be available, especially for vaccine platforms with no prior clinical experience.
- If possible, people at high risk of infection should be excluded from early clinical trials (e.g., healthcare workers).
- Sponsors should gather and assess at least preliminary clinical safety and immunogenicity data for each dose level and age group to enable the progression of clinical development to include greater numbers (e.g., hundreds) of participants and persons at higher risk of severe infection (e.g., younger vs. older adults).
- Preliminary immunogenicity data from early-phase development should include assessments of neutralizing vs. total antibody responses and Th1 vs. Th2 polarization.
- If available, preliminary evaluation of infection disease outcomes from earlier clinical development and results of nonclinical studies evaluating protection and/or histopathological markers of vaccine-associated ERD following virus challenge could be used to further inform potential vaccine-associated ERD risk and support clinical development.
- To meet the BLA approval standard, late-stage clinical trials to establish vaccination efficacy with formal hypothesis testing, including patients with medical comorbidities for trials attempting to measure protection against severe infection, will almost certainly require tens of thousands of participants.
- To prove universal safety, vaccination effectiveness potential, and a low risk of vaccine-associated ERD (e.g., in a few hundred people), late-phase trials should be preceded by adequate characterization of safety and immunogenicity for each vaccine candidate, dosage level, and age group to be examined).

- Nonclinical research examining vaccine-associated ERD protection and histopathological markers after the virus challenge and infection illness outcomes from earlier clinical development could be valuable sources of information for clinical trials involving thousands of people.
- While vaccine safety and efficacy in the virus-naive persons are vital, vaccine safety and infection results in individuals with prior virus infection, which may have been asymptomatic, should also be investigated. With the deployment of licensed vaccines, pre-vaccination screening for past infection is unlikely to occur in practice. As a result, participants with a history of virus infection or laboratory evidence of infection in the past do not need to be screened or excluded from the vaccine studies. Anyone with an acute illness should avoid vaccine trials (or another acute infectious condition).
- At all stages of immunization clinical studies, the FDA advocates the participation of different groups. This ensures that vaccines are safe and effective for all target population members.
- The FDA especially encourages affected populations, particularly racial and ethnic minorities, to enlist.
- In late-stage clinical trials, adequate representation of the elderly and those with medical comorbidities should be included in assessing vaccine safety and efficacy in adults.
- According to the FDA, pregnant women and women of reproductive potential who are not actively avoiding pregnancy should be included in pre-licensure clinical studies early in the development phase.
- Given the gravity of the public health crisis, vaccine developers must plan for pediatric safety and effectiveness evaluations, as well as assure compliance with the Pediatric Research Equity Act (PREA) (section 505B of the FD&C Act (21 USC 355c)). In addition, epidemiology and pathophysiology and the safety and efficacy of vaccines may differ between children and adults. Therefore, to ensure compliance with 21 CFR Part 50 Subpart D (Additional safeguards for children in clinical investigations), discussions on the likelihood of direct benefit and acceptable risk to support the initiation of pediatric studies, as well as the appropriate design and endpoints for pediatric studies, should be held in the context of specific vaccine development programs.
- Early phase trials usually try to down-select among several vaccine candidates and/or dosing regimens by randomly assigning participants to different treatment groups. While a placebo control or blinding is not required in early phase research, it may aid in evaluating preliminary safety outcomes.
- Efficacy trials, for example, should be randomized, double-blind, and placebo-controlled in the later stages.
- An individually randomized controlled trial with 1:1 randomization between vaccination and placebo groups is the most effective study for demonstrating vaccine efficacy. Other randomization approaches, such as cluster randomization, may be appropriate, but they require careful consideration of potential biases that individual randomization does not.

- As long as the study is well-designed and employs suitable statistical methods to assess efficacy, the trial comparing multiple vaccine candidates against a single placebo group could be a viable strategy to enhance efficiency.
- Suppose a safe and effective vaccine eliminates the requirement for an ethical placebo control group. Instead, the vaccine might be used as the control treatment in a study using noninferiority hypothesis testing to determine efficacy.
- Pre-specified criteria for adding or deleting vaccine candidates or dose regimens should be included in adaptive trial protocols. In addition, pre-specified criteria (e.g., safety and immunogenicity data) for progressing from one phase to the next should be included in seamless trial procedures.
- To evaluate the length of protection and the risk of vaccine-induced disease, study participants should be followed for infection outcomes (particularly severe illness symptoms) for as long as possible, ideally at least one to two years.
- Once appropriate preclinical evidence is available, healthy adult volunteers with a low risk of severe infection should be enrolled in FIH and other early phase studies (which typically expose 10–100 people to each vaccine candidate being examined). However, to reduce the possibility of vaccine-associated ERD, people at higher risk of severe infection should be excluded from early phase studies until more knowledge on the potential danger becomes available through continuous product development.
- Exclusion criteria should reflect the current understanding of risk factors for more severe infection, such as the CDC's, as infection pathophysiology advances.

6.10.4.3 Efficacy Considerations

- A vaccine effectiveness trial can use a specified virus infection as a primary outcome.
- Acute cases should be confirmed virologically (e.g., by RTPCR).
- Virologic approaches or serologic methods evaluating antibodies to the virus antigens not included in the vaccination can be used to monitor and confirm specific virus infections, including asymptomatic illness.
- Standardization of effectiveness endpoints across clinical trials may make it easier to compare vaccinations for deployment programs, as long as discrepancies in trial design and study demographics aren't thrown into the mix. For this purpose, FDA advises that virologically confirmed be specified as either the primary or secondary objective (with or without formal hypothesis testing). Symptoms of specific virus infections will be derived from clinical observation data.
- Sponsors should think about using efficacy trials to power formal hypothesis testing on a severe infection endpoint because a vaccine may be more effective at preventing severe infection than a mild infection. A serious infection should be evaluated as a secondary endpoint if not analyzed as

a primary endpoint (with or without formal hypothesis testing). The FDA proposes that a virologically proven virus with any following be categorized as a severe infection.

- At rest, clinical symptoms of severe systemic sickness (respiratory rate 30 minutes, heart rate 125 minutes, SpO2 93% on room air at sea level, or PaO2/FiO2 300 mm Hg) are present.
- Failure of the respiratory system (defined as needing high-flow oxygen, noninvasive ventilation, mechanical ventilation, or ECMO).
- Shock (systolic blood pressure > 90 mm Hg, diastolic blood pressure > 60 mm Hg, or need for vasopressors).
- Acute renal, hepatic, or neurologic impairment is severe.
- Admission to an intensive care unit.
- Death.
- If not evaluated as a primary outcome, specific-virus infection (symptomatic or not) should be evaluated as a secondary or exploratory endpoint.
- The aforementioned diagnostic criteria may need to be amended in some populations, such as pediatric patients and those with respiratory problems. Therefore, before beginning enrollment, sponsors should discuss their proposed case definitions with the Agency.

6.10.4.4 Statistical Considerations

- The primary efficacy endpoint should be at least 50% in placebo-controlled effectiveness research. In addition, the lower bound of the correctly alpha-adjusted confidence interval around the primary efficacy endpoint point estimate should be > 30% as the statistical success requirement.
- Early in any interim study, the same statistical success criterion should be employed to establish efficacy.
- A lower bound of 30% but greater than 0% as a statistical success requirement for a secondary efficacy endpoint may be acceptable if secondary endpoint hypothesis testing is dependent on significant endpoint success.
- The lower bound of the suitably alpha-adjusted confidence interval around the primary relative effectiveness point estimate should be >−10% for non-inferiority comparisons to a specific virus vaccination that has already been shown efficacious.
- Each vaccination candidate should utilize appropriate statistical methodologies to control type 1 error when conducting hypothesis testing on multiple endpoints and/or interim efficacy assessments.
- Interim analyses should be included in late-phase studies to assess the risk of vaccine-associated ERD and futility.
- Study sample sizes and interim analysis timing should be determined using statistical success criteria for primary and secondary efficacy analyses (if applicable) and realistic, data-driven estimates of vaccine efficacy and infection incidence for the populations and locations where the trial will be conducted.

6.10.4.5   Safety Considerations

- Vaccinations should be evaluated similarly to other preventative vaccines for infectious diseases, including the safety database size needed to justify vaccine licensure. During clinical development, safety assessments should cover the following:
- There are local and systemic adverse events in an adequate number of study participants for at least seven days following each study vaccination to evaluate reactogenicity (including a subset of participants in late phase efficacy trials).
- All trial participants who experienced unintentional adverse effects for at least 21–28 days following each study vaccination.
- After receiving all study vaccines, all trial participants had serious and other medically attended adverse effects for at least six months. Specific vaccine platforms may require more extensive safety monitoring (e.g., those that include novel adjuvants).
- Pregnancies in study participants who were conceived before vaccination or within 30 days of vaccination should be monitored for pregnancy outcomes such as miscarriage, stillbirth, or congenital defects.
- Preventive vaccinations for infectious illnesses normally include at least 3000 research participants who have been immunized with the dose regimen used for licensure. Therefore, if no significant safety concerns arise during clinical development that would warrant further pre-licensure evaluation, the FDA anticipates that adequately powered efficacy trials for vaccines will be sufficient to provide an acceptable safety database for younger adults and elderly populations.
- Vaccine trials should be monitored regularly for unfavorable imbalances in infective illness outcomes between the vaccine and control groups, especially for cases of severe infection that could indicate vaccine-associated ERD.
- Stopping a study based on signals of probable vaccine-associated ERD should be mentioned in advance.
- FDA recommends vaccine-associated ERD and other safety signal monitoring, using an independent data safety monitoring board (DSMB), especially during later stages of research.

6.10.5   Post-License Safety

6.10.5.1   General Considerations

Nine vaccine safety databases compiled from pre-licensure clinical investigations may have limitations, as with all licensed vaccines. Consider the following scenario:

- The number of people who received a vaccination in pre-licensure clinical trials may not be enough to detect some rare adverse responses.

- Some subpopulations likely to get a vaccination (e.g., pregnant women or people with medical comorbidities) may have limited pre-licensure safety data at the time of licensure.
- Before the vaccine is approved, the safety follow-up period for some vaccines may not have been completed for all patients involved in pre-licensure clinical studies to monitor for probable vaccination-associated ERD and other adverse effects.
- In the case of vaccinations, it is anticipated that a large population will be vaccinated in a short period during the early post-marketing phase. As a result, the FDA advises that pharmacovigilance actions be planned before approval.
- Manufacturers should explore creating specific Current Procedural Terminology (CPT) codes and using bar codes to designate the immediate container to make correct documentation and identification of vaccines in health records easier.

6.10.5.2 Pharmacovigilance Activities for Vaccines

- For licensed biological products, routine pharmacovigilance comprises the prompt reporting of serious and unexpected adverse events and periodic safety reports in compliance with 21 CFR 600.80 (post-marketing reporting of adverse experiences).
- The FDA recommends that applicants submit a Pharmacovigilance Plan (PVP) with their BLA submission for a vaccine, as described in the FDA Guidance for Industry; E2E Pharmacovigilance Planning. The content of a PVP for a vaccine will be determined by the vaccine's safety profile and based on data such as the pre-licensure clinical safety database, preclinical data, and existing safety information for comparable vaccines, among other things.
- The PVP should include steps to address all significant identified risks, significant prospective hazards, and significant gaps in knowledge. In addition, Pharmacoepidemiologic research or other activities should be considered to assess important concerns, such as vaccine-associated ERD. One or more of the following components of a PVP for a vaccine may be recommended by the FDA:
- Submission of adverse event report summaries at more frequent intervals than provided for routine required reporting, but reports of specific adverse events of interest in an expedited manner beyond routine required reporting immediately;
- Continued and extended safety surveillance (under an IND) for vaccine-related ERD in participants enrolled in pre-licensure clinical trials;
- A pregnant exposure registry actively gathers data about immunization during pregnancy and pregnancy and newborn outcomes. Pharmacoepidemiologic research to examine (an) important identified or possible risk(s) from the clinical development program, such as vaccine-associated ERD or other unusual or delayed-onset adverse events of special interest.

6.10.5.3 Required Post-Marketing Safety Studies

- The FDA may require such post-market studies or trials at the time of approval to assess a known serious risk associated with the drug's use, to assess signals of serious risk associated with the drug's use, or to identify an unexpected serious risk when available data indicate the potential for a serious risk. FDA may also require such studies or trials after approval if new safety information becomes available.
- When such studies or trials are needed, FDA may mandate post-marketing studies or trials for vaccines to analyze known or potential significant hazards.
- Diagnostic tests (e.g., RT-PCR) that support the pivotal efficacy analysis should be sensitive and accurate to confirm infection and be verified before use.
- Before being utilized in pivotal clinical trials, immunogenicity assays should be suitable for measuring meaningful immune responses to vaccination and verified.

6.10.6 ADDITIONAL CONSIDERATIONS

Efficacy testing in clinical trials must be validated in effectiveness trials based on real-world use of the product.

- Given the current level of information about a new infection, clinical endpoint efficacy trials that demonstrate illness protection are the most direct way to establish efficacy for a vaccine candidate.
- Suppose an applicant provides sufficient data and information to meet the applicable legal requirements. In that case, accelerated vaccine approval may be considered once a different understanding of the infecting virus immunology; specifically, vaccine immune responses that might be reasonably likely to predict protection against the infection are gained. It may be conceivable to approve a vaccine under these rules if adequate and well-controlled clinical studies show that the product affects a surrogate endpoint (e.g., immunological response) that is fairly expected to predict therapeutic benefit.
- The vaccine features, such as antigen structure, mechanism of delivery, and antigen processing and presentation in the vaccinated individual, would most likely identify a valid surrogate endpoint. However, given that the two vaccines transmit antigens in distinct ways and elicit different protective immune responses, an immunological marker developed for an adenovirus-based vaccine cannot be assumed to be transferable to a VSV-based vaccine.
- Because the virus is a novel virus, a surrogate endpoint that is reasonably likely to predict protection should preferably be generated from human effectiveness trials that look at clinical illness endpoints. Sponsors should

consult the FDA to establish an agreement on using the surrogate endpoint if it is derived from other data sources.

- An appropriate dataset evaluating the vaccine's safety in humans would be required for licensure consideration.
- Post-marketing confirmatory trials have been required for medications granted fast approval to verify and describe the projected effect on therapeutic benefit. Therefore, these studies should normally be ongoing when accelerated permission is granted, and they must be performed with care.
- If clinical disease endpoint efficacy studies cannot demonstrate vaccination efficacy, a controlled human infection model to generate evidence to support vaccine efficacy may be considered. However, several challenges would need to be adequately resolved, including logistical, human subject protection, ethical, and scientific concerns since the virus has yet to be established or defined in a controlled human infection scenario.

6.11 BIOSIMILAR mRNA VACCINES

Nucleic acid vaccines, such as mRNA and DNA vaccines, have been in development for decades, but there has never been an opportunity to quickly test their safety and efficacy; vaccines could take years or decades to offer sufficient proof of safety and efficacy. Now comes COVID-19 with its spread of the SARS-CoV2 virus that allowed fast data collection, securing approximately 150 infections among the study participants that, averaging about 30–40,000 in each study. Once there were about 150 infections, the double-blind coding was broken, and it unveiled a surprising 95%+ efficacy; the FDA would have approved the use at even 50% efficacy. In addition, the safety of the mRNA vaccine that had already been established was proven in multiple studies; however, the vaccine CureVac failed because of a lack of nucleoside modifications.

All biological goods, including preventive and therapeutic vaccines, whole blood and blood products, cellular products and exosomal preparations, gene therapies, tissue products, and live biotherapeutic agents, are regulated by the FDA's Center for Biologics Evaluation and Research (CBER). CBER is also in charge of regulating a variety of pharmaceuticals and technologies that are utilized in the testing and production of our biological goods. As part of that mission, products registered under a BLA with CBER comprise 351(a) filings. Suppose you're seeking something different (21 CFR 601.2). The BLA is governed by the federal regulations 21 CFR 600–680. The CDER oversees a broad spectrum of biological products, including biosimilars and interchangeable biologics. For example, insulin, glucagon, and human growth hormone were added to the CDER BLA program in March 2020 after being classified as medicines under the FDC Act.

mRNA vaccines are distinct because they are manufactured chemically rather than biologically, unlike many other vaccines. As a result, unlike therapeutic proteins, which require a full investigation of similarity to give biosimilar designation due to variations in secondary and tertiary structures and post-expression modifications, the vaccine structure is well understood. A potential biosimilar mRNA vaccine's sequencing might be 100 percent identical to that of a reference product. Biological therapeutic proteins are more akin to mRNA vaccines than generic chemical compounds.

mRNA vaccines are listed under CBER authority and approved as BLA; the 351(k) or biosimilar clause does not apply since it is restricted to therapeutic proteins. To make it clear, the FDA had issued a final guideline for the development of products for the treatment and prevention of COVID-19 (Feb 2021) that states:

> COVID-19 vaccine development may be accelerated based on knowledge gained from similar products manufactured with the same well-characterized platform technology. Similarly, with appropriate justification, some aspects of manufacture and control may be based on the vaccine platform and, in some instances, reduce the need for product-specific data. Therefore, FDA recommends that vaccine manufacturers engage in early communications with OVRR to discuss the type and extent of chemistry, manufacturing, and control information needed for the development and licensure of their COVID-19 vaccine.
>
> **(www.fda.gov/media/137926/download)**

This comment could imply that a "biosimilar" application for a licensed (BLA) product could be filed not under the BPCIA but by meeting its standards. For example, suppose a biosimilar mRNA vaccine sequence matches a reference product. In that case, toxicity and efficacy testing may be waived on a case-by-case basis, depending on other vaccine components, such as the formulation.

It is not always clear whether an mRNA vaccination should be classified as a biological or chemical product; however, we can obtain a sense of how the FDA will decide. The FDA has revised the BPCIA to apply 351(k) to biological goods, including therapeutic proteins:

> The Food and Drug Administration (FDA or the Agency) is proposing to amend its regulation that defines "biological product" to incorporate changes made by the Biologics Price Competition and Innovation Act of 2009 (BPCI Act) and to provide its interpretation of the statutory terms "protein" and "chemically synthesized polypeptide." Under that interpretation, the term protein would mean any alpha amino acid polymer with a specific, defined sequence greater than 40 amino acids in size. Likewise, a chemically synthesized polypeptide would mean any alpha amino acid polymer made entirely by chemical synthesis and greater than 40 amino acids but less than 100 amino acids in size. This proposed rule clarifies the statutory framework under which such products are regulated.

I don't see why the FDA won't change the BPCIA to allow chemically produced nucleic acids to be classified as 351(k) qualifying biologicals. A compelling argument will be that nucleic acids are the precursors to protein translation. As a result, they interact with the body's inherent protein expression system and are part of the DNA.

6.12   CONCLUSION

In the post-COVID-19 age, it is expected that the experience of the COVID-19 pandemic will also allow a better response to future pandemics. The regulatory approval of RNA products took years, and the traditional vaccines even decades; all of that has changed as the regulatory agencies are now providing guidelines that will allow faster development of RNA products. While the EU and US still have many differences, these are closing fast, but the core requirements remain unchanged. Therefore, as presented in this chapter, the developers are advised to plan the development program in close collaboration with the regulatory agencies and be prepared for what is considered essential and non-negotiable.

Appendix 1: COVID-19 mRNA Vaccine Manufacturing Feasibility

INTRODUCTION

The two mRNA vaccines against COVID-19 infection have proven better than any other type of vaccine ever approved by the US Food and Drug Administration FDA or European Medicines Agency. While the Western countries could spend over $100 B for protection, much of the world keeps waiting; the WHO estimates a current need of over 12 billion doses. Unlike traditional vaccines, mRNA vaccines can be manufactured quickly and at a lower cost. To promote this motivation, several non-profit and commercial organizations have put together their modeling, projections, and planning to manufacture billions of doses in a few months. While these exercises were timely, they also brought a better perception of the manufacturing technology of mRNA. In this appendix, I am condensing dozens of reports and outlining the steps for the production of the COVID-19 vaccine. Also included in this appendix is a regulatory plan to create biosimilar mRNA vaccines.

For example, in the case of the NIH-Moderna vaccine, it was estimated that producing eight billion doses in one year would cost $23 billion, using 842.1 kg of mRNA. This would require 4,620 employees working at 55 production lines, set up in 14 facilities. The capital cost for retrofitting facilities would be $3.2 billion, while the operating cost for the drug substance production campaign would be $17.5 billion. Fill and finish would cost $2 billion. Proportional costs are associated with other vaccines. The CVnCoV is an unmodified vaccine compared to the mRNA-1273 and BNT162b2, which have pseudouridine modification. The CVnCoV vaccine failed. (Table A.1)

Raw materials are the major cost component for mRNA vaccines. These materials currently cost more than materials for other kinds of vaccines. The significant difference in resource estimates between the three vaccines reflects differences in mRNA dose. mRNA-1273, which uses a 100 µg dose, is resource-intensive, followed by BNT162b2 (30 µg) and CVnCoV (12 µg). Raw material costs could come down with greater production volume and additional suppliers.

TABLE A.1

Summary of Crucial Resource Estimates for Producing Eight Billion Doses of mRNA Vaccine

Resource	mRNA-1273 (eight billion 100 µg doses)*	BNT162b2 (eight billion 30 µg doses)*	CVnCoV (eight billion 12 µg doses)*
Facilities	14	5	2
Production lines**	55	17	7
mRNA [kg]	842.1	252.6	101.1
Production batches	10,175	3,145	1,295
Personnel	4,620	1,386	554
Drug substance capital cost	3.19 billion	985 million	405.6 million
Drug substance operating cost¥	17.48 billion	5.40 billion	2.22 billion
Fill and finish operating cost¥	2.16 billion	3.04 billion	2.16 billion
Total cost‡	$22.83 billion	$9.43 billion	$4.38 billion

Notes: * The values of the production requirements were calculated based on producing eight billion vaccine doses within six months, as an additional six months are required beforehand to construct, equip, validate, and start up production.

** Drug substance production lines at the 30L bioreactor working volume scale.

¥ This operating cost is calculated for the six months required to produce eight billion doses, including the annualized facility-dependent capital costs.

‡ It was assumed there was sufficient drug product capacity, and new facilities did not need to be constructed.

A.1 MANUFACTURING PROCESS

There are two main phases in vaccine production:

- production of the drug substance (active ingredient production, bulk production, or primary manufacturing) and
- drug product manufacturing (fill and finish, or secondary manufacturing).

These two production processes usually happen at different locations, and they require different equipment, facilities, quality control methodologies, and expertise. Both the drug substance and drug product manufacturing processes follow strict regulatory guidelines. They must comply with current Good Manufacturing Practices (cGMP) to ensure product safety, efficacy, and quality. The steps required for producing mRNA vaccines are shown in Figure A.1.

Critically, mRNA vaccines offer several advantages over other vaccine platform technologies. Conventional cell-based expression technologies require growing cells

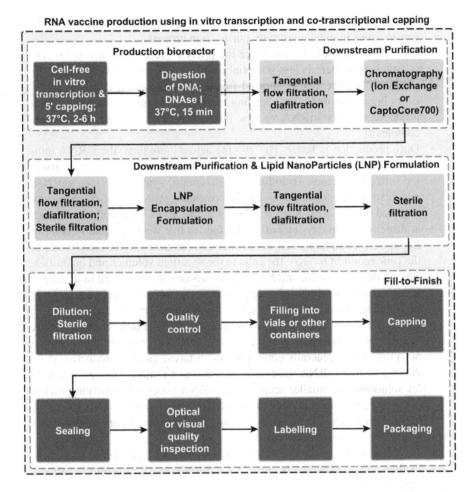

FIGURE A.1 Process flow diagram for mRNA drug substance production (aka. active ingredient production, bulk production, or primary manufacturing) and drug product manufacturing (aka. fill and finish or secondary manufacturing).

in large bioreactors (e.g., 2000L), which depends on carefully optimizing biological conditions. Cells introduce some variability. While mRNA production uses a novel process, it is cell-free and more akin to biochemical synthesis. There are at least seven distinct advantages:

- The process is more straightforward. mRNA vaccine production requires fewer steps than cell-based vaccine production, especially in the upstream processing section. The mRNA vaccine production reaction mix also uses fewer and more well-defined components than cell-based vaccine production as the mRNA vaccine production reaction mix does not contain nutrients for cells, cell debris, proteins, chromosomal DNA, lipids, and complex sugars that cells release. This simplicity of the reaction mix reduces the complexities in the downstream purification process.

- The process is more robust. Once the mRNA vaccine production process is established, there is less potential for biological variability. Living cells perform complex, interconnected functions. As a result, they can sometimes behave unpredictably, leading to unexpected results such as reduced production yields. mRNA vaccine production can essentially bypass this complexity.

- Dose production is faster. The vaccine active ingredient, the mRNA molecule, can be completed in two to six hours. The entire production batch for mRNA vaccines, including the enzymatic synthesis of the mRNA, purification, and formulation, can be completed within days, excluding the required quality control testing. For example, BioNTech produces batches at three- to seven-day intervals, with four to five weeks of quality control. In contrast, completing cell-based vaccines can take several months due to the time required to grow the cells to the specified volumes and quantities. The productivity of the mRNA vaccine production, expressed in doses per L of bioreactor working volumes per day, is two to four orders of magnitude higher than most cell-based vaccine production processes.

- The facilities and equipment can be an order of magnitude smaller. mRNA vaccine production can occur in much smaller bioreactors (e.g., 30L to 50L) than those generally employed in cell-based vaccine production (e.g., 2000L). While mRNA vaccine production can require high volume buffer solutions, the smaller scale of the mRNA vaccine production process means it can be implemented in smaller facilities. Multiple mRNA vaccine production processes, for example, can be placed into a conventional cell-based vaccine production facility.

- The capital costs are lower. Setting up the production process and covering facility-related expenses is cheaper for mRNA vaccines, given the small-scale nature.

- The process can be implemented in existing facilities. The number of facilities that can accommodate mRNA vaccine production is higher than the number of facilities that can be used to set up new cell-based vaccine production processes. In addition to its small-scale nature, mRNA vaccine production can be hermetically sealed from the environment. This can allow production in lower-grade clean rooms. mRNA vaccine production processes can, in principle, be set up in clean rooms in existing facilities used to produce other vaccines, monoclonal antibodies, insulin, veterinary vaccines, and other biologics and injectables.

- The process can be quickly repurposed for new variants or even new viral threats. mRNA vaccines involve rapid development and production timelines because the production platform is agnostic to the disease target. Different RNA sequences translating into other vaccines or candidate vaccine protein antigens can be produced using the same process. The only component in this production process that needs to be changed is the template DNA, based on which the RNA is enzymatically synthesized. The rest of the materials, equipment, consumables, unit operations, formulation components, fill and finish processes, quality control and quality assurance methods remain unchanged when switching to producing a new RNA sequence encoding for a new vaccine antigen. This flexibility can help ensure long-term sustainability.

Potential challenges with scaling up mRNA vaccines include the limited pool of production and quality experts with experience using the new technology—particularly compared to other kinds of vaccines—and challenges in quickly sourcing raw materials (e.g., the cationic lipid) at the quantities required.

A.1.1 PLASMID PRODUCTION

The template DNA is synthesized and amplified by PCR using the cDNA (complementary to the target RNA sequence) or any DNA comprising the cDNA (e.g., a plasmid vector consisting of the cDNA) as a template. In this case, the 5'-primer used for PCR is the sequence of a promoter of DNA-dependent RNA polymerase to generate a PCR product comprising at least a promoter for a DNA-dependent RNA polymerase and the DNA sequence encoding the target RNA sequence. This synthesized or amplified PCR product used as a template for in vitro transcription is template PCR.

The quality of the template PCR product is controlled by determining the identity of the DNA sequence encoding the target RNA sequence.

Synthesis of the template DNA by cloning of a DNA sequence encoding the RNA sequence into a plasmid DNA vector and subsequent amplification:

One alternative for using a PCR product as a template for in vitro transcription is plasmid DNA vectors comprising a DNA sequence encoding the RNA sequence ("insert DNA sequence") and a promoter of a DNA-dependent RNA polymerase. In this case, plasmids are chosen, which are amplified (e.g., in bacteria, particularly E. coli, by fermentation). This alternative has the advantage of producing fewer mutations in the amplified DNA compared to PCR. Alternatively, the insert DNA sequence is amplified by PCR, and therefore the PCR product is used as a template for in vitro transcription.

The production of plasmid DNA, its linearization, and preparation for IVT are presented in the cGMP mRNA Vaccine Manufacturing chapter.

A.1.2 UPSTREAM: IN VITRO TRANSCRIPTION (IVT)

mRNA vaccines represent an innovation in the drug substance production process. As shown in Figure A.1, the mRNA drug substance (DS) production process starts with the biochemical reaction whereby the mRNA is synthesized.

This in vitro transcription reaction for mRNA vaccine production starts with adding all the reaction components to the bioreactor. These reaction components include:

- Nucleotides (adenosine-5′-triphosphate (ATP), 1-methylpseudouridine-5′-triphosphate (mod-UTP), cytidine-5′-triphosphate (CTP), guanosine-5′-triphosphate (GTP));
- a linear template DNA (can be mass-produced in *Escherichia coli* and linearized using restriction enzymes);
- T7 RNA Polymerase enzyme (produced in *Escherichia coli*) and RNase enzyme inhibitors;
- 5′ cap analogue (e.g., CleanCap AG); and
- Spermidine, dithiothreitol (DTT), magnesium chloride ($MgCl_2$), optionally the pyrophosphatase enzyme (to break down the pyrophosphate by-product and consequently to maintain the Mg cofactor concentrations), nuclease-free purified water, and buffers to maintain the pH (e.g., Tris-HCl).

In this reaction, which takes about two to six hours to complete, the T7 RNA Polymerase enzyme links together the four RNA building blocks (ATP, mod-UTP, CTP, GTP) in the sequence provided by the linear template DNA (i.e., the Spike protein of the SARS-CoV- 2 viruses). The linear chain of nucleotides formed in this reaction constitutes the mRNA of the vaccine. In addition, a polyadenylated tail (poly(A) tail) is also encoded on the DNA and added to the mRNA during the in vitro transcription reaction.

The 5′ cap structure (e.g., CleanCap AG) at the beginning of the mRNA can be incorporated during the in vitro synthesis of the mRNA in an approach called co-transcriptional capping. (While capping can, in principle, also be done after synthesis, in this report, we modeled co-transcriptional capping.) The 5′ cap is essential for enabling the mRNA to work in the human body cells without being detected as an RNA of foreign (e.g., viral) origin.

The 1-methylpseudouridine-5′-triphosphate (mod-UTP) is used instead of the wild-type, unmodified uridine-5′-triphosphate (UTP) to reduce the immunogenicity and increase mRNA translational capacity and biological stability, which is advantageous for mRNA vaccinology. The Moderna and Pfizer vaccines use mod-UTP, but the CureVac candidate does not.

Following the 5′ capped mRNA synthesis, which contains mod-UTP, the linear template DNA is degraded by adding an enzyme that degrades DNA to the bioreactor. The Deoxyribonuclease I (DNase I) enzyme can be used. The activity of DNase I is highest in the presence of Calcium ions; thus, calcium chloride ($CaCl_2$) is also added to the bioreactor and the DNase I enzyme.

A.1.3 DOWNSTREAM: PURIFICATION

Following the digestion of the template DNA, the next task is to purify the product of interest, namely the full-length 5′ capped mRNA, out of the aqueous solution containing the above-described components and RNA fragments that were obtained by unsuccessful in vitro transcription or as a result of degradation. The downstream separation and purification of the mRNA can be achieved based on differences in size, electrical charge, hydrophobicity, binding affinity to specific ligands, and other properties. Following the digestion of the template DNA, the largest component by molecular mass is the mRNA product at a molecular mass of 2.5 MDa, followed by the enzymes, which are one order of magnitude smaller in molecular mass (e.g., the T7 RNA polymerase is $\approx$0.1 MDa, or $\approx$100 kDa, whereas DNase I is $\approx$0.03 MDa, or $\approx$30 kDa). Therefore, size-based separation, such as filtration, can be used.

The exact purification setup that mRNA COVID-19 vaccine production companies use is not disclosed publicly. However, possible purification unit operations include tangential flow filtration (TFF), ion-exchange chromatography, core bead chromatography (e.g., Capto Core 700), oligo dT affinity chromatography, size exclusion and hydroxyapatite chromatography. Out of these, TFF, ion-exchange chromatography, core bead chromatography (e.g., Capto Core 700), and oligo dT affinity chromatography are likely used.

A potential version of this downstream purification process is shown in Figure A.1. Based on this, a detailed process flow model was built in the SuperPro Designer bioprocess simulation tool.

In addition to washing away the impurities, in this TFF step, the mRNA is placed into a solution that is suitable for the next purification step. The solution retained by the TFF membrane is then flown into the Capto Core 700 chromatography unit operation, which is a core bead type chromatography whereby molecules can be separated based on both size and binding to hydrophobic and positively charged octylamine ligands. The advantage of using this chromatography approach is that lower amounts of chromatography medium/resin can purify the mRNA product more efficiently.

After the mRNA flows through the CaptoCore 700 chromatography column, it enters a second TFF unit operation whereby it is concentrated and then further washed using a 10x diafiltration volume. The impurities are washed away, and the buffer is again replaced with a sodium citrate buffer. Next, the mRNA in citrate buffer is sterile filtered. It then enters the formulation step, where the mRNA is enclosed into spheres of lipids called lipid nanoparticles (LNPs).

This LNP formulation step requires mixing a liquid stream containing four lipid components in ethanol with another liquid stream containing the mRNA in the water-based sodium citrate buffer. The four lipids are ionizable lipid (the most novel component), the phospholipid, cholesterol, and a polyethylene glycol (PEG)-lipid conjugate. The LNP formulation step can be carried out using microfluidics mixers, jet-impingement mixers (also known as T-junction mixers), or potentially in pressurized tanks. For fast and large-scale production, mixing in pressurized tanks is preferred, whereas microfluidics mixing is the least preferred option. In the model presented here, 14 hours were assumed for the LNP encapsulation reaction in a macro-scale process similar to the BioNTech/Pfizer approach. The entire formulation unit operation with setting up the equipment, transferring in solutions, performing the 14-hour long formulation reaction, and cleaning was modeled to take 19.24 hours.

The duration of this LNP formulation unit operation is not publicly available and can vary among the mRNA vaccine manufacturing companies. However, this step is considered the bottleneck in the mRNA drug substance production process.

Consequently, the duration of this step can impact the production performance of the process in terms of costs and annual production amounts.

The time required to complete one production batch was modeled at 58.78 hours. By optimizing the scheduling, batches can be completed at 22–25-hour intervals (i.e., if the production of a batch starts in the upstream section while the previous batch is being completed in the downstream and formulation sections of the production process). Following the LNP encapsulation step, the LNP-mRNA particles are first concentrated and washed in a diafiltration step. The ethanol and other impurities are washed away, and the buffer is replaced with the final formulation buffer, for example, by using 10x diafiltration volumes. After this, the LNP-mRNA-containing solution is sterile-filtered and filled into plastic bags (e.g., 10 L plastic bags), then sent to the fill and finish facilities.

The approach described here represents one possible way of purifying the synthesized mRNA and the LNP-mRNA complexes. Companies such as Moderna/Lonza, BioNTech/Pfizer, and CureVac might use different purification approaches; however, the goal remains the same: to separate the mRNA product of interest away from other impurities in the process to ensure product quality, safety, and efficacy, using cGMP-compliant processes (Figure A.2).

mRNA vaccine drug substance production process flow diagram obtained from SuperPro Designer. The production process consists of the following three key parts: 1) the in vitro transcription step, whereby the mRNA is capped co-transcriptionally using 5′ cap analogs (e.g., CleanCap AG); 2) the downstream purification step obtained by a series of tangential flow filtration steps and a Capto Core 700 chromatography step; 3) LNP formulation step followed by another tangential flow filtration step. The tangential flow filtration steps can perform both concentration and diafiltration of the mRNA product. A high-resolution version of the process flow diagram is available on the Public Citizen website.

A.1.4 FILL AND FINISH AND QUALITY CONTROL

The LNP-mRNA particles can be further purified and sterile filtered at the fill and finish facilities. At this point, quality control testing of the drug substance and the sterilized vials can also take place. Next, if required, the LNP-mRNA solution can be diluted to the concentration in which the solution is placed into glass vials. For example, NIH-Moderna (mRNA-1273) vaccine is filled into 10-dose glass vials, whereas the BioNTech-Pfizer (BNT162b2) vaccine is filled into six-dose glass vials. The sterile and clean glass vials are moved along a conveyor, and a liquid dispensing needle fills the formulated LNP-mRNA into the glass vials from the top in a sterile environment. Next, the vials are capped, sealed, and inspected for visual defects (this can be achieved using cameras and automated image processing). The vials without flaws are then labeled and packaged in several (e.g., two additional) layers of packaging.

Since both the drug substance and drug product manufacturing processes are compliant with cGMP, the raw materials, the in-process materials, and finished products are strictly monitored for their quality. As a result, the quality control and

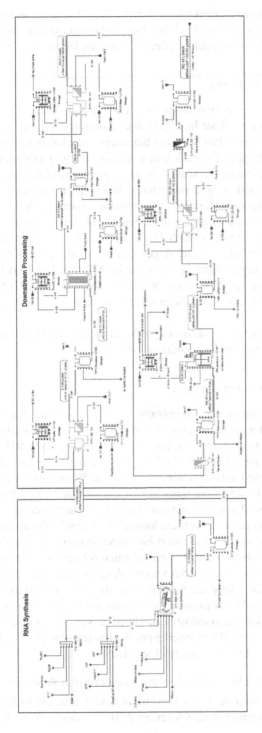

FIGURE A.2   In this process, the downstream purification starts with a dilution step followed by the TFF unit operation. The filter retains the mRNA molecule, and the other smaller components of the reaction mix flow through the TFF filter membrane. Then, an additional buffer solution (e.g., potassium chloride (KCl) buffer) is added to the solution retained by the filter to wash away the impurities through the filter membrane more effectively. The amount of added buffer solution is 10-fold the volume entering the TFF diafiltration step (i.e., 10x diafiltration volume). For the TFF steps presented here, ultrafiltration membranes with a molecular weight cut-off of 500 kDa or 300 kDa would be suitable.

batch release can take several weeks (e.g., four to five). To ensure uniform delays between production times and batch release, the production runs can be staggered, and the quality control for subsequent production runs can be carried out in parallel.

A.2   RESOURCE ANALYSIS

Modeling to produce eight billion doses in six months is done using SuperPro Designer Version 11, Build 2 from Intelligen, Inc, assuming batch operation mode. Industry experts use the SuperPro Designer bioprocess simulation tool to calculate material and energy balances for each unit operation in the production process. SuperPro Designer determines the size of the equipment, calculates labor requirements, schedules the functions and procedures, and performs economic calculations both for capital expenses (CapEx) and operating expenses (OpEx). SuperPro Designer is linked to chemicals, consumables, equipment, and other resources.

Producing eight billion doses of the NIH-Moderna COVID-19 vaccine (mRNA-1273), which contains 100 μg of mRNA per vaccine dose, requires 842.1 kg of mRNA to be produced. Eight billion doses of the BioNTech-Pfizer COVID-19 vaccine (BNT162b2) require the production of 252.6 kilograms of mRNA, whereas 101.1 kg of mRNA would yield eight billion doses of the CureVac (CVnCoV) mRNA vaccine.

The capital, annual operating, and doses produced per year expressed per production line, are shown below in the Appendix in Table A.2.

A.2.1   MATERIALS IN DS PRODUCTION

Materials represent the major cost component of mRNA vaccine drug substance production, accounting for approximately 73% of production costs. Based on process knowledge and input from other experts, we estimate that there are mRNA losses in the production process, including 30% in the downstream purification, 20% in the formulation and subsequent purification steps, and up to 5% in the processes occurring at the fill and finish sites. This translates to approximately 53% losses in the entire production process. Therefore, the raw material amounts used in the production process are higher to account for these losses. For example, the quantity of raw materials entering the in vitro transcription bioreactor is nearly double the amount needed to produce the equivalent mRNA amount when not accounting for the losses.

Some of the materials used for mRNA vaccine drug substances are new and lack a diversified supply chain. Many suppliers provide these key materials. We solely focus on these key materials. For example, we did not model plasmid DNA production because it is better known to industry, has been previously scaled compared to the production of some key mRNA vaccine production ingredients (e.g., CleanCap AG), and can be purchased from a variety of suppliers.

A.2.1.1   Raw Materials Used in the in vitro Transcription Reaction

The key raw materials used in the in vitro transcription reaction in limited supply include the 5′ cap analog (e.g., CleanCap AG) and modified nucleotides. In

TABLE A.2
Facility-Related Requirements for Producing Eight Billion mRNA Vaccine Drug Substance Doses

Name of facility-related resource	Facility-related requirements for producing 8 billion mRNA-1273 doses*	Facility-related requirements for producing 8 billion BNT162b2 doses*	Facility-related requirements for producing 8 billion CVnCoV doses*
Number of production lines‡	55	17	7
Number of facilities	14	5	2
Production lines per facility	4 production lines for 13 facilities; 3 production lines in 1 facility	4 production lines for 2 facilities; 3 production lines for 3 facilities	4 production lines for 1 facilities; 3 production lines for 1 facility
Total number of batches required	10,175	3,145	1,295
Total operating costs for drug substance ¥	17.48 billion	5.40 billion	2.22 billion
Total capital costs	3.19 billion	985 million	405.6 million

* The values of the production requirements were calculated based on producing eight billion vaccine doses within six months, as an additional six months are required beforehand to construct, equip, validate, and start-up production.
‡ Production lines at the 30L bioreactor working volume scale.
¥ This operating cost is calculated for the six months required to produce eight billion doses, and it includes the annualized facility-dependent capital costs.

addition, due to suddenly increased demand, suppliers might be struggling to produce sufficient quantities of the T7 RNA polymerase, the linearized template DNA, the DNase I enzyme, and the RNAse Inhibitor. However, the production of these components is based on well-established and scalable processes (e.g., fermentation in *Escherichia coli*). Therefore, if 5′ capping of the mRNA is carried out enzymatically, the amounts of capping enzymes should be considered instead of the 5′ cap analogs (e.g., CleanCap AG). The amounts of these materials required per production line (at the 30L bioreactor working volume scale) and the material amounts and the necessary costs for producing eight billion doses are shown below in Table A.3.

A.2.1.2 Raw Materials for LNP
Each of the three COVID-19 mRNA vaccines presented in this study is formulated in lipid nanoparticles (LNPs). These LNPs are spheres composed of four different lipids with the mRNA enclosed inside. The four types of lipids building up these spheres are ionizable lipids (i.e., cationic lipids), cholesterol, phospholipids, and polyethylene glycol (PEG) lipid. These classes of lipids are consistent for the 3 mRNA vaccines, as shown in Table A.4, however, the individual lipids vary among these

TABLE A.3
The Estimated Amounts and Costs of Key Raw Materials Used for mRNA Vaccine Production in the in vitro Transcription Reaction

Name of pure component	Amount per year per production line* [g/year]	Key material requirements for producing 8 billion mRNA-1273 doses		Key material requirements for producing 8 billion BNT162b2 doses		Key material requirements for producing 8 billion CVnCoV doses	
		Amounts [g / 8 billion doses]	Costs [USD / 8 billion doses]	Amounts [g / 8 billion doses]	Costs [USD / 8 billion doses]	Amounts [g / 8 billion doses]	Costs [USD / 8 billion doses]
CleanCap AG	50,972	1,471,906	5,887,608,320	441,572	1,766,282,496	176,629	706,512,998
Deoxyribonuclease I (DNase I)	28	809	426,336	243	127,901	97	51,160
RNase enzyme inhibitor	139	4,014	3,411,413	1,204	1,023,424	482	409,370
T7 RNA polymerase	185	5,342	728,176,702	1,603	218,453,011	641	87,381,204
linear template DNA	555	16,027	1,762,928,524	4,808	528,878,557	1,923	211,551,423
1-methylpseudouridine-5′-triphosphate (mod- UTP)	21,496	620,735	2,931,813,779	186,220	879,544,134	0	0

* Production line at 30L bioreactor working volume scale, producing 29,162 grams of mRNA per year. For further details, see Tables S3 and S4 in the appendix.

TABLE A.4

Estimated Lipid Components Required to Produce Eight Billion mRNA Vaccine Doses

mRNA Vaccine	Lipid Name	Lipid amount per dose [mg]	Lipid amount for 8 billion doses [metric tons] *
NIH-Moderna;	Ionizable lipid [a]	1.09	11.48
mRNA-1273	Phospholipid [b]	0.24	2.49
	Cholesterol	0.47	4.96
	PEG lipid [c]	0.13	1.42
	Total lipids	1.93	20.34
BioNTech-Pfizer;	Ionizable lipid [d]	0.43	4.54
BNT162b2	Phospholipid [e]	0.09	0.95
	Cholesterol	0.2	2.11
	PEG lipid [f]	0.05	0.53
	Total lipids	0.77	8.13
CureVac; CVnCoV	Ionizable lipid [g]	0.17	1.82
	Phospholipid [h]	0.04	0.38
	Cholesterol	0.08	0.84
	PEG lipid [i]	0.02	0.21
	Total lipids	0.31	3.25

[a] heptadecan-9-yl 8-((2-hydroxyethyl)(6-oxo-6-(undecyloxy)hexyl)amino)octanoate (SM-102);

[b] 1,2- distearoyl-sn-glycero-3-phosphocholine (DSPC);

[c] 1,2-dimyristoylrac-glycero-3-methoxypolyethylene glycol- 2000 (PEG2000 DMG);

[d] (4-hydroxybutyl)azanediyl)bis(hexane-6,1-diyl)bis(2-hexyldecanoate) (ALC-0315);

[e] 1,2-distearoyl-sn-glycero-3-phosphocholine;

[f] 2[(polyethylene glycol)-2000]-N,N-ditetradecylacetamide;

[g] probably (4-hydroxybutyl)azanediyl)bis(hexane-6,1-diyl)bis(2-hexyldecanoate) (ALC-0315);

[h] 1,2-distearoyl- sn-glycero-3-phosphocholine (DSPC);

[i] probably 2[(polyethylene glycol)-2000]-N,N-ditetradecylacetamide. It was assumed that 32% of the lipids are lost in the production process.

vaccines, as shown in the footnote below Table A.4. It is believed that BioNTech-Pfizer and CureVac use a similar formulation approach, based on the ionizable lipid (ALC-0315, (4-hydroxybutyl)azanediyl)bis(hexane- 6,1-diyl)bis(2-hexyldecanoate)). On the other hand, the NIH-Moderna candidate uses a different ionizable lipid ((SM-102, heptadecan-9-yl 8-((2-hydroxyethyl)(6-oxo-6 (undecyloxy)hexyl)amino)octanoate) and has a different lipid composition.

The NIH-Moderna (mRNA-1273) vaccine contains 1.93 mg of lipids in total per vaccine dose. However, the exact amount of the 4 constituent lipids is not disclosed. Here, the four lipids in the mRNA-1273 vaccine were estimated by assuming the same lipid ratios as in the BNT162b2 vaccine. The total amount of lipids required to produce eight billion doses of the mRNA-1273 was estimated at 20.34 metric tons, and over half of this amount consisted of the ionizable lipid.

The BioNTech-Pfizer (BNT162b2) vaccine contains 0.77 mg of lipids per vaccine dose, with known lipid types. The ratio of lipid to mRNA is higher in the BNT162b2 than in the mRNA-1273 vaccine. It is estimated that 8.13 metric tons of lipids would be required to produce eight billion BNT162b2 doses. The amounts of ionizable lipids, phospholipid, cholesterol, and PEG lipid for eight billion BNT162b2 were estimated at 4.54, 0.95, 2.11, and 0.53 metric tons, respectively.

The amount of lipids contained in a dose of CureVac (CVnCoV) was not available publicly. However, this was estimated based on similarity in lipid composition to the BNT162b2 vaccine and by taking into account the difference in the amount of mRNA per dose of these two vaccines. Thus, the total lipid per dose of CVnCoV was estimated at 0.31 mg. The total lipids required to produce eight billion CVnCoV doses were estimated at 3.25 metric tons. The amounts of ionizable lipids, phospholipid, cholesterol, and PEG lipid for eight billion CVnCoV were estimated at 1.82, 0.38, 0.84, and 0.21 metric tons, respectively.

It also is worth noting that approximately 17.8k metric tons of water for injection (RNAse-free purified water) is required per year per production line (Table A.5). This water for injection (WFI) requirement should be considered when designing the utilities and systems for generating the WFI. The total WFI requirements for producing eight billion doses are estimated at 514.4k metric tons, 154.3k metric

---

TABLE A.5
The Estimated Consumables Required to Produce Eight Billion mRNA Vaccine Doses

Name of key consumables and their unit of measurement for the amount	Key consumable requirements for producing 8 billion mRNA-1273 doses	Key consumable requirements for producing 8 billion BNT162b2 doses	Key consumable requirements for producing 8 billion CVnCoV doses
The tangential flow filtration membrane [m2]	505,262	151,579	60,631
Flow-through chromatography medium, e.g. Capto Core 700 [L] *	16,842	5,053	2,021
Oligo dT chromatography resin [L] *	467,836	140,351	56,140
Multimodal chromatography, hydrogen bonding and anion exchange chromatography, e.g. Prima S [L] *	168,421	50,526	20,210

* Out of these three types of chromatography resins, one or, potentially, two can be enough to purify the mRNA drug substance in combination with tangential flow filtration.

tons, and 61.7k metric tons for the mRNA-1273, BNT162b2, and CVnCoV vaccines, respectively.

The estimated annual purchase price of materials per production line at the 30L bioreactor working volume scale is $456.6 million per year, accounting for approximately 73% of the total production costs. Within this material cost amount, about 45% is the CleanCap AG purchase price. Therefore, the materials are estimated to cost $13.2 billion, $4 billion, and $1.6 billion when producing eight billion doses of the mRNA-1273, BNT162b2, and CVnCoV vaccines.

A.2.2   Consumables and Equipment for DS

The second highest cost component in the mRNA vaccine drug substance production. The cost of consumables accounts for approximately 24% of the total production costs. The mRNA vaccine production process can be based on single-use equipment and consumables, replaced after every production batch. Single-use equipment and consumables include:

- Single-use plastic bioreactor lining bags;
- Single-use plastic storage bags;
- Plastic (e.g., silicone) tubing, single-use aseptic connectors, clamps; and
- Disposable filter membranes, single-use filter assemblies, and chromatography columns.

In some cases, filter membranes and certain types of chromatography resins can be re-used, helping reduce costs. However, the re-use of these components has to be validated. The single-use consumables are usually held in place by more permanent structures (e.g., a single-use plastic bioreactor lining bag is placed inside a cylindrical steel support frame with glass or plastic windows).

The advantage of using single-use equipment is that the process can be assembled substantially faster than setting up stainless steel equipment. The upfront capital investment costs for single-use equipment are lower than the permanent stainless-steel equipment. Still, the operating costs could increase in the case of single-use equipment compared to stainless steel equipment. In addition, because single-use-based production requires substantially less cleaning, it can reduce labor costs and water and cleaning agent requirements, minimize cleaning validation, and increase production speeds.

mRNA vaccine production at the 30L bioreactor working volume scale would require around US$150 million worth of consumables per year based on the process-cost modeling results obtained with SuperPro Designer, using the model presented in Figure A.1. The consumables required to produce eight billion doses of the mRNA-1273, BNT162b2, and CVnCoV vaccines is estimated at $4.3 billion, $1.3 billion, and $520 million, respectively.

The amounts of chromatography resins and TFF membranes were also estimated, assuming that 5 g of mRNA can be purified per m^2 of TFF membrane;

50 g of mRNA can be purified per L of flow-through chromatography medium (e.g., Capto Core 700); 1.8 g of mRNA can be purified per L of oligo dT resin 62; and that 5 g/L of mRNA can be purified per L of multimodal chromatography resin that combines hydrogen bonding and anion exchange chromatography (e.g., Prima S). These values were obtained from the consumables suppliers and from discussions with biomanufacturing experts. For TFF, it was also taken into account that 3 different TFF unit operations were used for mRNA purification and post-formulation purification. The amount of these consumables required to produce eight billion doses are shown below in Table A.5. It is worth noting that some of these consumables (e.g., TFF membranes, oligo dT resins, and Prima S resins) can be reused for multiple batches, reducing the required amounts for these consumables. However, re-using these consumables needs to be rigorously tested and validated.

A.2.3 Labor for DS

The labor cost in the mRNA vaccine production process represents less than 3% of the total production costs. The cost of labor can vary among the different geographical locations, countries, and continents. Still, the cost of labor is not expected to have a substantial impact on the overall production costs. The SuperPro Designer modeling tool also assumed that 60% of the labor hours are used directly for producing the product, and the remaining 40% is used for other activities.

A.2.4 Another Resource for DS

The remaining resource requirements include 1) laboratory, quality control, and quality assurance; 2) utilities; 3) sales resources; 4) waste treatment and disposal, failed product disposal; 5) transportation and miscellaneous. These were estimated to account for less than 1% of the total production costs. Out of these, laboratory, quality control, and quality assurance costs are the highest cost components and were assumed to account for 50% of the total labor costs. In addition, assessing royalties and licensing fees for some components, including the cationic lipids used in the LNP formulation, was outside the scope of this report.

A.2.5 Fill and Finish Requirements

After producing the mRNA vaccine drug substance, this active ingredient is filled into plastic bags and shipped to the fill and finish facilities. It is filled into vials using aseptic filling lines operating under cGMP guidelines. The filling COST into vials depends on the filling technology and vial or container size. The cost per dose tends to decrease as the vial size increases. For example, the NIH-Moderna mRNA-1273 is filled into 10-dose vials, whereas the BioNTech-Pfizer BNT162b2 vaccine is filled into 5-dose vials, which were eventually approved as 6-dose vials. While the vial size for CureVac's CVnCoV is not known, given its thermostability, larger

TABLE A6
Key Fill and finish Resource Requirements for Producing Eight Billion mRNA Vaccine Doses

Name of fill and finish resource	Fill and finish requirements for producing mRNA-1273 vaccines	Fill and finish requirements for producing BNT162b2 vaccines	Fill and finish requirements for producing CVnCoV vaccines
Doses per vial	10	6	10**
Total number of filling lines for producing 8 billion doses*	15	25	15
Number of empty glass vials for producing 8 billion doses, with 5% losses	842.1 million	1.684 billion	842.1 million
Total operating fill and finish costs for producing 8 billion doses***	2.16 billion	3.04 billion	2.16 billion

* The values of the production requirements were calculated based on producing eight billion vaccine doses within six months;

** The vial size for CureVac's CVnCoV is not available publicly and it was assumed at ten doses per vial due to the higher thermostability of this vaccine;

*** Includes the cost of the empty glass vials, however, the cost of the drug substance is not included in this estimate. This consists of the annualized capital cost for the fill and finishes facilities.

* Production at the 30L bioreactor working volume scale produces 29162 grams of mRNA per year.

multidose vials (e.g., 10-dose vials or higher) would be more cost-effective. The fill and finish production cost (including the cost of the vial) was estimated at $0.27 per dose and $0.37 per dose for filling into 10-dose vials and 5-dose vials, respectively. The cost estimates were obtained using the SuperPro Designer bioprocess modeling tool. Filling eight billion mRNA-1273 vaccine doses into 10-dose vials is estimated to cost $2.16 billion. Filling eight billion BNT162b2 vaccine doses into 5-dose (or 6-dose) vials is estimated to cost $3.04 billion, as shown below in Table A.6.

A.3 APPENDIX

Tables S1–S3 list additional costing information for the manufacturing of mRNA vaccines. Several lower price options are now available as shown in Table S4 (www.hzymes-global.com); no conflict of interest.

TABLE S1

The Estimated Costs and Doses Produced Per Year Per Per Drug Substance Production Line for the NIH-Moderna (mRNA-1273), BioNTech-Pfizer (BNT162b2), and CureVac (CVnCoV) Vaccines

Name of indication	Amount per production line for mRNA-1273 vaccine drug substance production *	Amount per production line for BNT162b2 vaccine drug substance production *	Amount per production line for CVnCoV vaccine drug substance production *
Capital cost, CapEx [USD]	57,947,000	57,947,000	57,947,000
Operating cost, OpEx [USD/year]	635,690,000	635,690,000	635,690,000
Doses per year	291,620,000	972,066,667	2,430,166,667

TABLE S2

Estimated Amounts of Raw Materials Used in the mRNA-LNP Vaccine Drug Substance Production Process Based on the Manufacturing Process (Figure A.2)**

Name of pure component	Material amounts per year per production line* [g / year]	Material amount for producing 8 billion mRNA-1273 doses [g / 8 billion doses]	Material amount for producing 8 billion BNT162b2 doses [g / 8 billion doses]	Material amount for producing 8 billion CVnCoV doses [g / 8 billion doses]
Acetic acid	9,926,646	286,649,349	85,994,805	34,397,922
Adenosine-5'-triphosphate (ATP)	22,519	650,276	195,083	78,033
Calcium chloride (CaCl2)	5,977	172,596	51,779	20,712
Cholesterol	187,675	5,419,445	1,625,834	650,333
Citric acid	1,357,085	39,188,214	11,756,464	4,702,586
CleanCap AG	50,972	1,471,906	441,572	176,629
cytidine-5'-triphosphate (CTP)	21,452	619,464	185,839	74,336
Deoxyribonuclease I (DNase I)***	28	809	243	97
Disodium phosphate (Na2HPO4)	17,130,535	494,674,304	148,402,291	59,360,916
Dithiothreitol (DTT)	18,193	525,355	157,606	63,043
Ethyl alcohol (ethanol)	93,049,356	2,686,963,682	806,089,105	322,435,642
Guanosine-5'-triphosphate (GTP)	23,229	670,778	201,233	80,493
Ionizable lipid	434,380	12,543,486	3,763,046	1,505,218
Linear template DNA	555	16,027	4,808	1,923
Magnesium chloride (MgCl2)	30,890	892,003	267,601	107,040
Monopotassium phosphate (KH2PO4)	31,146	899,395	269,819	107,927
Phospholipid	94,139	2,718,429	815,529	326,211

(Continued)

TABLE S2 (CONTINUED)

Estimated Amounts of Raw Materials Used in the mRNA-LNP Vaccine Drug Substance Production Process Based on the Manufacturing Process (Figure A.2)**

Name of pure component	Material amounts per year per production line* [g / year]	Material amount for producing 8 billion mRNA-1273 doses [g / 8 billion doses]	Material amount for producing 8 billion BNT162b2 doses [g / 8 billion doses]	Material amount for producing 8 billion CVnCoV doses [g / 8 billion doses]
Polyethylene glycol (PEG) lipid	53,576	1,547,101	464,130	185,652
Potassium chloride (KCl)	30,119,051	869,740,530	260,922,159	104,368,864
Pyrophosphatase***	888	25,643	7,693	3,077
RNase enzyme inhibitor	139	4,014	1,204	482
Sodium acetate	46,324,346	1,337,696,902	401,309,071	160,523,628
Sodium chloride (NaCl)	124,585,712	3,597,631,384	1,079,289,415	431,715,766
Sodium citrate	7,291,590	210,557,476	63,167,243	25,266,897
Sodium hydroxide (NaOH)	8,795,066	253,972,987	76,191,896	30,476,758
Spermidine	3,225	93,128	27,938	11,175
Sucrose	761,772	21,997,505	6,599,252	2,639,701
T7 RNA polymerase***	185	5,342	1,603	641
Tris hydrochloride (Tris HCl)	272,325	7,863,863	2,359,159	943,664
Water for injection (WFI), RNase free	17,811,917,463	514,350,419,836	154,305,125,951	61,722,050,380
1-methylpseudouridine-5′- triphosphate (mod-UTP)	21,496	620,735	186,220	0

* Production line at 30L bioreactor working volume scale produces 29162 grams of mRNA per year;

** For calculating the material requirements for producing eight billion doses, additional 5% losses were assumed to occur in the fill and finish process. This is the list of all materials used in the production process, including materials used for cleaning;

*** The amount of enzymes required depends on the specific activity of the enzymes, and this can vary between different suppliers.

TABLE S3

Estimated Cost of Raw Materials Used in the mRNA-LNP Vaccine Drug Substance Production Process Based on the Manufacturing Process (Figure A.2)**

Name of solution or material	Material amounts per year per production line* [kg/year]	Annual material cost per production line* [USD/year]	Material costs for producing 8 billion mRNA-1273 doses [USD / 8 billion doses]	Material costs for producing 8 billion BNT162b2 doses [USD / 8 billion doses]	Material costs for producing 8 billion CVnCoV doses [USD / 8 billion doses]
0.1 M CaCl2 solution	23	133	3,841	1,152	461
0.1 M Spermidine solution	221	27,112	782,907	234,872	93,949
1 M DTT solution	126	109,170	3,152,476	945,743	378,297
1 M MgCl2 solution	66	204	5,891	1,767	707
1 M NaOH solution	13,616	1,571	45,365	13,610	5,444
1 M Tris HCl solution	961	98,887	2,855,536	856,661	342,664
1 mg/ml DNA template solution	552	61,050,086	1,762,928,524	528,878,557	211,551,423
100 mM ATP solution	442	5,549,985	160,265,571	48,079,671	19,231,868
100 mM CleanCap AG	449	203,887,446	5,887,608,320	1,766,282,496	706,512,998
100 mM CTP solution	442	5,538,693	159,939,494	47,981,848	19,192,739
100 mM GTP solution	442	5,549,984	160,265,542	48,079,663	19,231,865
100 mM mod-UTP solution	442	101,528,497	2,931,813,779	879,544,134	351,817,654
250 mM KCl solution	1,621,076	551,973	15,939,190	4,781,757	1,912,703
Cholesterol	188	4,691,877	135,486,194	40,645,858	16,258,343
DNase I	11	14,764	426,336	127,901	51,160
Ethyl Alcohol	93,049	744,395	21,495,714	6,448,714	2,579,486

(Continued)

TABLE S3 (CONTINUED)

Estimated Cost of Raw Materials Used in the mRNA-LNP Vaccine Drug Substance Production Process Based on the Manufacturing Process (Figure A.2)**

Name of solution or material	Material amounts per year per production line* [kg/year]	Annual material cost per production line* [USD/year]	Material costs for producing 8 billion mRNA-1273 doses [USD / 8 billion doses]	Material costs for producing 8 billion BNT162b2 doses [USD / 8 billion doses]	Material costs for producing 8 billion CVnCoV doses [USD / 8 billion doses]
Ionizable lipid	434	21,719,000	627,174,294	188,152,288	75,260,915
Sodium Citrate buffer	405,377	200,225	5,781,849	1,734,555	693,822
PBS solution	15,573,214	1,877,842	54,225,988	16,267,796	6,507,119
PEG lipid	54	1,071,520	30,942,023	9,282,607	3,713,043
Phospholipid	94	1,412,086	40,776,465	12,232,939	4,893,176
Pyrophosphatase solution	468	14,714,660	424,911,667	127,473,500	50,989,400
RNase enzyme inhibitor solution	276	118,137	3,411,413	1,023,424	409,370
Sodium acetate	330,888	766,536	22,135,074	6,640,522	2,656,209
Sucrose	762	3,809	109,992	32,997	13,199
T7 RNA polymerase solution	184	25,216,706	728,176,702	218,453,011	87,381,204
Tris-HCl 1x buffer	102,680	162,239	4,684,936	1,405,481	562,192
Water for injection (WFI), RNAse free	6,178	741	21,398	6,419	2,568
TOTAL	18,152,715	456,608,278	13,185,366,482	3,955,609,944	1,582,243,978

* Production line at 30L bioreactor working volume scale, producing eight billion doses, producing 29162 grams of mRNA per year;

** For calculating the material requirements for producing eight billion doses and additional 5% losses were assumed to occur in the fill and finish process. This is the list of materials used in the production process which come in direct contact with the mRNA product, excluding auxiliary materials (e.g., materials used for cleaning); In addition to these costs, there might also be additional licensing costs for using the lipids in the LNP formulation step, especially for the ionizable lipid.

TABLE S4
Lower Price Options for Raw Materials

Product Quotation

Order	Product	Concentration	Unit	Packing Specs (KU)	Package Volume (μL)	Quantity		Price
HMD5501	UltraNuclease (Endotoxin-free)	250U/μL	KU	5	20	1	piece	$48
				50	200	1	piece	$468
				500	2000	1	piece	$2,704
				5000	20000	1	piece	$21,247
HMD5501-GMP	UltraNuclease (GMP Class)	250U/μL	KU	5	20	1	piece	$95
				50	200	1	piece	$936
				500	2000	1	piece	$5,408
				5000	20000	1	piece	$42,494
HMD5501T	UltraNuclease Assay kit	96T	box	96 test/box		1	kit	$1,067
HMD5502	Trypsin	70mg/mL	mg	0.1	1.4	1	piece	$10
				1	14	1	piece	$99
				10	140	1	piece	$891
				100	1400	1	piece	$7,924
HMD5502T	Trypsin Assay kit			96 test/box		1	kit	$1,067
EN-1001	T7 RNA Polymerase	50U/μL	KU	5	100	1	piece	$105
				25	1000	1	piece	$482
EN-1001B	10ÍT7 Buffer			50T		1	piece	$0
EN-1002	Vaccinia Capping Enzyme	10U/μL	KU	0.5	50	1	piece	$206
				2	200	1	piece	$817
EN-1002B	10ÍCapping Buffer			50T		1	piece	$0
EN-1003	mRNA Cap-2'-O Methyltransferase	50U/μL	KU	2	40	1	piece	$109
				10	200	1	piece	$499
EN-1003B	10ÍCapping Reaction Buffer			50T		1	piece	$0
EN-1004	Poly (A) Polymerase	5U/μL	KU	0.1	20	1	piece	$97
				0.5	100	1	piece	$443
EN-1005	RNase Inhibitor (Recombinant)	40U/μL	KU	2.5	62.5	1	piece	$30
				10	250	1	piece	$109
EN-1006	DNase I	2U/μL	KU	0.1	50	1	piece	$17
				1	500	1	piece	$104
EN-1006B	10ÍDNase I Buffer				150	1	piece	$0
EN-1007	RNase III	2U/μL	KU	0.25	125	1	piece	$452
				1	500	1	piece	$1,657
EN-1008	T4 RNA Ligase	10U/μL	KU	1	100	1	piece	$103
				5	500	1	piece	$471
EN-1009	Pyrophosphatase Inorganic (yeast)	0.1U/μL	U	10	100	1	piece	$83
				50	500	1	piece	$380
EN-1010	Alkaline Phosphatase	5U/μL	KU	0.5	100	1	piece	$94
				2.5	500	1	piece	$422
EN-2001B	10ÍTranscription Buffer			50T		1	piece	$0

SUGGESTED READING

Citizen.org, How to Make Enough Vaccine for the World in One Year. https://www.citizen
.org/article/how-to-make-enough-vaccine-for-the-world-in-one-year/

Demetri Petrides, *SuperPro Designer User Guide: A Comprehensive Simulation Tool for the Design, Retrofit & Evaluation of Specialty Chemical, Biochemical, Pharmaceutical, Consumer Product, Food, Agricultural, Mineral Processing, Packaging AND Water Purification, Wastewater* (Scotch Plains, 2013). http://www.intelligen.com/downloads/SuperPro_ManualForPrinting_v10.pdf (accessed on Mar.2020)

Demetri Petrides, 'Bioprocess Design and Economics', in *Bioseparations Science and Engineering*, 2nd Edition (Oxford, UK: Oxford University Press, 2015), pp. 1–83. http://www.intelligen.com/downloads/BioProcessDesignAndEconomics_March_2015.pdf (accessed on 12 May 2020)

E P Wen, R J Ellis, and N S Pujar, *Vaccine Development and Manufacturing, Wiley Series in Biotechnology and Bioengineering* (Hoboken: John Wiley & Sons, Inc., 2015). https://doi.org/10.1002/9781118870914; Kis, Shattock, Shah, and others.

Edmond Girasek and others, 'Headcount and FTE Data in the European Health Workforce Monitoring and Planning Process', *Human Resources for Health*, 14.Suppl 1 (2016), 42. https://doi.org/10.1186/s12960-016- 0139-2

Ellis Wen, Kis Pujar, Shah Shattock, and others; Joanna Sugden, 'Oxford-Astra Zeneca's Covid-19 Vaccine Helps U.K. Lead Race to Reach Nursing Homes', *The Wall Street Journal*, 2021. https://www.wsj.com/articles/oxford-astrazenecas-covid-19-vaccine-helps-u-k-lead-race-to-reach-nursing- homes-11611138601 (accessed 28 April 2021).

Michael D Buschmann and others, 'Nanomaterial Delivery Systems for MRNA Vaccines', *Vaccines*, 2021. https://doi.org/10.3390/vaccines9010065

Norbert Pardi and others, 'mRNA Vaccines: A New Era in Vaccinology', *Nature Reviews. Drug Discovery*, 17.4 (2018), 261–79. https://doi.org/10.1038/nrd.2017.243

Zoltán Kis, Cleo Kontoravdi, Antu K Dey, and others, 'Rapid Development and Deployment of High-volume Vaccines for Pandemic Response', *Journal of Advanced Manufacturing and Processing*, 2.3 (2020), e10060. https://doi.org/10.1002/amp2.10060

Zoltán Kis, Cleo Kontoravdi, Robin Shattock, and others, 'Resources, Production Scales and Time Required for Producing RNA Vaccines for the Global Pandemic Demand', *Vaccines*, (2021), 1–14. https://doi.org/10.3390/vaccines9010003

Appendix 2: Pharmacopeial Testing

B.1 PHARMACOPEIAL EVOLUTION

The new era of mRNA therapeutics, particularly the vaCines, will soon culminate into regulatory plans that will require quality testing as the major component to assure safety and efficacy of these products. Whereas several suggestions by researchers and proofs of testing protocols in the regulatory filing are available to developers, there remains a significant gap in the understanding of the methodologies to test RNA products. Recently, the US Pharmacopeia (USP) issued a first draft of suggestions based on analytical procedures and best practices to support the assessment of common quality attributes of mRNA vaCines. This draft chapter also builds on best practices described in general chapters of VaCines for Human Use—General Considerations and VaCines for Human Use—Viral VaCines. Methods in the USP draft chapter were adapted from publicly available sources but have not been verified or validated by USP (https://www.uspnf.com/sites/default/files/usp_pdf/EN/USPNF/usp-nf-notices/mrna-vaccine-chapter.pdf).

B.1.1 TESTING METHODS

The quality of mRNA drug substances is determined by their design, development, and specifications applied to them during the development and manufacturing process. These draft guidelines provide methods for assessment of quality attributes for identity, purity, quantity, physical state (integrity) and safety of the bulk purified mRNA drug substance, as listed in Table B.1. These methods can also be applied for drug product following extraction of the mRNA from LNP.

B.1.2 IDENTITY

B.1.2.1 Method A: Identity of Encoded RNA Sequence by NGS

Multiple commercial instruments are available for mRNA sequencing. A common form of this technique involves library preparation, cluster generation, sequencing, and bioinformatic data analysis, including quality control determinations. Library preparation involves mRNA enrichment and isolation through the hybridization of the mRNA poly(A) tail to a poly(T) oligomer attached to a solid support, typically a magnetic bead. The isolated mRNA is fragmented in the presence of divalent cations and at high temperature, or through other appropriate mechanical cleavage methods.

TABLE B.1
Quality Attributes for mRNA Drug Substance

Quality	Attribute	Method
Identity	Sequence confirmation	Next generation sequencing (NGS)
		Sanger sequencing
		Reverse Transcriptase–PCR
Content	RNA content	RT-qPCR and RT–dPCR, Ultraviolet Spectroscopy
Integrity	Percentage of intact mRNA and fragment mRNA	Capillary gel electrophoresis
	5' cap	IP–RP–HPLC
	3' poly(A)	RP–HPLC
	mRNA Integrity	Gel electrophoresis
Purity	Product related impurities -dsRNA	Immunoblot
	Residual DNA template	qPCR
Safety	Endotoxin	USP <85>
	Bioburden	USP <61>, <62>, <1115>
	Sterility	USP <71>
Other	Appearance	USP, <790>
	pH	USP <791>

The mRNA fragments are then used as the templates to make double-stranded (ds) complementary DNA (cDNA) using reverse transcriptase and random primers. DNA adapters and indexes are then ligated onto the ends of the ds cDNA that are in preparation for amplification. The constructed library of cDNA fragments is then subjected to amplification using specific primer sets that are complementary to those used during library construction along with fluorescent labeled deoxynucleoside triphosphates (dNTPs) and dideoxynucleotides triphosphates (ddNTPs). The ddNTPs act as terminators that prohibit any further attachment of nucleotides at the 3' end. Once completed, most sequencing instruments use optical detection to determine nucleotide incorporation during DNA synthesis, while others may use electrical detection. Appropriate software and bioanalytical tools are then used to determine the sequence of the starting mRNA molecule:

Purification and fragmentation of mRNA: One of the key processes in next-generation sequencing (NGS) is the enrichment of mRNA for the subsequent library construct
SDS lysis buffer: 1% SDS, 10 mM of EDTA
RNA fragmentation buffer (10X): 1M Tris, pH 8.0 and 100 mM of $MgCl_2$
Stop solution: 200 mM of EDTA, pH 8.0

For the RNA purification step, for each reaction, add the following mixture in each well of the 96 well plate. Mix 14.5 μL of SDS lysis buffer, 48 μL of 6M GuHCl and

7.25 µL of proteinase K (20mg/mL). Add 1–10 µg of mRNA sample. Mix well and incubate at room temperature for 10 min and then heat at 65°C for 10 min prior to the addition of 145 µL of RNA clean-up beads. Wash beads twice in 70% ethanol using a magnetic bead strand and then elute RNA into the 30 µL resuspension buffer. Assess the quality of RNA by using the Agilent Fragment Bioanalyzer system or CGE method (integrity methods provided below).

Alternatively, mRNA-sequencing (mRNA-Seq) protocol can be applied using the poly(A)-selection strategy for purifying mRNA by filtering RNA with 3′ polyadenylated (poly(A)) tails to include only mRNA. All other non-polyadenylated transcripts such as rRNA, tRNA, and degraded RNA all gets washed away in the final step.

For mRNA fragmentation, mix 1–18 µL of purified mRNA, 2 µL of RNA fragmentation buffer (can be prepared fresh or purchased) and nuclease-free water to final volume of 20 µL in a sterile PCR tube. Incubate in a preheated thermal cycler for 5 min at 94°C. Transfer the tube to ice and add 2 µL of Stop solution. Clean fragmented RNA using ethanol precipitation. Mix 22 µL of fragmented RNA, 2 µL of 3M sodium acetate at pH 5.2, 1–2 µL of 10 mg/mL linear acrylamide and 60 µL of 100% ethanol in a sterile 1.5 mL microcentrifuge tube. Mix well and incubate at −80°C for 30 min. Centrifuge the tube in a microcentrifuge at 14,000 rpm for 25 min at 4°C. Carefully remove ethanol and wash the pallet with 300 µL of 70% ethanol. Repeat the wash step and remove 70% ethanol. Air dry the pellet for up to 10 min at room temperature to remove residual ethanol and resuspend in 14.5 µL of nuclease-free water.

> **Synthesis of first strand cDNA:** RNA fragments are reverse transcribed to cDNA because the DNA is more stable and allows for amplification using DNA polymerases. mRNA can be transcribed from the coding strand (has the same sequence as mRNA) or template strand (used for transcription). This process will use the cleaved RNA fragments into the first strand of cDNA using random primers and reverse transcriptase.
>
> **First strand buffer (5X):** Mix 250 mM of Tris-HCl at pH 8.3, 375 mM of KCl, and 15 mM of $MgCl_2$
>
> **Second strand buffer (2X):** Mix 0.2 M of HEPES at pH 6.9, 20 mM of $MgCl_2$, 5 mM dithiothreitol and 0.14 M KCl
>
> **10 mM dNTP mix:** Mix 10 mM of each nucleotide (dATP, dCTP, dGTP and dTTP) in 0.6 mM of Tris-HCl

In a 200 µL PCR tube, add 1 µL of gene specific primers and 11.1 µL of mRNA. Incubate the sample in a PCR thermal cycler at 65°C for 5 min and then on ice immediately. Set the thermal cycler to 25°C. Per reaction, mix the following reagents in the order listed in a separate PCR tube. Add 4 µL of first strand buffer prepared fresh or from a kit,4 2 µL of 100 mM DTT, 0.4 µL of 25 mM dNTP mix (prepared fresh or from a kit), 0.5 µL RNase Inhibitor to final volume of 6.9 µL per reaction. Add 6.9 µL of mixture to the PCR tube and mix well. Heat the sample in the preheated PCR thermal cycler at 25°C for 2 min. Add 1–2 µL of reverse transcriptase enzyme (1 µL for less than 5 kb cDNA and 2 µL for longer) to the sample and incubate the sample in a thermal cycler with programed at 25°C for 10 min, 42°C for 50 min, 70°C for 15 min then hold at 4°C. Then place the tube on ice.

Synthesize second strand cDNA: This process removes the RNA template and generates double-stranded cDNA.

To the first strand of cDNA mix, add 62.8 μL of ultra-pure water. To this mixture, add 10 μL of second strand buffer, and 1.2 μL of 25 mM dNTP mix. [25 mM dNTP mix can be obtained from Thermo, Product Code R1122 or equivalent] Mix well and incubate on ice for 5 min. Add 1.0 μL of RNaseH, and 5.0 μL of DNA Polymerase I. Mix well and incubate at 16°C in a thermal cycler for 2.5 h. Purify the sample using a PCR purification kit, following the instructions provided by the manufacturer, and elute in 50 μL of elution buffer supplied in the kit. Final product will be in the form of double-stranded DNA. Here, samples can be stored at –15°C to –25°C or on ice before moving on to performing the end repair protocol.

End repair: This process removes 3′ overhangs into blunt ends. Preheat two heat blocks, one at 20°C and the other 37°C. In a 1.5 mL RNase-free tube, add 50 μL of eluted DNA, 27.4 μL of RNase-free water, 10 μL of 10X end repair buffer, 1.6 μL of 25 mM dNTP mix, 5 μL T4 DNA Polymerase, 1 μL of Klenow DNA Polymerase, and 5 μL T4 PNK to a total volume of 100 μL. Incubate the sample in a heat block at 20°C for 30 min. Purify the sample using PCR purification kit, following the instructions provided by the manufacturer, and elute in 50 μL of elution buffer supplied in the kit. Final product will be in the form of double-stranded DNA. Here, samples can be stored at –15°C to –25°C or on ice before moving on to performing end repair protocol.

Adenylate 3′ ends: This process adds an "A" base to the 3′ end of the blunt phosphory-lated DNA fragments. In a 1.5 mL RNase-free tube add 32 μL of eluted DNA, 5 μL of A-tailing buffer, [Fast DNA End Repair Kit can be obtained from ThermoFisher, Product Code K0771 or equivalent]10 μL of 1 mM dATP, and 3 μL of Klenow exo (3′ to 5′ exo minus) to a total volume of 50 μL. [Klenow Exo can be obtained from Illumina, Product Code 11318090 or equivalent] Incubate the sample in a 37°C heat block for 30 min. Purify the sample using PCR purification kit following the instructions provided by the manufacturer, [MinElute PCR Purification Kit can be obtained from QIAGEN, Product Code 28004 or equivalent] and elute in 23 μL of elution buffer. Final product will be in the form of double- stranded DNA. Here, samples can be stored at –15°C to –25°C or on ice before moving on to performing end repair protocol.

Ligate adapters: This procedure ligates multiple indexing adapters to the ends of the ds cDNA, preparing them for hybridization onto a flow cell.

In a 1.5 mL RNase-free tube, add 23 μL of eluted DNA, 25 μL of 2X Rapid T4 DNA Ligase buffer, 1 μL of PE Adapter Oligo Mix, [PE Adapter Oligo Mix can be obtained from Illumina, Product Code 1001782 or equivalent] and 1 μL of T4 DNA Ligase to a total volume of 50 μL. Incubate the sample at room temperature for 15 min, then purify the sample using a PCR purification kit following the instructions provided by the manufacturer and elute in 10 μL of elution buffer. Ensure complete removal of ethanol. Here, samples can be stored at –15°C to –25°C or on ice before moving on to performing end repair protocol.

Purification of cDNA templates: This process purifies the products of the ligation reaction on a gel to select a size for enrichment.

Prepare a solution with 2% agarose gel in distilled water and 1X TAE buffer (final concentration) to a final volume of 50 mL. Load the samples onto the gel. On the first and the third wells, load 2 μL 100 bp DNA ladder, and on second well load 10 μL DNA elute from the ligation step mixed with 2 μL of 6X DNA Loading Dye. [6X DNA Gel Loading Dye can be obtained from ThermoFisher, Product Code R0611 or equivalent]. Run the gel at 120 V for 60 min. Remove the gel slice by using a clean gel excision tip before following instructions in the Gel Extraction Kit, to purify the sample and elute in 30 μL of elution buffer. Here, samples can be stored at –15°C to –25°C or on ice before moving on to performing end repair protocol.

Enrichment of purified cDNA templates: This procedure uses PCR to selectively enrich those DNA fragments that have adapter molecules on both ends and to amplify the amount of DNA in the library.

In a 200 μL PCR tube, per reaction add 10 μL of 5X phusion buffer, 1.0 μL of PCR primer PE 1.0, 1.0 μL of PCR Primer PE 2.0, 0.5 μL of 25 mM dNTP mix, 0.5 μL of Phusion DNA Polymerase, and 7.0 μL of nuclease-free water to a total volume of 20 μL per reaction. Add 30 μL of the purified ligation mixture to the PCR tube before amplification. PCR amplification can be done by 30 s at 98°C, then 15 cycles of 10 s at 98°C, 30 s at 65°C, 30 s at 72°C, 5 min at 72°C and hold at 4°C. Purify the sample using a PCR purification kit, following the instructions provided by the manufacturer, and elute in 30 μL of elution buffer. Here, samples can be stored at –15°C to –25°C or on ice.

Validation of library: Quantify your libraries using qPCR, ddPCR, Bioanalyzer, or microchip. Check the size and purity of the sample.

Analysis of the sequencing data: Vendor supplied software is used to analyze the run data files and determine the sequence of the starting mRNA molecule. Alternatively, tools such as Sailfish, RSEM, and BitSeq can also help quantify the expression levels, while MISO can help quantify spliced genes. There are three steps to NGS analysis. First is the FASTQ "raw" data file generation using the vendor supplied software. Second, using the trimming and alignment tool for BAM/SAM files which have reads that are aligned to genome, and finally, identification of mutations/variants.

B.1.2.2   Method B: Identity by Sanger Sequencing

Sanger sequencing is a standard sequencing technique that yields information about the identity and order of the four nucleotide bases in a segment of DNA. It is a technique that uses dye-labeled chemical analogs that are missing the hydroxyl group required for extension of the DNA chain called dideoxyribonucleotides triphosphates (ddNTPs) of the nucleotide bases.

TE buffer solution: 10 mM of Tris-Cl, 1 mM of EDTA, pH 8.0

cDNA synthesis (prior to Sanger Sequencing): Combine 10 µL of master mix (containing hexamer and oligo-dT primers, dNTPs, RNase Inhibitor and reverse transcriptase), 1–15 µL of sample (15 µL sample expected to have low titer), and water to final volume of 50 µL. Vortex the mixture briefly and centrifuge for 5–10 s at 1,000 x g. Put samples in the thermal cycler and run the program detailed in Table A.2. Samples can be held at 4°C for up to 8 h or freeze at –20°C for longer storage.

PCR amplification: Primers should be in pairs consisting of forward primer and reverse primer, which focus on specific regions of the target gene. Resuspend dried and desalted primers to final concentration of 100 µM with TE buffer solution. Next, add 492 µL of TE buffer solution to each labeled microcentrifuge tube for each primer pair. Add 4 µL each of both the forward and reverse primer pairs to the appropriate microcentrifuge tubes. Each one should be 0.8 µM in this amplification primer mix.

In each well of a 96-well PCR plate, combine 1.5 µL of amplification primer mix in duplicate, 5 µL of PCR dye mix, 1 µL of cDNA sample (20–40 ng of cDNA), and water to final volume of 10 µL. Make sure to include a positive and a negative control (no-template). Seal the plate, vortex the mixture briefly and centrifuge for 5–10 s at 1000 x g. Put samples in the thermal cycler and run the program detailed in Table B.3.

| | | Cycling (40 cycles) | | | |
	Polymerase Activation	Deactivation	Annealing	Extension	Hold
Temperature (°C)	95	96	62	68	4
Time	10 min	3 s	15 s	30 s	Indefinitely

TABLE B.2
Thermal Cycler Conditions (Prior to Sanger Sequencing)

| | Steps | | | |
	Annealing	Polymerase Extension	Polymerase Inactivation	Hold
Temperature (°C)	25	50	80	4
Time (min)	10	15	10	Indefinitely

TABLE B.3
Thermal Cycler Conditions (Amplification)

		Steps			
	Polymerase Activation	Cycling (40 cycles)			
		Denaturation	Annealing	Extension	Hold
Temperature (°C)	95	96	62	68	4
Time	10 min	3 s	15 s	30 s	Indefinitely

TABLE B.4
Thermal Cycler Conditions (Cycle Sequencing)

				Steps			
	Post PCR Cleanup	Post PCR Inactivation	Polymerase Activation	Cycling (25 cycles)			
				De-naturation	An-nealing	Exten-sion	Hold
Temperature (°C)	37	80	96	96	50	60	4
Time	15 min	2 min	1 min	10 s	5 s	75 s	Indefinitely

Cycle sequencing: Remove the seal from the plate and add 2 µL dye sequencing master mix, 1 µL of dye tagged forward, and tagged reverse primer. [NOTE—Add tagged forward primer to one of the duplicate PCR reactions, and the tagged reverse primer to the other reaction.]

Seal the plate, vortex the mixture briefly, and centrifuge for 5–10 s at 1000 x *g*. Put samples in the thermal cycler and run the program as detailed in Table B.4.

Sequencing clean-up: Centrifuge the reaction plate for 1 min at 1000 x *g*. Prepare a mixture aCording to the kit. There are several kits available to support removal of unincorporated terminators and salts. [NOTE—Make sure solutions are homogeneous with no particulates before using.]

Add 55 µL of this mixture to each well. Seal the plate, vortex the reaction plate for 40 min, and centrifuge the plate for 2 min at 1000 x *g*.

Collection of data: Load the plate into the genetic analyzer such as the capillary electrophoresis (see integrity methods below). Select or create an appropriate run module aCording to capillary length, number of capillaries, and polymer type on the instrument. The electrophoresis will separate the labeled chain-terminated fragments by length with single-nucleotide resolution. Once the run is finished, the instrument will generate a file that can be converted into a sequence.

Data analysis: Use a sequence scanner software to generate a report. Software should be able to call low frequency somatic variants at a detection level below 5%.

B.1.2.3   Method C: Identity by RT-PCR

Reverse transcription PCR (RT-PCR) can be used to identify and quantify mRNA and is performed in two steps: reverse transcription (first strand of cDNA synthesis), and PCR amplification.

10 mM dNTP mix: Mix 10 mM of each nucleotide (dATP, dCTP, dGTP and dTTP) in 0.6 mM Tris-HCl.
First strand buffer (5X): Mix 250 mM of Tris-HCl at pH 8.3, 375 mM of KCl, and 15 mM of $MgCl_2$.
PCR buffer (10X): 200 mM of Tris HCl at pH 8.4 and 500 mM of KCl.
First strand cDNA synthesis: Prepare the following mixed solution. (Table B.5)

Heat the mixture at 65°C for 5 min and then quickly cool on ice for 2 min. Centrifuge for 5–10 s at 1,000 x g. Next, prepare a reverse transcription reaction system by combining the following solutions. (Table B.6)

Gently vortex the mixture for a few minutes. If random primers are used, incubate at 25°C for 2 min, then add 1 μL (200 U) of Reverse Transcriptase to the reaction tube and mix gently with pipette. Incubate at 42–50°C for 50 min.

[NOTE—If reverse primer of PCR is used as a reverse transcription primer, it is recommended to perform the reaction at 45–50°C; otherwise, it is generally recommended to perform the reaction at 42°C.]

TABLE B.5
First-Strand cDNA Solution

Component	Volume
Gene specific primer (2 pmole)	1 μL
mRNA (1–500 ng)	X μL
10 mM dNTP mixture	1 μL
RNase-free water	Final volume to 12 μL

TABLE B.6
Reverse Transcription Reaction Solution

Component	Volume
cDNA mixture from above	12 μL
First strand buffer (5X)	4 μL
RNase-free water	20 μL

Inactivate and stop the reverse transcription reaction by heating at 70°C for 15 min. Sample can be used immediately for subsequent PCR reactions or can be stored at –20°C for short-term storage and –80°C for long-term storage.

RT-PCR: Using Table B.7 prepare a 50 μL reaction solution.

[NOTE—There are 4 different fluorescent DNA probes that are available for RT-PCR product detection. These products are SYBR Green, TaqMan, Molecular Beacons, and Scorpions. All these probes allow the detection of PCR products by generating a fluorescent signal. Follow manufacturers' protocols for each.]

Gently mix the reaction and place it in the thermal cycler using the following program. (Table B.8)

> **Preparation of cDNA for standard curve:** Standard curve is necessary to quantitate the results. Dilute stock plasmid 1:1000 to a dilution of 1 ng/μL. Prepare standards as described below.

[NOTE—Avoid using a plasmid that contains a gene of interest to avoid contamination.] (Table B.9)

TABLE B.7
RT-PCR Reaction Solution

Component	Volume
PCR buffer (10X)	5 μL
50 mM MgCl2	1.5 μL
10 mM dNTP mixture	1 μL
Forward primer (10 μM)	1 μL
Reverse primer (10 μM)	1 μL
Taq DNA polymerase (5 Units/μL)	0.4 μL
cDNA from first strand reaction	2 μL
ddH2O (PCR-grade water)	Final volume to 50 μL

TABLE B.8
Thermal Cycler Conditions (First-Strand Synthesis)

Temperature (°C)	Time	Cycles
94	2 min	1
94	30 s	15–40
Tm – 5	30 s	
72	1 min	
72	5 min	1
4	Hold	1

TABLE B.9
cDNA Standard Curve Preparation

Concentrations	Dilutions
1 ng	Dilute 1 ng/μL stock solution 1:8 (70 μL of stock DNA solution + 490 μL of PCR-grade water)
0.1 ng	Dilute 1 ng/8 μL standard solution 1:10 (50 μL of standard + 450 μL of PCR-grade water)
0.01 ng	Dilute 0.1 ng/8 μL standard solution 1:10 (50 μL of standard + 450 μL of PCR-grade water)
0.001 ng	Dilute 0.01 ng/8 μL standard solution 1:10 (50 μL standard + 450 μL PCR-grade water)

TABLE B.10
First-Strand cDNA Solution

Component	Volume
Gene specific primer (2 pmole)	1 μL
mRNA (1–500 ng)	X μL
10 mM dNTP mixture	1 μL
RNase-free water	Final volume to 12 μL

B.1.3 QUANTITATION

B.1.3.1 Method A: Quantitation by Digital PCR

Digital PCR can be used for mRNA quantification without a standard curve. Genomic RNA is reverse transcribed to cDNA and amplified, followed by quantitation on a digital or droplet digital PCR System.

10 mM dNTP mix: Mix 10 mM of each nucleotide (dATP, dCTP, dGTP, and dTTP) in 0.6 mM of Tris-HCl.

First strand buffer (5X): Mix 250 mM of Tris-HCl at pH 8.3, 375 mM of KCl, and 15 mM of $MgCl_2$.

Primer/probe mix (20X): Mix 10 μL of 100 μM of forward primer, 10 μL of 100 μM of reverse primer, 5 μL of 100 μM labeled probe, and 75 μL of PCR-grade water.

First strand cDNA synthesis: Prepare the following mixed solution.

[NOTE—To increase the efficiency of cDNA synthesis, the reverse transcription reaction should include a target gene-specific primer that is the same primer used as reverse primer for each target in the ddPCR reaction.] (Table B.10)

Heat the mixture at 65°C for 5 min, and then quickly cool on ice for 2 min. Centrifuge for 5–10 s at 1000 x g. Next, prepare a reverse transcription reaction system by preparing the following mixed solution. (Table B.11)

Gently vortex the mixture for few seconds. If random primers are used, incubate at 25°C for 2 min then add 1 μL (200 U) of reverse transcriptase to the reaction tube and mix gently with pipette. Incubate at 42–50°C for 50 min.

[NOTE—If reverse primer of PCR is used as a reverse transcription primer, it is recommended to perform the reaction at 45–50°C, otherwise, general recommendation is to perform the reaction at 42°C.]

Inactivate and stop the reverse transcription reaction by heating at 70°C for 15 min. Sample can be used immediately for subsequent PCR reactions or can be stored at –20°C for short-term storage and –80°C for long-term storage.

Expression by dPCR: Thaw all components including primer/probe mix. Additionally, primer/probe mix can also be purchased. Mix thoroughly by vortexing each tube for 30 s at maximum speed to ensure homogeneity. Centrifuge briefly to collect contents at the bottom. Prepare the following reaction mixture on ice. (Table B.12)

Mix thoroughly by vortexing each tube for 10 s at maximum speed. Centrifuge briefly and allow the reaction tubes to equilibrate to room temperature for no more than 10 min.

TABLE B.11
Reverse Transcription Reaction Solution

Component	Volume
cDNA mixture from above	12 μL
First strand buffer (5X)	4 μL
RNase-free water	20 μL

TABLE B.12
dPCR Reaction Mixture

Component	Volume per Reaction (μL)	Final Concentration
Supermix	5	1x
Reverse transcriptase	2	20 U/ μL
300 mM DTT	1	15 mM
Target primers/probe	Variable	900 nM/ 250 nM
RNA/Dnase-free water	Variable	NA
Total RNA	Variable	100 pg–100 ng per reaction
Total volume	20	NA

Droplet generation: Load 20 µL of each reaction mixture from above into a
  sample well of a DG8 cartridge. Add 70 µL of Droplet Generator Oil to the
  bottom row of the cartridge designed for "oil." Fit rubber DG80 Gasket onto
  the Cartridge and place it on the Droplet Generator. This process should
  take about 1 min. Droplets are held in the top row. Using a multi-channel
  pipettor, transfer 45 µL droplets into 96-well PCR plate and cover the plate
  with foil sheet immediately. Seal the plate using the PCR Plate Sealer at
  180°C for 5 s.

  Run the plate on thermocycler using the following cycling conditions.
  Table B.13

  [NOTE—To determine aCeptable temperature ranges for reverse transcription, perform a thermal gradient from 42°C to 51.5°C while fixing the
  annealing/extension step at 52°C. Using the optimized reverse transcription temperature, perform a thermal gradient from 50°C to 63°C to identify
  aCeptable annealing/extension temperature ranges.]

Data analysis: Follow instructions for data acquisition and analysis based on
  the system used.

B.1.3.2   Method B: RNA Concentration by Ultraviolet Spectroscopy

This method is used to calculate RNA concentration in the bulk solution. The absorbance of a diluted RNA sample is measured at 260 nm and 280 nm, and the concentration is calculated using the Beer-Lambert Law equation. The A260/A280 ratio is
used to assess RNA purity. The absorbance ratio of the *Sample solution* of 1.8–2.1 is
indicative of highly purified RNA.

[NOTE—The A260/A280 ratio is dependent on both pH and ionic strength. As
pH increases, the A280 decreases while the A260 is unaffected.]

Buffer solution: 0.01 M solution of Tris(hydroxymethyl)aminomethane and
  0.001 M disodium ethylenediaminetetraacetic acid solution in water. Adjust
  with hydrochloric acid to a pH of 8.0.
Sample solution: Mix RNA bulk solution with *Buffer solution* to obtain a
  solution with an absorbance value between 0.5 and 1.0 at the wavelength of
  maximum absorbance at 260 nm.

TABLE B.13
Thermal Cycler Conditions

Cycling Step	Temperature (°C)	Time	Cycles
Reverse transcription	42–63	60 min	1
Enzyme activation	95	10 min	1
Denaturation	95	30 sec	40
Annealing/extension	52	1 min	40
Enzyme deactivation	98	10 min	1
Hold	4	Infinite	1

Perform sample readings in quartz cuvettes. Perform a background correction by making readings from a blank (Buffer solution only) at 320 nm, 260 nm, and 280 nm.

[NOTE—Dirty cuvettes and dust particles cause light scatter at 320 nm which can impact absorbance at 260 nm.]

Analysis: Determine the absorbance of the *Sample solution* using Beer-Lambert Law equation, by calculating the concentration with the cell path length of 1 cm.

B.1.3.4 Beer-Lambert Law Equation

$$A = \varepsilon bC$$

A = absorbance
ε = molar extinction coefficient
b = path length, 1 cm
C = concentration

[NOTE—The molar extinction coefficient of RNA is: $40(\mu g/mL)^{-1}cm^{-1}$ (absorbance max at 260 nm).]

B.1.4 RNA Integrity

A high-resolution analytical method that can measure the integrity of RNA molecules by size and length is crucial for quality assurance, understanding potency, and for optimization of manufacturing processes. Most commonly, this evaluation is performed using capillary gel electrophoresis. A common form of this technique involves filling a capillary with a separation gel matrix with a fluorescent dye. A microliter size injection is made on the capillary using voltage injection and the RNA fragments bind the fluorescent dye as they migrate through the capillary by size using electrophoretic separation. Size comparison is performed against a reference ladder sample that has RNA fragments of defined size. The instrument software determines the size and concentration of the RNA fragments present in the sample. There are two common platforms, one using an Agilent system and the other using SCIEX system.

B.1.4.1 Method A: Capillary Gel Electrophoresis Using Agilent System

RNA ladder: Use a suitable RNA ladder.
RNA diluent marker solution: Use a suitable RNA diluent marker solution. **Intercalating dye solution:** Use a suitable intercalating dye solution. **Separation gel:** Use a suitable separation gel.
Capillary conditioning solution (5X): Use a suitable 5X capillary conditioning solution.

Capillary conditions solution (1X): Mix 1-part *Capillary conditioning solution (5X)* with 4 parts sub-micron filtered Type I water. **Capillary gel solution:** Prepare by mixing *Intercalating dye solution, Separation gel*, and *1X Capillary conditioning solution* in 0.1:1:1 proportion to create a sufficient volume depending on the number of samples to be analyzed.

RNA ladder solution: Prepare a 3 μL (25 ng/μL) *RNA ladder* aliquot and store on ice. Transfer 2 μL of the 25 ng/μL ladder to a 0.5 mL tube. Dilute to the working concentration of 2 ng/μL with RNase-free water. Heat-denature the ladder at 70°C for 2 min, immediately cool to 4°C, and keep on ice.

Blank solution: Use a suitable blank solution.

mRNA sample preparation: Heat-denature the RNA samples at 70°C°C for 2 min, immediately cool to 4°C, and keep on ice before use. The mRNA input sample must be within a total concentration range of 250 pg/μL to 5000 pg/μL. If the concentration of the sample is above this range, dilute with RNase-free water. Prepare each sample in duplicate.

Sample plate preparation: Using a fresh RNase-free 96-well sample plate, pipette 18 μL of the *RNA diluent marker solution* to each well in a row that is to contain sample or *RNA ladder solution*. Fill any unused wells within the row of the sample plate with 20 μL of *Blank solution*. Pipette 2 μL of each denatured RNA sample into the assigned well on the plate containing 18 μL of *RNA diluent marker solution*. Mix the contents of the well by pipetting up and down. The *RNA ladder solution* must be run in parallel with the samples for each experiment to ensure aCurate quantification. Pipette 2 μL of denatured *RNA ladder solution* into the 18 μL of *RNA diluent marker solution* in the designated ladder well. Mix the contents of the well by pipetting up and down. After mixing each well, centrifuge the plate to remove any air bubbles. Check the wells of the sample plate to ensure there are no air bubbles trapped in the bottom of the wells. The presence of trapped air bubbles can lead to injection failures.

Separation procedure and analysis: Run experiment in reverse polarity at −29 kv and 25°C on an Agilent system equipped with DAD and 260 nm optical filter. Run current at 6.9 uA and introduce sample into the capillary inlet electrokinetically at −20 kV for 10 s with UV detection at 260 nm. The sample plate is loaded in the instrument. Capillary washes and filling with *Separation gel* are performed automatically by the instrument. Samples and *RNA ladder solution* are injected onto the capillary using electrokinetic injection followed by electrophoretic separation through the capillary based on fragment size. Instrument software analyzes the samples by comparison to the *RNA ladder solution* to determine the size and quantitation of the RNA fragments present in the sample.

B.1.4.2 Method B: Capillary Gel Electrophoresis Using SCIEX System

A high-resolution analytical method that can measure the integrity of RNA molecules by size and length is crucial for quality assurance, understanding potency, and for optimization of manufacturing processes. The following method uses PA800 plus

Pharmaceutical Analysis System from SCIEX with LIF detection to evaluate the total RNA integrity. The instrument software determines the size and concentration of the RNA fragments present in the sample.

1X TBE buffer: 89 mM Tris, 89 mM boric acid, 2 mM EDTA, pH 8.3

Separation buffer: 1% Polyvinylpyrrolidone (PVP) at 1.3 MDa in 1X TBE buffer with 4 M Urea and 50,000x dilution or 0.002% SYBR green dye

RNA ladder and marker: Dilute RNA ladder in ddH_2O to 25 ug/mL, and spike with 1.2 K RNA marker, then denature the solution for 5 min at 65°C and cool on ice for 5 min before loading.

Sample preparation: Dilute sample in the separation buffer (RNA size ranging from 200 bases to 6500 bases)

Cartridge: EZ cartridge preassembled with bare fused-silica capillary (50 μm I.D., 30 cm total length, 20 cm effective length).

Capillary gel electrophoresis: Carry out electrophoresis experiment with reverse polarity with 200 V/cm electrical field (6 kV) at 25°C. Introduce sample into the inlet of the capillary electrokinetically at 5k V for 3 s. Sample tray temperature should be kept at 4°C with LIF detector configured to 488 nm laser with an emission filter of 520 nm.

Generate a calibration curve from the RNA ladder to estimate the size of an unknown sample peaks. Introduce the remaining of the samples into the inlet of the capillary. All samples should be analyzed in duplicate.

Data analysis: Process data using the 32 Karat software.

B.1.4.3   Quantitation of mRNA 5'- Cap by IP–RP–HPLC

A cap is required at the 5' end of the mRNA molecule to protect the molecule from degradation and to facilitate suCessful protein translation. Capping efficiency is a critical quality attribute for a therapeutic mRNA vaccine. Capped and uncapped mRNA fragments can be separated and quantitated using ion pair reversed-phase high performance liquid chromatography (IP-RP-HPLC). It may be necessary to perform site-specific cleavage of the mRNA molecule using ribonuclease H to produce smaller specific mRNA fragments in the sample that can be adequately resolved using IP RP-HPLC.

Solution A: 100 mM of triethylammonium acetate buffer, pH 7.0, is prepared by mixing 2.21 mL of glacial acetic acid in 350 mL of water. While mixing, 5.58 mL of triethylamine is added slowly. The pH is adjusted to pH 7.0 by addition of either triethylamine or acetic acid.

Solution B: Solution A with 25% (v/v) acetonitrile

Mobile phase: See the gradient table. (Table B.14)

RNase cleavage buffer: Prepare a solution of 20 mM of HEPES-KOH 50 mM of KCl and 10 mM of $MgCl_2$, pH 9.0.

Sample solution: To increase the resolution, select a site-specific RNA cleavage probe with 2'-O-methyl modifications, except at the 3' end which has 4 to 6 deoxyribonucleic acids (DNA) at the cleavage site. The RNA cleavage

---

TABLE B.14
IP-RP-HPLC Gradient Table

Time (min)	Solution A (%)	Solution B (%)
0	90.0	10.0
36	85.5	14.5

---

probe is product specific and should be chosen to produce a 5'-cap fragment of sufficient size for the IP–RP–HPLC analysis. The RNA cleavage probe-RNA complex mixture should be between 0.5 and 2.0 mM in *RNase cleavage buffer.* Anneal the RNA cleavage probe to mRNA by heating to 90°C and then cooling slowly to room temperature. The RNA cleavage probe concentration should be 120% of the mRNA concentration to ensure complete hybridization of the mRNA. Add RNase H to a final concentration of 20 units per 100 μL reaction volume. Incubate the reaction at 37°C for 3 h.

B.1.4.4   Chromatographic System
(See *Chromatography <621>, System Suitability.*)

Mode: LC
Detector: UV 260 nm
Column: Xterra C18 4.6-mm × 7.5-cm; packing L1
Column temperature: 50°C Flow rate: 0.5 mL/min Injection volume: 15 μL

B.1.4.5   Analysis

Sample: *Sample solution*

Measure the areas of the 5' capped mRNA peak and of the uncapped mRNA peaks. Calculate the percentage of uncapped mRNA:

$$Result = \left[AU / (AU + AC) \right] \times 100$$

A U = area of the uncapped mRNA peak A C = area of the 5' capped mRNA peak

System suitability requirements: (See *Chromatography <621>, System Suitability.*)
ACeptance criteria: As determined by regulatory authorities.

B.1.4.6   Percent Poly(A) Tailed RNA by RP-HPLC
A poly(A) tail is required at the 3' end of the mRNA molecule to protect the molecule from degradation and to facilitate suCessful protein translation. The presence

of a poly(A) tail is a critical quality attribute for a therapeutic mRNA vaccine. mRNA molecules with and without a poly(A) tail (tailless) can be separated and quantitated using ion pair reversed-phase high performance liquid chromatography (IP-RP-HPLC). It may be necessary to perform site-specific cleavage of the mRNA molecule using ribonuclease H to produce smaller specific mRNA fragments in the sample that can be adequately resolved using IP-RP-HPLC.

[NOTE—Poly(A) tail is dependent upon the manufacturing process and the design of the mRNA itself and could fall under characterization and not drug substance.]

Solution A: 100 mM of triethylammonium acetate buffer, pH 7.0, is prepared by mixing 2.21 mL of glacial acetic acid in 350 mL of water. While mixing, 5.58 mL of triethylamine is added slowly. The pH is adjusted to pH 7.0 by addition of either triethylamine or acetic acid.

Solution B: *Solution A* containing 25% acetonitrile.

Mobile phase: See the gradient table. (Table B.15)

RNase cleavage buffer: Prepare a solution of 20 mM of HEPES-KOH, 50 mM of KCl, and 10 mM of $MgCl_2$, pH 9.0.

Sample solution: To increase the resolution, select a site-specific RNA cleavage probe with 2′-O-methyl modifications, except at the 3′ end which has 4 to 6 deoxyribonucleic acids (DNA) at the cleavage site. The RNA cleavage probe is product specific and should be chosen to produce a 5′-cap fragment of sufficient size for the IP–RP–HPLC analysis. The RNA cleavage probe- NA complex mixture should be between 0.5 and 2.0 mM in *RNase cleavage buffer*. Anneal the RNA cleavage probe to mRNA by heating to 90°C and then cooling slowly to room temperature. The RNA cleavage probe concentration should be 120% of the mRNA concentration to ensure complete hybridization of the mRNA. Add RNase H to a final concentration of 20 units per 100 μL reaction volume. Incubate the reaction at 37°C for 3 h.

TABLE B.15
RP-HPLC Gradient Table

Time (min)	Solution A (%)	Solution B (%)
0	62	38
1	60	40
16	40	60
22	34	66
22.5	30	70
23	0	100
24	0	100
25	62	38
27	62	38

B.1.4.7   Chromatographic System

(See *Chromatography* <621>, *System Suitability.*)

Mode: LC
Detector: UV 260 nm
Column: DNASep, 7.8-mm × 5-cm; packing nonporous, alkylated polysty-
rene divinylbenzene matrix, packing LXX
Column temperature: 75°C Flow rate: 0.9 mL/min Injection volume: 15 µL

B.1.4.8   Analysis

Samples: *Sample solution*

Measure the areas of the poly(A) mRNA peak and of the tailless mRNA peak.
Calculate the percentage of poly(A) mRNA:

$$\text{Result} = \left[A_U / \left(A_U + A_c \right) \right] \times 100$$

A_U = area of the poly(A) mRNA peak A_c = area of the tailless mRNA peak

System suitability requirements: (See *Chromatography* <621>, *System
Suitability.*)

B.1.5   INTEGRITY OF MRNA BY GEL ELECTROPHORESIS

HT stock solution (50X): Prepare a HEPES–triethanolamine (HT) solution
by pouring 1.5 M triethanolamine in a beaker placed on a balance, then
add 35.7 g (1.5M) of HEPES. Add high quality deionized water to ~0.9%
of the final volume. Dissolve reagents completely using a magnetic stirrer
and bring to 100 mL final volume. The pH of the buffer should be 7.6 ± 0.2
without adjustment. Filter the solution through a high-protein binding filter
of 0.2 µm pore size.
Electrophoresis buffer (5X): Dissolve 54 g of tris base, 27.5 g of boric acid,
and 20 mL of 0.5 M EDTA in water to final volume of 1000 mL. Place the
solution in a hot water bather with a magnetic stir bar to dissolve.
Running buffer (1X): Dilute *HT stock solution* with deionized water, 1:50.
Loading dye: Add *HT stock solution*, 0.5M EDTA (pH 8.0) and bromophenol
blue to deionized water to the final concentration of 2.1X electrophoresis
buffer, 1mM EDTA and 0.04% bromophenol blue. Add ethidium bromide
for a final concentration of 10 µg/ mL. Filter through a 0.2 µm syringe filter.
Loading buffer (2X): Prepare sufficient amount of the master mix by combining 14 volumes of loading dye with 1 volume of 37% formaldehyde

[NOTE—Loading dye mixed with formaldehyde is not stable upon storage and must
be used within a few hours.]

Add the freshly prepared 2X master mix to each RNA sample (1:1 v/v). Close tubes tightly, mix the contents, and spin briefly in a microcentrifuge. Denature the sample by heating at 70°C for 5 min, then cool to room temperature.

mRNA sample preparation: Dissolve 1–3 µg of mRNA in 50% formaldehyde.
RNA markers (0.5–9 kb long): Dilute 2 µL of the marker with 3 µL of nuclease-free water and mix with 15 µL of loading dye.
Analysis: Heat 1 g of agarose in 72 mL of deionized water until dissolved. Cool agarose to 60°C. Add 10 mL of *HT stock solution* and 0.4 M formaldehyde. Pour the gel in the tank and add enough *Running buffer* to cover the gel by a few millimeters. Tightly cover the gel casting assembly with plastic wrap during agarose solidification to prevent formaldehyde losses from the gel.

Remove the comb.

Load the gel and electrophoresis at 6 V/cm until the bromophenol blue has migrated as far as two-thirds the length of the gel. Visualize the gel on a UV transilluminator. The bands can also be quantified by densitometry using the known RNA standards. ACeptance criteria: Visual observation of the marker should show distinct bands and a single band for the intact RNA sample, similar to those of the in-house control standard.

B.1.5.1 dsRNA by Immunoblot

If dsRNA is present in the mRNA vaccine, it has the potential of being immunogenic. For that reason, dsRNA content should be determined and controlled.

[NOTE—dsRNA is dependent upon the manufacturing process and the design of the mRNA itself and could fall under characterization and not for drug substance.]

TBS-T buffer: Prepare a solution of 50 mM Tris–HCl, 150 mM NaCl, and 0.05 % of Tween-20, pH 7.4.
Blocking buffer: Prepare a solution 5 % nonfat dried milk in *TBS-T buffer*.
Incubation buffer: Prepare a solution 1 % nonfat dried milk in *TBS-T buffer*.
dsRNA antibody solution: Dilute the reconstituted antibody 1:5000 in *Incubation Buffer*.
Detection antibody solution: Dilute the reconstituted HRP-conjugated donkey anti-mouse IgG 1:5000 in *Incubation Buffer*.
Detection reagent: Chemiluminescent Western Blotting Detection Reagent

Procedure and Analysis: Blot 200 ng of the mRNA test sample and a dsRNA reference sample at the limit of detection onto a positively charged nylon blotting membrane and dry for 30 min. Incubate membrane with *Blocking Buffer* for 1 h. Rinse membrane with *TBS-T buffer* twice. Incubate membrane with *dsRNA Antibody Solution* at room temperature for 1 h. Rinse membrane 4 times and wash 6 times, 5 min per wash, with *TBS-T buffer*. Incubate membrane with *Detection Antibody Solution* at room temperature for 1 h. Rinse membrane 4 times and wash 6 times, 5 min per wash, with *TBS-T buffer*. Detect membrane with *Detection Reagent*. Capture images with an appropriate digital imaging system.

B.1.5.2   Residual DNA Template (qPCR)

The following method is suitable for measurement of residual host cell DNA in mRNA vaCines drug substance. Extraction is not required for drug substance; therefore, a quantitative polymerase chain reaction (qPCR)-based method can be directly used for the measurement of residual host cell DNA. For discussion of the principles and best practices for this type of testing, see USP: Nucleic Acid-Based Techniques— Approaches for Detecting Trace Nucleic Acids (Residual DNA Testing), which may be a helpful resource.

Sample preparation: There are several procedures for nucleic acid extraction that may be appropriate for biopharmaceutical sample testing. One such procedure is described in detail below and validated for starting DNA concentrations ranging from
0.01 to 50 pg/μL.

Resuspension solution: Dissolve tris(hydroxymethyl)aminomethane hydrochloride (Tris-HCl) and ethylenediaminetetraacetic acid (EDTA) to obtain a solution of 10 mM and 1.0 mM, respectively. Add hydrochloric acid or sodium hydroxide to adjust to a pH of 8.0.

DNA standard stock solution: Dilute reference material to a concentration of 1 μg/mL in *Resuspension solution.*

Sample solutions: Samples for testing may require dilution or reconstitution to 1) overcome matrix interference affecting the DNA recovery, 2) yield an appropriate starting volume, or 3) bring the analyte concentration within the quantitative range of the *qPCR method. Sample solutions* may be diluted in water or in *Resuspension solution* if necessary. For drug substance samples, *Sample solutions* should contain sufficient starting material to allow determination of the residual DNA content, if present at the specification limit.

Positive control solution: Prepare by spiking *DNA standard stock solution* to *Sample solutions* at a concentration appropriate for the *assay* (specification, or otherwise justified).

Negative control solution: Water or *Resuspension solution* is used in place of *Sample solutions* in the extraction procedures and will be extracted with any samples (if extraction is necessary). The *Negative control solution* is tested using the qPCR-based method to determine the DNA content contributed by the background and to demonstrate that there is no potential cross-contamination during the assay. This is also known as the no-template control.

B.1.5.3   qPCR Analysis

2X Master mix: A suitable buffer containing magnesium chloride, deoxyadenosine triphosphate, deoxyguanosine triphosphate, deoxycytidine triphosphate, deoxyuridine triphosphate, deoxythymidine triphosphate, and highly purified DNA polymerase. Mix well immediately before use.

DNA stock primers and probes: Determine the fragment of the DNA template that needs to be amplified and design the forward and reverse primers. Prepare individual 10 μM solutions of the primer pairs and probe specific to mRNA vaccines, using DNAse-free water.

DNA probe solution: Dilute *DNA stock probe* to 2.5 μM with DNAse-free water.

Standard solutions: Dilute the *DNA standard stock solution* to obtain 5 or more suitable standards within the concentration range of 0.001–100 pg/μL.

Analysis of samples: *Sample solutions, Positive control solution, Negative control solution,* and *Standard solutions.*

[NOTE—If samples are extracted, then extracted *Sample solutions* and extracted *Control solutions* will be used.]

Transfer 25 μL of the 2X Master mix to each well of a 96-well qPCR plate. Add 5 μL each of the *DNA stock forward primer,* the *DNA stock reverse primer,* and the *DNA probe solution* of the appropriate species to each well. Add 10 μL of either (extracted) *Sample solutions, Standard solutions,* (extracted) *Negative control solution,* or (extracted) *Positive control solution* to their respective wells.

[NOTE—The qPCR reaction volume may be scaled as appropriate to aCommodate different instruments.]

Mix, seal the plate tightly, and centrifuge for 1 min at $1000 \times g$. Place the plate in a suitable qPCR thermal cycler. Incubate for 2 min at 50°C, then for 10 min at 95°C, followed by 40 cycles, with each cycle consisting of 95°C for 15 s and 60°C for 1 min.

[NOTE—Some instruments and reagents require a preincubation step. Carefully follow specific instrument/reagent recommendations.]

Monitor the signal of the labeled probe using a suitable fluorescence detector. Determine the threshold value using the instrument-specific recommendations. Record the cycle thresholds (C_t) for each sample.

B.1.5.4   Calculations

Plot the log quantity of DNA of the Standard solutions versus the C_t. Calculate the slope and the intercept.

Using these values and the following equation, calculate the quantity of DNA in each well: Result=10 ($C_t - b/m$)

C_t = cycle threshold of the Sample solutions

b = intercept of the line for the Standard solutions m = slope of the line for the Standard solutions. Calculate the quantity of DNA in each of the Sample solutions. Correct for any dilution or concentration of the sample.

B.2   CONCLUSION

Development of RNA products requires extensive quality testing for safety and efficacy. The testing methods used for biological drugs, traditional vaccines, and gene therapy are widely available and applicable to the development of mRNA products.

Recently, the USP has proposed quality control methods that should soon evolve into specific chapters in the USP; these are presented above, though they are still not finalized. Several books on this subject are available, and so is a vast volume of data in the patent applications and publications to establish optimal testing protocol.

REFERENCE

United States Pharmacopeia, Analytical Procedures for mRNA vaccine Quality. *Draft Guideline*. https://go.usp.org/e/323321/-vaccine-Chapter-2022-03-3-pdf/6rxsm7/466863544?h =HNPNnrqz_I2UHnOxui45tzRUrVIX4yMFpyCtQuaMhCg

Appendix 3:
Suggested Reading

Pityriasis rosea-like rash after messenger RNA COVID-19 vaccination: A case report and review of the literature: 10.1016/j.jdin.2022.01.009

Factors influencing SARS-CoV-2 RNA concentrations in wastewater up to the sampling stage: A systematic review: 10.1016/j.scitotenv.2022.153290

Globally Vibrio cholera antibiotics resistance to RNA and DNA effective antibiotics: A systematic review and meta-analysis: 10.1016/j.micpath.2022.105514

Snapshots of RNA polymerase III in action - A mini review: 10.1016/j.gene.2022.146282

Global prevalence of RNA-positive horses for hepacivirus (EqHV): systematic review and meta-analysis: 10.1016/j.jevs.2022.104003

A review of non-coding RNA related to NF-κB signaling pathway in the pathogenesis of osteoarthritis: 10.1016/j.intimp.2022.108607

RNA-based therapy in the management of lipid disorders: a review: 10.1186/s12944-022-01649-3

Genetic and RNA-related molecular markers of trastuzumab-chemotherapy-associated cardiotoxicity in HER2 positive breast cancer: a systematic review: 10.1186/s12885-022-09437-z

A novel concept of human antiviral protection: It's all about RNA (Review): 10.3892/br.2022.1512

Telomeric Repeat-Containing RNA (TERRA): A Review of the Literature and First Assessment in Cutaneous T-Cell Lymphomas: 10.3390/genes13030539

A Systematic Review of Common and Brain-Disease-Specific RNA Editing Alterations Providing Novel Insights into Neurological and Neurodegenerative Disease Manifestations: 10.3390/biom12030465

Clinicopathological and prognostic significance of long non-coding RNA EWSAT1 in human cancers: A review and meta-analysis: 10.1371/journal.pone.0265264

Emerging Potential of Exosomal Non-coding RNA in Parkinson's Disease: A Review: 10.3389/fnagi.2022.819836

A brief review of machine learning methods for RNA methylation sites prediction: 10.1016/j.ymeth.2022.03.001

Potential diagnostic and prognostic value of the long non-coding RNA SNHG3 in human cancers: A systematic review and meta-analysis: 10.1177/03936155221077121

Temporary exacerbation of pre-existing psoriasis and eczema in the context of COVID-19 messenger RNA booster vaccination: A case report and review of the literature: 10.1016/j.jdin.2021.11.004

Long Non-Coding RNA in Esophageal Cancer: A Review of Research Progress: 10.3389/pore.2022.1610140

Diagnostic accuracy of assays using point-of-care testing or dried blood spot samples for the determination of HCV RNA: a systematic review: 10.1093/infdis/jiac049

A narrative review of long noncoding RNA: insight into neural ischemia/reperfusion mediated by two pathophysiological processes of injury and repair: 10.21037/atm-22-268

Review: RNA-based diagnostic markers discovery and therapeutic targets development in cancer: 10.1016/j.pharmthera.2022.108123

Immunogenicity and clinical features relating to BNT162b2 messenger RNA COVID-19 vaccine, Ad26.COV2.S and ChAdOx1 adenoviral vector COVID-19 vaccines: a systematic review of non-interventional studies: 10.1186/s43094-022-00409-5

Potential Candidates against COVID-19 Targeting RNA-Dependent RNA Polymerase: A Comprehensive Review: 10.2174/1389201022666210421102513

Diagnostic value of exosome derived long noncoding RNA in gastric cancer in Chinese population: A PRISMA-compliant systematic review and meta-analysis: 10.1097/MD.0000000000028153

Association of three micro-RNA gene polymorphisms with the risk of cervical cancer: a meta-analysis and systematic review: 10.1186/s12957-021-02463-4

Interactions between long non-coding RNAs and RNA-binding proteins in cancer (Review): 10.3892/or.2021.8207

A review on detection of SARS-CoV-2 RNA in wastewater in light of the current knowledge of treatment process for removal of viral fragments: 10.1016/j.jenvman.2021.113563

Molecular Insight into the Therapeutic Potential of Long Non-coding RNA-Associated Competing Endogenous RNA Axes in Alzheimer's Disease: A Systematic Scoping Review: 10.3389/fnagi.2021.742242

[Regulatory mechanism of long noncoding RNA in the occurrence and development of leukemia: a review]: 10.13345/j.cjb.210139

Micro-RNA Implications in Type-1 Diabetes Mellitus: A Review of Literature: 10.3390/ijms222212165

Systematic review on the current knowledge and use of single-cell RNA sequencing in head and neck cancer: 10.1111/apm.13173

Cancer driver gene and non-coding RNA alterations as biomarkers of brain metastasis in lung cancer: A review of the literature: 10.1016/j.biopha.2021.112190

Controversial roles of cold-inducible RNA-binding protein in human cancer (Review): 10.3892/ijo.2021.5271

A Systematic Review of Transcriptional Dysregulation in Huntington's Disease Studied by RNA Sequencing: 10.3389/fgene.2021.751033

A Review on the Role of Small Nucleolar RNA Host Gene 6 Long Non-coding RNAs in the Carcinogenic Processes: 10.3389/fcell.2021.741684

Status of diagnosis and treatment of esophageal cancer and non-coding RNA correlation research: a narrative review: 10.21037/tcr-21-687

Application of single-cell RNA sequencing technology in liver diseases: a narrative review: 10.21037/atm-21-4824

[Research Progress of Non-coding RNA in Multiple Myeloma with Heart Disease---Review]: 10.19746/j.cnki.issn.1009-2137.2021.05.051

SARS-CoV-2 spike protein and RNA dependent RNA polymerase as targets for drug and vaccine development: A review: 10.1016/j.bsheal.2021.07.003

Clinicopathological and Prognostic Significance of Long Non-coding RNA MIAT in Human Cancers: A Review and Meta-Analysis: 10.3389/fgene.2021.729768

New Therapeutics in Endometriosis: A Review of Hormonal, Non-Hormonal, and Non-Coding RNA Treatments: 10.3390/ijms221910498

CRISPR/Cas13-Based Platforms for a Potential Next-Generation Diagnosis of Colorectal Cancer through Exosomes Micro-RNA Detection: A Review: 10.3390/cancers13184640

Changes in RNA expression levels during antidepressant treatment: a systematic review: 10.1007/s00702-021-02394-0

Long intergenic non-protein coding RNA 460: Review of its role in carcinogenesis: 10.1016/j.prp.2021.153556

PIWI-interacting RNA in cancer: Molecular mechanisms and possible clinical implications (Review): 10.3892/or.2021.8160

A systematic review on COVID-19: urological manifestations, viral RNA detection and special considerations in urological conditions: 10.1007/s00345-020-03246-4

Review of machine learning methods for RNA secondary structure prediction: 10.1371/journal.pcbi.1009291

Long non-coding RNA as a potential biomarker for prognosis of glioma: A protocol for systematic review and meta-analysis: 10.1097/MD.0000000000026921

Non-coding RNA Activated by DNA Damage: Review of Its Roles in the Carcinogenesis: 10.3389/fcell.2021.714787

Wastewater Based Epidemiology Perspective as a Faster Protocol for Detecting Coronavirus RNA in Human Populations: A Review with Specific Reference to SARS-CoV-2 Virus: 10.3390/pathogens10081008

Circular RNA: A novel type of biomarker for glioma (Review): 10.3892/mmr.2021.12240

SARS-CoV-2 RNA detection in cerebrospinal fluid: Presentation of two cases and review of literature: 10.1016/j.bbih.2021.100282

Aptima HPV messenger RNA testing and histopathologic follow-up in women with HSIL cytology: A study emphasizing additional review of HPV-negative cases: 10.1002/cncy.22421

A Review on the Development of Gold and Silver Nanoparticles-Based Biosensor as a Detection Strategy of Emerging and Pathogenic RNA Virus: 10.3390/s21155114

Association between frailty phenotype, quantification of plasma HIV-1 RNA, CD4 cell count and HAART in HIV-positive subjects: a systematic review and meta-analysis of observational studies: 10.1080/09540121.2021.1956414

A comprehensive review of m6A/m6Am RNA methyltransferase structures: 10.1093/nar/gkab378

Clinicopathological and prognostic significance of long non-coding RNA-ROR in cancer patients: A systematic review and meta-analysis: 10.1097/MD.0000000000026535

Prevalence of SARS-CoV-2 RNA on inanimate surfaces: a systematic review and meta-analysis: 10.1007/s10654-021-00784-y

Roles of long non-coding RNA in osteoarthritis (Review): 10.3892/ijmm.2021.4966

Long noncoding RNA network: Novel insight into hepatocellular carcinoma metastasis (Review): 10.3892/ijmm.2021.4967

Long and short non-coding RNA and radiation response: a review: 10.1016/j.trsl.2021.02.005

Circulating serum and plasma levels of micro-RNA in type-1 diabetes in children and adolescents: A systematic review and meta-analysis: 10.1111/eci.13510

Extracellular Vesicles and Host-Pathogen Interactions: A Review of Inter-Kingdom Signaling by Small Noncoding RNA: 10.3390/genes12071010

A review on the interaction of nucleoside analogues with SARS-CoV-2 RNA dependent RNA polymerase: 10.1016/j.ijbiomac.2021.03.112

Importance of N(6)-methyladenosine RNA modification in lung cancer (Review): 10.3892/mco.2021.2290

Molecular techniques for the genomic viral RNA detection of West Nile, Dengue, Zika and Chikungunya arboviruses: a narrative review: 10.1080/14737159.2021.1924059

Role of C14orf166 in viral infection and RNA metabolism and its relationship with cancer (Review): 10.3892/mmr.2021.12039

The Biological Function, Mechanism, and Clinical Significance of m6A RNA Modifications in Head and Neck Carcinoma: A Systematic Review: 10.3389/fcell.2021.683254

What are the applications of single-cell RNA sequencing in cancer research: a systematic review: 10.1186/s13046-021-01955-1

A review of the presence of SARS-CoV-2 RNA in wastewater and airborne particulates and its use for virus spreading surveillance: 10.1016/j.envres.2021.110929

Effects of long noncoding RNA on prognosis of oral squamous cell carcinoma: A protocol for systematic review and meta-analysis: 10.1097/MD.0000000000025507

Multiple Functions of RNA Methylation in T Cells: A Review: 10.3389/fimmu.2021.627455

Prevalence and Persistent Shedding of Fecal SARS-CoV-2 RNA in Patients With COVID-19 Infection: A Systematic Review and Meta-analysis: 10.14309/ctg.0000000000000343

Environmental Detection of SARS-CoV-2 Virus RNA in Health Facilities in Brazil and a Systematic Review on Contamination Sources: 10.3390/ijerph18073824

Circular RNA as a Potential Biomarker for Melanoma: A Systematic Review: 10.3389/fcell.2021.638548

mTOR inhibition in COVID-19: A commentary and review of efficacy in RNA viruses: 10.1002/jmv.26728

Systematic review and meta-analysis of factors associated with re-positive viral RNA after recovery from COVID-19: 10.1002/jmv.26648

Relationship between long non-coding RNA polymorphism and the risk of coronary artery disease: A protocol for systematic review and meta-analysis: 10.1097/MD.0000000000025146

Key Factors That Enable the Pandemic Potential of RNA Viruses and Inter-Species Transmission: A Systematic Review: 10.3390/v13040537

Corrigendum: CSF HIV RNA Escape in Opsoclonus-Myoclonus-Ataxia Syndrome: Case Report and Review of the Literature: 10.3389/fneur.2021.665996

Long non-coding RNA review and implications in acute lung inflammation: 10.1016/j.lfs.2021.119044

A brief review of RNA modification related database resources: 10.1016/j.ymeth.2021.03.003

Underlying metastasis mechanism and clinical application of exosomal circular RNA in tumors (Review): 10.3892/ijo.2021.5179

Research progress review on long non-coding RNA in colorectal cancer: 10.4149/neo_2020_201012N1073

The Potential Therapeutic Effect of RNA Interference and Natural Products on COVID-19: A Review of the Coronaviruses Infection: 10.3389/fphar.2021.616993

Anti-Tumor Mechanisms Associated With Regulation of Non-Coding RNA by Active Ingredients of Chinese Medicine: A Review: 10.3389/fonc.2020.634936

Circulating RNA biomarkers in diffuse large B-cell lymphoma: a systematic review: 10.1186/s40164-021-00208-3

Salivary Micro-RNA and Oral Squamous Cell Carcinoma: A Systematic Review: 10.3390/jpm11020101

Long non-coding RNA signatures as predictors of prognosis in thyroid cancer: a narrative review: 10.21037/atm-20-8191

Candidate RNA biomarkers in biofluids for early diagnosis of ovarian cancer: A systematic review: 10.1016/j.ygyno.2020.11.018

The Application of Single-Cell RNA Sequencing in Studies of Autoimmune Diseases: a Comprehensive Review: 10.1007/s12016-020-08813-6

Detection of RNA viruses from influenza and HIV to Ebola and SARS-CoV-2: a review: 10.1039/d0ay01886d

Evolution of RNA viruses from SARS to SARS-CoV-2 and diagnostic techniques for COVID-19: a review: 10.1186/s43088-021-00150-7

THE PECULIARITY OF COVID-19 GENOME AND THE CORONAVIRUS RNA TRANSLATION PROCESS AS APOTENTIAL TARGET FOR ETIOTROPIC MEDICATIONSWITH ADENINE AND OTHER NUCLEOTIDE ANALOGUES (REVIEW):

Small nucleolar RNA and its potential role in breast cancer - A comprehensive review: 10.1016/j.bbcan.2020.188501

Role of small interfering RNA (siRNA) in targeting ocular neovascularization: A review: 10.1016/j.exer.2020.108329

Recurrence of SARS-CoV-2 viral RNA in recovered COVID-19 patients: a narrative review: 10.1007/s10096-020-04088-z

The Functional Role of Long Non-coding RNA UCA1 in Human Multiple Cancers: a Review Study: 10.2174/1566524020666200619124543

Relationship between long non-coding RNA and prognosis of patients with coronary heart disease after percutaneous coronary intervention: A protocol for systematic review and meta-analysis: 10.1097/MD.0000000000023525

De Novo Nucleic Acids: A Review of Synthetic Alternatives to DNA and RNA That Could Act as Bio-Information Storage Molecules: 10.3390/life10120346

Relationship between long non-coding RNA TUG1 and prognosis of patients with gastric carcinoma: A protocol for systematic review and meta-analysis: 10.1097/MD.0000000000023522

Research progress of circular RNA in digestive tract tumors: a narrative review: 10.21037/tcr-20-2708

Sumera A, Radhakrishnan AK, Aziz Baba A, George E. A link between long non-coding RNA (lncRNA) and thalassaemia: A review. *Malays J Pathol.* 2020 Dec;42(3):323–332. PMID: 33361713.

Role of m6A RNA methylation in cardiovascular disease (Review): 10.3892/ijmm.2020.4746

The role of long intergenic noncoding RNA 00511 in malignant tumors: a meta-analysis, database validation and review: https://doi.org/10.1080/21655979.2020.1795384

A systematic review and meta-analysis of long noncoding RNA linc-UBC1 expression and prognosis and clinicopathological phenotypes in human cancers: 10.1080/21691401.2020.1770776

Recurrent SARS-CoV-2 RNA positivity after COVID-19: a systematic review and meta-analysis: 10.1038/s41598-020-77739-y

CSF HIV RNA Escape in Opsoclonus-Myoclonus-Ataxia Syndrome: Case Report and Review of the Literature: 10.3389/fneur.2020.585527

Emerging evidence on noncoding-RNA regulatory machinery in intervertebral disc degeneration: a narrative review: 10.1186/s13075-020-02353-2

Antiviral activity of chlorpromazine, fluphenazine, perphenazine, prochlorperazine, and thioridazine towards RNA-viruses. A review: 10.1016/j.ejphar.2020.173553

Recent Clinical and Preclinical Studies of Hydroxychloroquine on RNA Viruses and Chronic Diseases: A Systematic Review: 10.3390/molecules25225318

Definition and review on a category of long non-coding RNA: Atherosclerosis-associated circulating lncRNA (ASCLncRNA): 10.7717/peerj.10001

Review of Single-Cell RNA Sequencing in the Heart: 10.3390/ijms21218345

Prognostic significance of long intergenic non-protein-coding RNA 511expression in malignant tumors: A systematic review and meta-analysis: 10.1097/MD.0000000000023054

Prognostic Value of Long Noncoding RNA SPRY4-IT1 on Survival Outcomes in Human Carcinomas: A Systematic Review and Meta-Analysis with TCGA Database: 10.1155/2020/5868602

Prognostic and Clinicopathological Significance of Long Non-Coding RNA BLACAT1 in Cancer: An Updated Meta-Analysis and TCGA Data Review: 10.7754/Clin.Lab.2020.200310

A review on kinases phosphorylating the carboxyl-terminal domain of RNA polymerase II-Biological functions and inhibitors: 10.1016/j.bioorg.2020.104318

The role of long noncoding RNA SNHG7 in human cancers (Review): 10.3892/mco.2020.2115

Dynamics of the RNA polymerase I TFIIF/TFIIE-like subcomplex: a mini-review: 10.1042/BST20190848

Circular RNA Signature in Lung Adenocarcinoma: A MiOncoCirc Database-Based Study and Literature Review: 10.3389/fonc.2020.523342

The relationship between Long Noncoding RNA (lncRNA) Small Nucleolar RNA Host Gene
   12 (SNHG12) expression in solid malignant tumors and prognosis of tumor patients: A
   systematic review and meta-analysis: 10.1097/MD.0000000000022247
Emerging role of circular RNA in intervertebral disc degeneration: Knowns and unknowns
   (Review): 10.3892/mmr.2020.11437
Review: Long non-coding RNA in livestock: 10.1017/S1751731120000841
Comprehensive review and assessment of computational methods for predicting RNA post-
   transcriptional modification sites from RNA sequences: 10.1093/bib/bbz112
Corrigendum to: Comprehensive review and empirical analysis of hallmarks of DNA-, RNA-
   and protein-binding residues in protein chains: 10.1093/bib/bbz102
Association of Silicone Breast Implants, Breast Cancer and Anti-RNA Polymerase III
   Autoantibodies in Systemic Sclerosis: Case-Based Review: 10.2147/OARRR.S262428
Control Measures for SARS-CoV-2: A Review on Light-Based Inactivation of Single-
   Stranded RNA Viruses: 10.3390/pathogens9090737
High expression of long noncoding RNA LUCAT1 correlates with a poor clinical outcome in
   solid tumors: A systematic review and meta-analysis: 10.1016/j.prp.2020.153047
Diagnostic and prognostic value of circular RNA CDR1as/ciRS-7 for solid tumours: A sys-
   tematic review and meta-analysis: 10.1111/jcmm.15619
Long non-coding RNA (lncRNA) and epithelial-mesenchymal transition (EMT) in colorectal
   cancer: a systematic review: 10.1080/15384047.2020.1794239
Successful recovery of recurrence of positive SARS-CoV-2 RNA in COVID-19 patient with
   systemic lupus erythematosus: a case report and review: 10.1007/s10067-020-05230-0
The Role of RNA and DNA Aptamers in Glioblastoma Diagnosis and Therapy: A Systematic
   Review of the Literature: 10.3390/cancers12082173
Systemic Sclerosis Sine Scleroderma Manifested with Gastrointestinal Bleeding,
   Antiphospholipid Syndrome and Positive Anti-RNA Polymerase III Antibody: Case
   Report and Literature Review: 10.2147/IMCRJ.S254859
Targeting RNA With Antisense Oligonucleotides and Small Interfering RNA: JACC State-
   of-the-Art Review: 10.1016/j.jacc.2020.05.070
[New Advane of Research on Relationship between Long Noncoding RNA and Acute
   Myeloid Leukemia--Review]: 10.19746/j.cnki.issn.1009-2137.2020.04.057
Advances in the role of exosomal non-coding RNA in the development, diagnosis, and treat-
   ment of gastric cancer (Review): 10.3892/mco.2020.2068
The circular RNA HIPK3 (circHIPK3) and its regulation in cancer progression: Review:
   10.1016/j.lfs.2019.117252
Long non-coding RNA MEG3 is involved in osteogenic differentiation and bone diseases
   (Review): 10.3892/br.2020.1305
Circular RNA is a popular molecule in tumors of the digestive system (Review): 10.3892/
   ijo.2020.5054
Circular RNA; a new biomarker for breast cancer: A systematic review: 10.1002/jcp.29558
The Processing, Gene Regulation, Biological Functions, and Clinical Relevance of
   N4-Acetylcytidine on RNA: A Systematic Review: 10.1016/j.omtn.2020.01.037
Prognostic value and therapeutic potential of the long noncoding RNA TP73-AS1 in cancers:
   A systematic review and meta-analysis: 10.1038/s41598-020-65726-2
Role of Micro-RNA for Pain After Surgery: Narrative Review of Animal and Human Studies:
   10.1213/ANE.0000000000004767
Association of long non-coding RNA and leukemia: A systematic review: 10.1016/j.
   gene.2020.144405
Detection of viral RNA in diverse body fluids in an SFTS patient with encephalopathy, gas-
   trointestinal bleeding and pneumonia: a case report and literature review: 10.1186/
   s12879-020-05012-8

Prognostic value of long non-coding RNA GHET1 in cancers: a systematic review and meta-analysis: 10.1186/s12935-020-01189-9

[Research Progress on Non-Coding RNA in Multiple Myeloma --Review]: 10.19746/j.cnki .issn.1009-2137.2020.02.061

A technical review and guide to RNA fluorescence in situ hybridization: 10.7717/peerj.8806

Prevalence and characteristics of hepatitis C virus infection in Shenyang City, Northeast China, and prediction of HCV RNA positivity according to serum anti-HCV level: retrospective review of hospital data: 10.1186/s12985-020-01316-y

Letter to the Editor on the article "Long non-coding RNA MALAT1 as a valuable biomarker for prognosis in osteosarcoma: A systematic review and meta-analysis" (Int J Surg 2019; Nov 15;72:206-213. doi: 10.1016/j.ijsu.2019.11.004. [Epub ahead of print]): 10.1016/j.ijsu.2019.11.035

A commentary on "Long non-coding RNA MALAT1 as a valuable biomarker for prognosis in osteosarcoma: A systematic review and meta-analysis" (Int J Surg 2019;72:206-213): 10.1016/j.ijsu.2019.12.008

A Mini-review of the Computational Methods Used in Identifying RNA 5-Methylcytosine Sites: 10.2174/2213346107666200219124951

Association of Micro RNA and Postoperative Cognitive Dysfunction: A Review: 10.2174/1389557520666200621182717

A Review on the Progress and Prospects of Dengue Drug Discovery Targeting NS5 RNA-Dependent RNA Polymerase: 10.2174/1381612826666200523174753

Micro-RNA and the Features of Metabolic Syndrome: A Narrative Review: 10.2174/1389557520666200122124445

Prognostic Values of Long Noncoding RNA linc00152 in Various Carcinomas: An Updated Systematic Review and Meta-Analysis: 10.1634/theoncologist.2018-0358

Recent Advances on the Semi-Supervised Learning for Long Non-Coding RNA-Protein Interactions Prediction: A Review: 10.2174/0929866526666191025104043

Functions, mechanisms and regulation of Pumilio/Puf family RNA binding proteins: a comprehensive review: 10.1007/s11033-019-05142-6

Comparison of 16S Ribosomal RNA Targeted Sequencing and Culture for Bacterial Identification in Normally Sterile Body Fluid Samples: Report of a 10-Year Clinical Laboratory Review: 10.3343/alm.2020.40.1.63

Long Non-Coding RNA in Drug Resistance of Non-Small Cell Lung Cancer: A Mini Review: 10.3389/fphar.2019.01457

Prognostic and clinical significance of long non-coding RNA HNF1A-AS1 in solid cancers: A systematic review and meta-analysis: 10.1097/MD.0000000000018264

Defining cerebrospinal fluid HIV RNA escape: editorial review AIDS: 10.1097/QAD.0000000000002252

Long non-coding RNA MALAT1 as a valuable biomarker for prognosis in osteosarcoma: A systematic review and meta-analysis: 10.1016/j.ijsu.2019.11.004

A systematic review of MERS-CoV seroprevalence and RNA prevalence in dromedary camels: Implications for animal vaccination: 10.1016/j.epidem.2019.100350

Interpretation of differential gene expression results of RNA-seq data: review and integration: 10.1093/bib/bby067

Clustering single cells: a review of approaches on high-and low-depth single-cell RNA-seq data: 10.1093/bfgp/ely001

A systematic review of FTA cards® as a tool for viral RNA preservation in fieldwork: Are they safe and effective?: 10.1016/j.prevetmed.2019.104772

Global status of synchronizing Leishmania RNA virus in Leishmania parasites: A systematic review with meta-analysis: 10.1111/tbed.13316

Analysis of RNA in the estimation of post-mortem interval: a review of current evidence: 10.1007/s00414-019-02125-x

The prognostic value of long noncoding RNA SNHG16 on clinical outcomes in human cancers: a systematic review and meta-analysis: 10.1186/s12935-019-0971-2

A review of the relationship between long noncoding RNA and post-stroke injury repair: 10.1177/0300060519867493

Comprehensive review and empirical analysis of hallmarks of DNA-, RNA- and protein-binding residues in protein chains: 10.1093/bib/bbx168

Systematic review of computational methods for identifying miRNA-mediated RNA-RNA crosstalk: 10.1093/bib/bbx137

A homozygous mutation of alanyl-transfer RNA synthetase 2 in a patient of adult-onset leukodystrophy: A case report and literature review: 10.1002/brb3.1313

A review on native and denaturing purification methods for non-coding RNA (ncRNA): 10.1016/j.jchromb.2019.04.034

Systematic review of the performance and clinical utility of point of care HIV-1 RNA testing for diagnosis and care: 10.1371/journal.pone.0218369

Two Old Dogs, One New Trick: A Review of RNA Polymerase and Ribosome Interactions during Transcription-Translation Coupling: 10.3390/ijms20102595

Prognostic Value of Long Noncoding RNA CRNDE as a Novel Biomarker in Solid Cancers: An Updated Systematic Review and Meta-Analysis: 10.7150/jca.31088

Prognostic value of long noncoding RNA ROR in patients with cancer in China: A systematic review and meta-analysis: 10.1097/MD.0000000000015758

Accuracy of Messenger RNA Human Papillomavirus Tests for Diagnostic Triage of Minor Cytological Cervical Lesions: A Systematic Review and Meta-Analysis: 10.1097/OLQ.0000000000000970

New tools for pathology: a user's review of a highly multiplexed method for in situ analysis of protein and RNA expression in tissue: 10.1002/path.5223

Biological and Clinical Relevance of Long Non-Coding RNA PCAT-1 in Cancer, A Systematic Review and Meta-Analysis: 10.31557/APJCP.2019.20.3.667

Pivotal prognostic and diagnostic role of the long non-coding RNA colon cancer-associated transcript 1 expression in human cancer (Review): 10.3892/mmr.2018.9721

Critical review on engineering deaminases for site-directed RNA editing: 10.1016/j.copbio.2018.08.006

The prognostic role of long noncoding RNA CRNDE in cancer patients: a systematic review and meta-analysis: 10.4149/neo_2018_180320N191

Mini review: Revisiting mobile RNA silencing in plants: 10.1016/j.plantsci.2018.10.025

Primary transcripts: From the discovery of RNA processing to current concepts of gene expression - Review: 10.1016/j.yexcr.2018.09.011

Prognostic values of long noncoding RNA PVT1 in various carcinomas: An updated systematic review and meta-analysis: 10.1111/cpr.12519

Coexistence of mucosa-associated lymphoid tissue lymphoma and systemic sclerosis showing positive for anticentromere antibody and anti-RNA polymerase III antibody: A case report and published work review: 10.1111/1346-8138.14480

Long noncoding RNA HOXD-AS1 in various cancers: a meta-analysis and TCGA data review: 10.2147/OTT.S184303

Effect of micro-RNA on tenocytes and tendon-related gene expression: A systematic review: 10.1002/jor.24064

Long non-coding RNA: its evolutionary relics and biological implications in mammals: a review: 10.1186/s40781-018-0183-7

Diagnostic efficacy of long non-coding RNA in lung cancer: a systematic review and meta-analysis: 10.1136/postgradmedj-2018-135862

Circular RNA, a novel marker for cancer determination (Review): 10.3892/ijmm.2018.3795

Long non-coding RNA CRNDE in cancer prognosis: Review and meta-analysis: 10.1016/j.
cca.2018.07.003

Modeling and analysis of RNA-seq data: a review from a statistical perspective: 10.1007/
s40484-018-0144-7

The prognostic value of long noncoding RNA Sox2ot expression in various cancers: A systematic review and meta-analysis: 10.1016/j.cca.2018.05.038

Clinicopathological and prognostic significance of long noncoding RNA MALAT1 in human
cancers: a review and meta-analysis: 10.1186/s12935-018-0606-z

The Prognostic Value of Expression of the Long Noncoding RNA (lncRNA) Small Nucleolar
RNA Host Gene 1 (SNHG1) in Patients with Solid Malignant Tumors: A Systematic
Review and Meta-Analysis: 10.12659/MSM.911687

Long noncoding RNA CYTOR in cancer: A TCGA data review: 10.1016/j.cca.2018.05.010

Long noncoding RNA LINC00152 as a novel predictor of lymph node metastasis and survival
in human cancer: a systematic review and meta-analysis: 10.1016/j.cca.2018.03.034

Index